Accountable Care

Bridging the
Health Information Technology
Divide

First Edition

D1451631

EDITORS
Bill Spooner
Bert Reese
Colin Konschak

FOREWORD BY
John D. Halamka, MD

This publication is intended to provide accurate and authoritative information in regard to the subject matter covered. The statements and opinions expressed in this book are those of the authors.

ISBN-13:   978-0-9834824-7-5
ISBN-10:   0983482470

Convurgent Publishing, LLC
4445 Corporation Lane, Suite #227
Virginia Beach, VA 23462
Phone: (877) 254-9794, Fax: (757) 213-6801
Web Site: www.convurgent.com
E-mail: info@convurgent.com

Special Orders.
Bulk Quantity Sales. Special discounts are available on quantity purchases of 25 or more copies by corporations, government agencies, academic institutions, and other organizations. Please contact Convurgent Publishing's Sales Department at sales@convurgent.com or at the address above.

Library of Congress Control Number: 2012943475
Bibliographic data:

Executive Editors
Accountable Care: Bridging the Health Information Technology Divide / Ed. Bill Spooner, Bert Reese, Colin Konschak
p. cm.

1. Health policy. 2. Accountable care. 3. Electronic health records. 4. Health information exchange. 5. Healthcare quality. 6. Health information technology. 7. Data analytics. 8. Comparative effectiveness research. 9. Network transitions.

ISBN: 978-0-9834824-7-5

Corresponding editor, J.M. Bohn
jb@convurgent.com

Praise for *Bridging the Divide*

"Healthcare reform is underway, and it is clear that we are moving toward reimbursement models that reward quality over quantity. As managing the health of populations becomes more important, effective health information technologies are required across the continuum of care. The authors have identified all of the relevant technological components required in an accountable care model and provide clear direction on how to move your organization in this direction. This book is a must read for anyone in the health information technology industry. Providers, vendors, and researchers alike."

Charles Wagner
System Vice President of Applications
OhioHealth

"As healthcare leaders, we are in the midst of our dynamic industry facing a shifting focus of how our delivery systems are viewed, measured, and ultimately reimbursed. This new world, based on population health management and outcomes-based reimbursement, will require us to reassess the technological infrastructure needed to succeed. This text provides a succinct overview and plan that will be essential for delivering accountable care to the communities we serve."

Michael Mayo, FACHE
Hospital President
Baptist Medical Center-Jacksonville

"A "must have" text for healthcare executives. Truly global in perspective, "Bridging the Divide," shows healthcare leaders what they should expect from information and technology in the 21st century and how to go about getting it."

Rick Skinner
Vice President and Chief Information Officer
Cancer Care Ontario

"The authors have laid out a very clear roadmap of health information technologies required by the accountable care model. Chapter 1 introduces a very thorough Accountable Care Organization Reference Model (ACORM) that sets up discussions of various technologies and capabilities throughout the rest of the book. This text will be very helpful for those responsible for developing the infrastructure required for success in an era of accountable care."

Chris Belmont
Chief Information Officer
Ochsner Health System

"An insightful assessment of both literature and regulatory issues impacting the landscape of health information technology issues being faced by healthcare leaders across the globe in the 21st century. An important text to have on every healthcare CIO's desk."

Beth Lindsay Wood
Chief Information Officer
Tampa General Hospital

"As clinically integrated networks are setting foundations across the country for future ACOs, the underpinning technologies are crucial to successful population management. This book provides a comprehensive assessment of technology issues that healthcare leaders need to address in mapping strategies for selection, implementation, and adoption of health information technology solutions for CINs and ACOs."

Bruce Flareau, MD
President
BayCare Physician Partners

ACKNOWLEDGEMENTS

During the 17-month process of developing this book, many people have participated in its unfolding. As the healthcare industry and its health information technology sector have been impacted by sweeping reforms in recent years, bringing *Accountable Care: Bridging the Health Information Technology Divide, First Edition*, to the market required input from a number of executives, peers, stakeholders, and family members to support the authors and other contributors throughout this development process. On behalf of the executive editor team and the book's authors, there are a few key people we wish to express sincere appreciation to for their support and involvement.

John D. Halamka, MD provided an early review of the manuscript and the foreword statement for this book. As one of the nation's leading health IT physician executives, serving as Chief Information Officer of Beth Israel Deaconess Medical Center, Chairman of the New England Healthcare Exchange Network (NEHEN), Co-Chair of the HIT Standards Committee, a full Professor at Harvard Medical School, and a practicing Emergency Physician, we recognize how valuable his time is, and we were extremely grateful for his contribution.

Numerous case studies are found throughout this book, but three in particular required significant involvement from key contributors. First was the case study on Cornerstone Healthcare (Cornerstone) in Chapter 2. We owe special thanks to Cornerstone's Chief Executive Officer, Grace E. Terrell, MD, and Cornerstone's Chief Medical Officer, John J. Walker, MD, for participating in development of their case study. Second, we give thanks to two executives from Microsoft Corporation who provided their case study and valuable insights for the conclusion of Chapter 3, Hector Rodriguez, MBA, Director, HLS Industry Technology Unit, (Microsoft U.S. Public Sector Health & Life Sciences) and Kevin Rapp, Director of Healthcare Strategy, Louisville, KY (Microsoft Enterprise Partner Group. In Chapter 9, Rick Skinner, Vice President and Chief Information Officer of Cancer Care of Ontario, provided a case study on his organization's experience with mobile application development for which we greatly appreciate.

Regarding the subject of network transitions, Judah Thornewill, PhD, of Group Plus LLC, was a significant contributor as subject matter expert and collaborator, with Robert Esterhay, MD, on developing content on the importance of the network transition occurring in healthcare today and for the future with accountable care organizations. For his time and efforts we extend sincere appreciation.

Last, and most importantly, we are grateful to the families and colleagues of all the authors and editors. Collectively this group has invested thousands of hours in the development of this book and, in healthcare, we understand that time is a precious commodity that we cannot get back after it is gone. For the encouragement to drive this project to completion, we appreciate all those who have supported us along the way.

PREFACE

The definition of a revolution: it destroys the perfect and enables the impossible.

Seth Godin (1960-)
Author, innovator, and entrepreneur
February 25, 2012

A revolution in healthcare is upon us. The ecosystem that comprises the United States healthcare system has evolved over time, but for many years was un-impacted by the technological revolution that ascended upon many other industries. A cottage industry was in place, bound by the tradition of medicine, but there was a need for disruption to advance our ability to improve the quality of care delivered. A technological revolution has been embraced, and the pace of change is accelerating. Our ability to transform processes, systems, organizations and the way we help people heal has been impacted by waves of innovation cascading from the field of information technologies over the last five decades. The changes we have seen have been transformational and have altered the landscape of care delivery in America and abroad. The ability of physicians, caregivers, and administrators to share needed healthcare information, both clinical and administrative, to improve the health of populations has improved and advanced beyond what was unimaginable earlier in history.

Accountable Care: Bridging the Health Information Technology Divide, First Edition, is a book, 17 months in the making, that touches on many elements of this technological journey with a focal point of clinically integrated accountable care organizations (ACOs) at the epicenter. There is an array of technological and organizational issues effecting positive change in this era of accountable care. As the nation and global health system shifts focus from volume-driven care to performance and quality-driven care, leadership is returning to the provider. This is resulting in a greater emphasis on clinical and administrative performance and on the priority of improving population health.

Changes in the economic, societal, political, and clinical dimensions are impacting and driving the need for new technological solutions. Three overarching influential factors touched on throughout the book are the aging of our US and global population (e.g., Baby Boomers, Generation X, and Generation Y), complexity of the healthcare system, and the continuous drive for new innovation. Each of these factors will continue to have a profound effect on the future development of how we deliver and administer care for patients in America and abroad.

Purpose of the Book

As a first edition text, *Accountable Care: Bridging the Health Information Technology Divide* starts a series that will focus on various aspects of health information technologies that are part of the future for accountable care organizations and other care delivery organizations. Many chapters were developed as an anthology of independent works by the authors, with the final chapter, The New Horizon, offering the reader a degree of integration with a predictive view, drawing upon many of the issues covered throughout the earlier chapters. The book helps meet educational needs, as well as provide a text to help set strategic direction for organizations seeking to understand how the many moving parts fit together in the complex adaptive system of healthcare. Key topics covered include:

➢ State of affairs and landscape of the industry

➢ Electronic health records

➢ Data analytics and business intelligence

➢ Standards and interoperability

➢ Health information exchange

➢ Personal health records and mobile health

➢ Quality and patient safety

➢ Meaningful Use of electronic health records

➢ Revenue cycle management and other financial implications for ACOs

➢ Comparative effectiveness research

➢ A capstone chapter dedicated to strategy, policy, and network transition implications

Intended Audience

The intended audience is broad in nature. A historical perspective is provided for students of healthcare seeking to get a holistic sense of the information technology transformation underway. For the healthcare executive, physician, and caregiver audience, material is provided with depth of evidence to validate points made throughout each chapter. For policy makers, researchers, and those evaluating the direction of the industry, this work is offered as a reference manual and to provide insights on the complex nature of the healthcare system in this renaissance era that is certain to continue well beyond the foreseeable horizon. Additional information on this work, its future second edition, and related materials can be found at www.bridgingthedivide.info.

Health information technologies are driving our industry forward and helping meet the challenges of care delivery in the 21st century. As the Institute of Medicine noted in its 2001 report, *Crossing the Quality Chasm: A New Health System for the 21st Century*, "IT has enormous potential to improve the quality of health care with regard to all six of the aims set forth."

Over the past decade, this point has helped drive efforts for change throughout the US healthcare system—an industry that continues to make progress and works toward continuous improvement in the quality of care delivered for all patients.

Bill Spooner
Bert Reese
Colin Konschak

Table of Contents

Foreword

The Horizon for Accountable Care Organizations

In a world of healthcare reform and impending changes in reimbursement approaches, everyone wants to become an accountable care organization (ACO), but few know what this really implies.

A senior executive recently told me, "We need a comprehensive community-wide business intelligence platform to support care management, population health, and cost analytics."

No problem!

Creating an ACO depends upon on a foundation of IT systems, business processes, and behavioral change. However, clinical and IT leaders have lacked a roadmap for this journey, and many are still trying to formulate a strategy.

This book provides the background they will need to navigate the challenges ahead.

I believe that a successful ACO requires five tactics, all of which are addressed in detailed chapters written by experts.

Universal Adoption of EHRs—Meaningful Use is not enough. An ACO needs to think beyond today's disconnected hospitals, clinics, labs, pharmacies, and long-term care facilities. Organizations should use IT to remove the chaos and heterogeneity caused by incomplete communication and missed handoffs. Rather than allow "a thousand wildflowers to bloom," IT should be used strategically across the community, minimizing the number of different vendors so that it is easier to create a "model office" that standardizes work and encourages the capture of healthcare information using uniform data dictionaries.

Healthcare Information Exchange—The culture of the ACO must move from data silos to a knowledge ecosystem, ensuring every member of the care team has access to and contributes to the patient's lifetime healthcare record. Data is no longer a competitive asset; it is a community currency that raises the tide for all participants. Yes, privacy must be protected, but, at the same time, healthcare delivery organizations must become patient-centered electronic medical homes that collect data about their patients from all sites of care.

Business Intelligence/Analytics—You cannot improve what you do not measure. Clinician level report cards are needed to identify variations in care processes and outcomes. Data from multiple sources needs to be cleansed, normalized, and maintained in a form that supports ad hoc queries and repeatable reports. Novel technologies are needed that turn data into information, knowledge, and wisdom. Registries and community-wide repositories are needed.

Universal Availability of PHRs—Patients and families must be partners in their care. It is challenging for patients with multiple caregivers to coordinate appointments, diagnostic testing, and therapies. Personal Health records enable patients or their proxies to take an active role in the navigation of our healthcare system. As data is shared openly with patients, educational materials will become increasingly important so that patients understand their care plans and how to be good stewards of their own wellness.

Decision Support for Care Management—Medicine has traditionally been an apprenticeship combining art and science. IT enables best practices to be widely circulated, actionable alerts/reminders to be routed to appropriate caregivers, and evidence-based education to be delivered just in time during care processes. Care Management requires thinking about wellness, not just sickness, and gathering data from novel sources, such as via sensors in the home. Decision support helps identify the right care for the right patient at the right time.

I believe you will find this book to be an essential reference as you carefully balance the transition between the fee for service and capital global payment systems, which will exist in parallel for the next few years. Building the necessary management and IT infrastructure to thrive in the future requires urgent action. If you move too fast, you could take risks that jeopardize the organization's financial stability before it is ready to support new care models. If you move too slowly, your opportunities for future success may disappear. This book will help you decide what to do and when.

John D. Halamka, MD
Chief Information Officer
Harvard Medical School

Chapter 1. Introduction

David Shiple and Shane Danaher

Technology—which has the potential to improve quality and safety of care as well as reduce costs—is rapidly evolving, changing the way we deliver health care.[1]

Institute of Medicine
Committee on Patient Safety and Health Information Technology (2011)

State of Affairs

The information technology renaissance of the last four decades has led to the rapid growth of new knowledge management and information sharing applications, data warehouses, artificial intelligence, analytics, and other tools that are aiding organizations in industries throughout the world in their daily operations and long-term planning. Quantum leaps have been taken in society's ability to share and distribute information globally and to use it to improve processes, document events, to help save lives, create new career fields, and advance our abilities to communicate across boundaries that were once considered inconceivable. As an example, from 1986 to 2007, global capacity for bidirectional technologies and information diffusion capability grew at 28% annually, along with a 23% annual increase in globally stored information.[2] This growth has fueled the evolving landscape of technologies, particularly those that process, disseminate, and enable the more efficient and effective use of information for the betterment of the global community.

In light of the global emersion in information technologies, the need for increased acquisition and adoption of medical and health information technology (HIT) has gained strength and garnered support for the past three decades in the United States (US) healthcare system. Regulatory support, financing of system implementations and evaluations, and focusing on the "safety, costs, and social affects"[3] have been central factors in understanding how we as a system can make best use of new tools and applications to improve the quality of care in America.

For the US healthcare system, trends such as these have resulted in an acceleration of the pace of technological change in support of improving the quality of healthcare services delivered in America. In fact, in 2007, it was noted in the *New England Journal of Medicine* that "Sophisticated observers and advocates of computerizing medical information view the adoption of HIT as the opening wedge into, indeed a fundamental catalyst of, widespread change in the practice of medicine."[4]

In 2001, the Institute of Medicine (IOM) addressed the importance of information technology in the future of healthcare noting that "it must play a central role in the redesign of the health care system" in order to achieve significant improvement in the care delivered by healthcare organizations and providers.[5] While strides have been made in the redesign, new challenges have emerged with the deployment of new systems and capabilities throughout the US healthcare system. Some of the challenges have been:

➢ Need for greater investment of resources (e.g., financial capital to fund equipment and staff for system implementations) that often reaches beyond the budgets of healthcare organizations;[6]

➢ Occurrence of new types of errors and complications (e.g., unintended consequences) with system implementations and adoption;[7]

➢ Resistance to change by organizations delivering care, patient populations, and those who provide care;

➢ A decade of effort to drive the enactment of transformational federal healthcare reform legislation;[8]

➢ Disruption to the clinician workflow and administrative processes; and

➢ Planning for information security and system interoperability in a market environment driven by freedom of choice and the economic underpinnings of a democratic society.

Many of these challenges will be addressed throughout this book in the ensuing chapters, but even with their influence, the United States has established a strong and learning healthcare system that continues to make improvements on a daily basis. It is a system with a data-driven culture that continuously feeds the evolutionary development of this healthcare system in the modern era.[9] It is a complex system where the information generated by healthcare professionals and patients populates the system with increasingly more meaningful data, leading to newfound opportunities for growth and improvement in the care delivered throughout the United States and around the globe. The growth of this system has not come without a cost. National health expenditures (NHE) were $27.2 billion in 1960 and, since 2002, NHE have exceeded 15% of gross domestic product (GDP) , with spending exceeding $2 trillion since 2005.[10] Figure 1-1 illustrates this historical trend.

Figure 1-1. National Health Expenditures 1960-2010

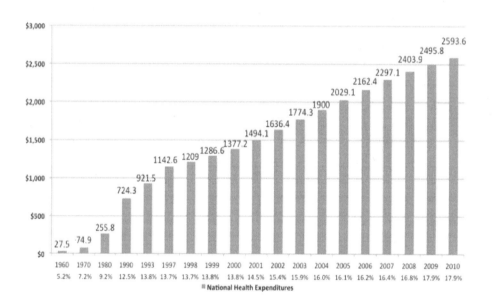

This path of escalating healthcare costs as illustrated above, started back in the 1960s with the beginning of the Medicare program in 1965. Over the past 25 years, the Medicare Advantage (Part C) program has witnessed a key challenge in dealing with

> ...the inevitable errors in traditional Medicare's administered price system, by allowing the health plans and providers to negotiate prices or, in some cases, to integrate the finance and delivery functions.[11]

This path of cost escalation has included accelerated growth in premiums and out-of-pocket costs for consumers during the past two decades that has contributed to the need for change in the financing and delivery system of care. In addition, a retreat from the Medicare Advantage program has been seen as part of the perceived consumer resistance to the program

> Medicare Advantage (formerly Medicare+Choice) reflects, in part, the belief that competition among health plans will help constrain costs.[3] Although evidence supports the premise that managed care organizations (MCOs) have lower spending compared with indemnity fee-for-service systems, debate persists over whether the rate of health care spending growth differs among diverse delivery systems.[4] Rather, evidence suggests that although managed competition slows health care cost growth, the effects are not large enough to stem the rising share of GDP devoted to health care.[12]

The need for acquisition and adoption of new technologies has been necessary to mitigate safety and quality concerns throughout the US healthcare system, and these costs for new technologies have contributed nearly half of the increases seen in the overall rise in national health expenditures between 1940 and 1990.[13] Other underlying issues identified by the Congressional Budget Office in 2008 that have influenced this cost escalation have included:[14]

- Aging population and demographic shifts,
- Changes in third-party payment,
- Growth in personal income,
- Price growth for services and products in the healthcare sector, and
- Administrative cost burdens.

In addition, our historical volume-driven healthcare system that is transitioning to a performance-driven and value-driven system has contributed to the cost growth, along with the transformation of the nation's healthcare workforce (e.g., physicians, nurses, pharmacists, administrators) as it is impacted by new technologies, reforms in healthcare laws, training requirements, and new tools to be adopted. From a cost comparison perspective with other industrialized nations, the cost of healthcare in the United States is among the highest globally. Compared to our five closest trading partners, the United States spends one dollar on healthcare services and products for every 47 cents expended by our international partners in covering their citizens' cost of healthcare.[15] Yet when patients in other countries seek specialized care for complex medical conditions, they often find their path leading to the United States for the best quality of care available.

These challenges in healthcare have evolved over time, and the US private and public markets have introduced systemic changes as potential solutions. The 1970s-80s brought the introduction of health maintenance organizations (HMOs). Then consumer-centric healthcare plans in the 1990s,[16] the increased adoption of patient-centered medical home[17] models over the past decade, along with clinically integrated networks[18] and other care delivery system-based solutions, were introduced to try and mitigate the challenge of cost growth. However, each model has come with new dilemmas to be addressed by its stakeholders in regards to cost, quality, and access to care. In light of these efforts and the continued presence of the above issues, along with the focus for meeting national priorities for quality of care[19] and the IOM's six aims for improvement of healthcare in America,[20] new solutions have still been sought that achieve efficient, safe, high-quality, and affordable cost of care.

A Convergence of Trends

Escalating costs are one of the key trends in the US healthcare system's evolution to its current state. Despite the high costs and having the best care delivery system in the world by many standards, quality is not as good as it can be. Throughout the system, there are tremendous opportunities for improvement. For many decades, the system was volume driven, and today there is a much greater focus on quality-driven and performance-driven care than ever before in history.

But we know there are other trends and factors that have played a critical role in how the system has reached this stage in maturity. So what are they?

In addition to the factors noted by the Congressional Budget Office in 2008, three other critical factors have and will continue to impact the development of our nation's healthcare system. Each serves as an impetus for several of the changes that we see occurring today. Figure 1-2 identifies these three factors.

- ➢ With fewer primary care physicians in the market, access to primary care becomes problematic when relocating or changing health plans;

- ➢ Commercial plans covering fewer medical needs; and

- ➢ Evaluating care delivery options for meeting needed healthcare services (e.g., increased number of retail clinics and integrative or alternative medicine services).

The effect of these two segments of the population, and most significantly the Baby Boomers, has and will continue to have a profound effect on systemic changes made to our nation's care delivery system and how care is delivered around the globe.

Continuous Need for Innovation

Healthcare is changing rapidly, and there is a constant need for innovations, some sustaining and some disruptive, as defined by Clayton Christensen and colleagues in *The Innovator's Prescription*.[23] As information technology has evolved, consumers, patients, and other stakeholders of the healthcare system are putting innovations to use on a regular basis. Sustaining innovations bring about incremental change, while those that are disruptive hold the power to cause paradigm shifts. Think of the introduction of electronic medical records (EMRs) into the care delivery and clinical workflow processes. Though introduced decades ago, adoption was slowed due to several systemic barriers that are being mitigated through regulatory reforms, financial incentives, and a stronger understanding of the impact to clinical workflow and transformation that must occur with their implementation.

Innovative ideas are needed to advance therapies, therapeutic delivery systems, care delivery models, and health information technologies that are much of the focus of the chapters to follow. Innovations have the capacity to drive competition in the market and to bring to the forefront new capabilities that improve the quality of care in America's healthcare system.

Health System Complexity

Understanding and bringing order to the ecosystem that is the US healthcare system has been a key challenge for lawmakers, healthcare leaders, and researchers throughout the 20th and now into the 21st century. The advent of new information technologies has brought about new capabilities that bring sense-making tools and concepts into a system riddled with challenges as major changes occur in the national operating structure (e.g., introduction of Medicare in the 1960s, growth of the managed care sector with the Health Maintenance Organization Act of 1973 and, most recently, the Affordable Care Act). Connections have emerged in both linear and nonlinear relationships[24] across our nation's health system as new information technology systems have opened portals for new pathways to solving problems, both in the medical science realm and the systems engineering perspectives on the structure and function of organizations. Complexity science is multi-disciplinary and, when examining the ecosystem that our nation's health system has evolved into, it introduces many concepts that help achieve the IOM's six aims for improvement: safety, effectiveness, equitable, efficiency, patient-centered, and timely.

The US healthcare system has evolved as a complex adaptive system, and increasing our understanding of some inherent characteristics of these types of systems is crucial. A few of these characteristics are:[25]

➢ Nonlinear and dynamic;

➢ Involve independent and intelligent agents;

➢ Agents adhere to rules, laws, and policies but may or may not have a centralized command and control authority presiding over their roles or actions;

➢ The system is adaptable and self-learning;

➢ Complexity is a result of the evolving interactions of all the system elements;

➢ They can function as an open system structure with feedback loops; and

➢ System behaviors are often unpredictable.

Each of these characteristics can be seen throughout various elements of our nation's healthcare system. Influential individuals or organizations can represent agents in the structure of the healthcare ecosystem, and dynamic change is part of the norm in today's healthcare operating environment. Throughout this book, these three factors will be referred to by a number of the chapter authors as common issues of importance related to the topics they address. Each factor is unique, but they are all interrelated and have contributed to the development, lessons learned, and growth of our modern day healthcare system in the United States.

Dawn of the Network Transition

As healthcare delivery advances in the 21st century, on both the clinical patient care delivery side and the field of academic medical research, we are embracing a new frontier—one that some scholars refer to as a "world of networks."[26]

The Network Transition in Healthcare

Scholars studying the rapid emergence of new kinds of networks in society are finding increasing evidence for the idea that the key driver of change in the global economy of the 21st century will not be large organizations, but, rather, networks of individuals and organizations collaborating through information and communications technology.

One way to think about this is Wikipedia. In the 1990s, the worldwide encyclopedia market was led by a few large capital-backed organizations such as Encyclopedia Britannica. Today, the encyclopedia market is driven by a radically new kind of global collaborative—created and used by millions of people. This is an example of a network transition in the global encyclopedia market.

Will a similar network transition occur in healthcare? Might ACOs improve the connections of providers, payers, and patients through interoperable health IT platforms and advanced health information exchanges? Can these new information technology–enabled structures of care act as bridges for a network transition across the healthcare industry?

Network Level Action Research (NLAR)

One research approach that can be used to develop answers to these kinds of questions is "Network Level Action Research" (NLAR) .[27]

NLAR is a network-level approach to conducting participatory action research.[28] It brings practitioners and researchers together into a network level collaborative where they work to achieve a shared goal. Networks in an NLAR project can be small scale (e.g., a few individuals and organizations) or large scale (e.g., many individuals and organizations of multiple types). NLAR differs from other types of action research by involving both researchers and practitioners in a formally organized network level collaborative.

In the context of healthcare system challenges being addressed today, NLAR is an important method for making sense of underlying complexities involved in:

➢ Population health management for the Baby Boomers, Generation X, and Generation Y;

➢ Identifying new health IT innovations at an accelerated pace; and

➢ Meeting the socioeconomic and public welfare goals of our nation's health system.

NLAR can provide a new lens for addressing hard problems (such as relevance and dissemination) that cannot be solved by researchers or practitioners working on their own at individual or organizational levels. NLAR has potential to increase relevance of research and speed up dissemination of results.

Comparative effectiveness research (to be addressed in Chapter 10) is one kind of research that could be included in NLAR projects. Researchers and practitioners benefit by focusing on relevant problems and lowering barriers to dissemination. Other kinds of research in an NLAR project could include adoption research (factors affecting individual or organizational level adoption of health information technologies and use of such given innovations and novel medical technologies identified through comparative effectiveness research); organizational outcomes research (effect on organizations trying to implement the innovation), or network research (effects of network patterns on participation and outcomes).

In the concluding chapter of this book, the network transition and NLAR concepts will be further explored in light of current health policy, the issue of complexity in our US healthcare system, and its potential influence on future health IT and delivery system model innovation.

Dawn of Accountable Care

Regulatory Path

Accountable care organizations (ACOs) represent an important step in the journey to collaborative healthcare. Efforts of Henry J. Kaiser and Sindney R. Garfield, MD in establishing Kaiser Permanente (nation's first HMO) along with Paul M. Ellwood, MD in development the "modern health maintenance organization concept"[29] that served as other evolutionary steps in the journey. The origin of the accountable care organization (ACO) model can be traced to efforts by policy researchers at the Dartmouth-Brookings Institute and the Medicare Physician Group Practice Demonstration Project that started in 2005 and ended in 2010.[30] The early results of the project provided evidence to prompt the federal government's efforts to support the advancement of the ACO model in the Affordable Care Act. In 2006, Dr. Elliot Fisher introduced the accountable care organization model concept to the Medicare Payment Advisory Commission (MedPAC) .[31] In recent years, ACO pilots have also been established between private insurance payers and care provider organizations in efforts to continue the move toward shared savings program structures. Central to the establishment of ACOs, both public and private, are three key design principles:[32]

➤ **Accountability**. Establish local organizational accountability and have physician leadership in place.

➤ **Performance Measurement**. Ensure there are comprehensive and transparent measures of outcomes, quality, and costs.

➤ **Payment Reform**. Improve system and processes to pay for value and performance around improved health outcomes for the patient population.

With these points in mind, Flareau and colleagues provide a definition of accountable care organizations

> Accountable care organizations are collaborations between physicians, hospitals, and other providers of clinical services that will be clinically and financially accountable for healthcare delivery for designated patient populations in a defined geographic market. The ACO is provider led with a focus on population-based care management and providing services to patients under both public and private payer programs.[33]

The importance of ACOs being provider led cannot be understated. In fact, the growth and development of physician leaders is a focal point for many ACOs as America's healthcare enterprise is reformed. In Terrell and Bohn's *M.D. 2.0: Physician Leadership for the Information Age. From Hero to Duyukdv*, it was noted that

> If physicians are to take leadership roles in 21st Century health care, they will need to collaborate with others to take co-responsibility for costs,

resource utilization, quality, patient safety, and the other health care macroeconomic problems that are driving healthcare system changes.[34]

Collaborative management and leadership will be essential in the era of accountable care. While ultimate accountability for ACOs will rest with provider leadership, collaborative models for engaging with, empowering, and embracing leaders from the fields of nursing and ancillary disciplines are required to maximize the full potential of each ACO's technology, clinical, and administrative resources.

These principles have aided and functioned as lynchpins in the development of federal health reform policy for ACOs. With these historical points as a foundation, a number of legislative acts have been enacted since 2009 (as illustrated in Figure 1-3) that related to and have led to the final Medicare Shared Savings Program rules (e.g., the CMS ACO program) being published in October 2011.

Figure 1-3. Paths of Recent Legislative Acts

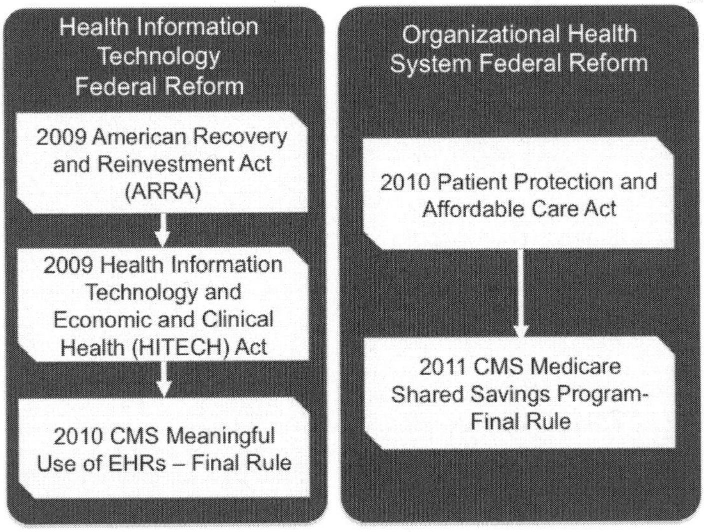

Health Information Technology Federal Reform

- 2009 American Recovery and Reinvestment Act (ARRA)
- 2009 Health Information Technology and Economic and Clinical Health (HITECH) Act
- 2010 CMS Meaningful Use of EHRs – Final Rule

Organizational Health System Federal Reform

- 2010 Patient Protection and Affordable Care Act
- 2011 CMS Medicare Shared Savings Program- Final Rule

The two columns presented represent two important paths in recent legislative acts. The left column is focused on key acts with a focus on health information technology. In the 1990s, the challenges with using paper-based medical records as part of the culture of medical care started coming to the forefront, and the journey toward increasing adoption of electronic health records began. The 2009 American Recovery and Reinvestment Act (ARRA) established the 2009 Health Information Technology and Economic and Clinical Health (HITECH) Act. HITECH set the stage for the $19 billion CMS Meaningful Use of Electronic Health Records program and the needed financial incentives to propel the acquisition and adoption of electronic health records (EHRs), which shall be discussed in depth in later chapters.

The right column represents organizational system reforms. While there are many changes initiated under the Affordable Care Act, the final CMS Medicare Shared Savings Program rules are the legislative impetus that finally established the legislative framework for public sector ACOs and a framework that will be applicable for private sector ACOs as they evolve as well. In CMS's proposed and final rule for the Medicare ACO program, an important overarching set of principles was identified that links to the national quality strategy to be discussed in Chapter 6. These principles were identified as the *Three-Part Aim*: better care for individuals, better health for populations, and lower growth in expenditures. A guiding focus is provided with these principles for all initiatives under the auspice of healthcare leaders charged with establishing a Medicare ACO. Recognizing the importance of applying the Medicare ACO rules to multiple payer relations with various healthcare providers who have established advanced care coordination and infrastructure (e.g., health information technologies, administrative processes, risk management, staff) necessary to take on greater degrees of risk and to move toward a stronger value and performance-driven care delivery model, CMS established the Pioneer ACO program.[35] Thirty-two healthcare provider organizations from across the country were selected and are identified in Table 1-1.

Table 1-1. Organizations Participating in Pioneer ACO Program

Organization	Service Area
Allina Hospitals & Clinics	Minnesota and Western Wisconsin
Atrius Health	Eastern and Central Massachusetts
Banner Health Network	Phoenix, Arizona, Metropolitan Area (Maricopa and Pinal Counties)
Bellin-Thedacare Healthcare Partners	Northeast Wisconsin
Beth Israel Deaconess Physician Organization	Eastern Massachusetts
Bronx Accountable Healthcare Network (BAHN)	New York City (the Bronx) and Lower Westchester County, New York
Brown & Toland Physicians	San Francisco Bay Area, California
Dartmouth-Hitchcock ACO	New Hampshire and Eastern Vermont
Eastern Maine Healthcare System	Central, Eastern, and Northern Maine
Fairview Health Systems	Minneapolis, Minnesota, Metropolitan Area
Franciscan Alliance	Indianapolis and Central Indiana
Genesys PHO	Southeastern Michigan
Healthcare Partners of Nevada	Clark and Nye Counties, Nevada

Organization	Service Area
Heritage California ACO	Southern, Central, and Coastal California
JSA Medical Group, a division of HealthCare Partners	Orlando, Tampa Bay, and Surrounding South Florida
Michigan Pioneer ACO	Southeastern Michigan
Monarch Healthcare	Orange County, California
Mount Auburn Cambridge Independent Practice Association (MACIPA)	Eastern Massachusetts
North Texas ACO	Tarrant, Johnson, and Parker Counties in North Texas
OSF Healthcare System	Central Illinois
Park Nicollet Health Services	Minneapolis, Minnesota, Metropolitan Area
Partners Healthcare	Eastern Massachusetts
Physician Health Partners	Denver, Colorado, Metropolitan Area
Presbyterian Healthcare Services – Central New Mexico Pioneer Accountable Care Organization	Central New Mexico
Primecare Medical Network	Southern California (San Bernardino and Riverside Counties)
Renaissance Medical Management Company	Southeastern Pennsylvania
Seton Health Alliance	Central Texas (11-County Area Including Austin)
Sharp Healthcare System	San Diego County, California
Steward Health Care System	Eastern Massachusetts
TriHealth, Inc.	Northwest Central Iowa

Organization	Service Area
University of Michigan	Southeastern Michigan

With the final CMS ACO rules also came important waivers from the Department of Health and Human Services (DHHS) Office of the Inspector General (OIG) , Federal Trade Commission (FTC) , Department of Justice (DOJ) , and the Internal Revenue Service (IRS) that were "...designed to provide added flexibility for industry participants and help reduce potential regulatory barriers to Medicare ACO formation."[36]

The Model

As the industry movement to accountable care has gained momentum over the past several years, there has been a transition from the cottage industry that once existed within the primary and specialty care areas of the industry. Figure 1-4 illustrates the transformation that has been underway as the industry has garnered lessons from the multitude of pilot projects, managed care operations, and care provider organization initiatives. This model builds off the "learning system" model discussed by the Institute of Medicine in its landmark 2001 report, *Crossing the Quality Chasm: A New Health System for the 21st Century.* [37]

Figure 1-4. Ascension to Accountable Care

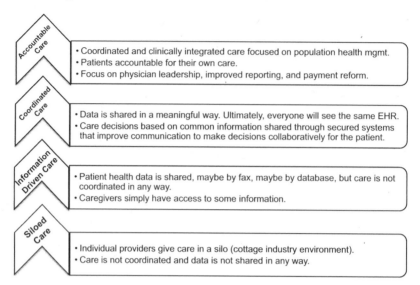

The four stages described touch on the transition that has been underway from a disjointed and fragmented system of care delivery to one that is embracing the use of health information technology tools and applications to achieve greater levels of clinically integrated care coordination, patient engagement, and physician leadership. As the industry has progressed, quality has continued to improve, wasted resources have been reduced, and patients are receiving improved care at the population level. Many improvements are still needed, and there are a number of basic models for ACOs, as shown in Figure 1-5.

Figure 1-5. Potential ACO Models[38]

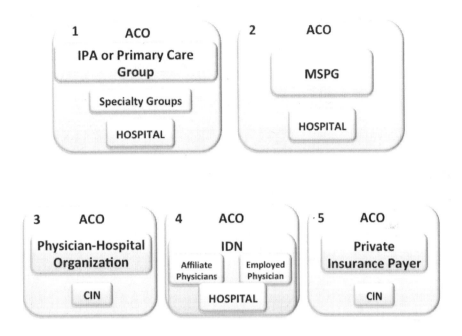

This model illustrates a number of potential configurations for ACO development and operation. As new configurations are tested among industry participants, lessons will be learned, benefits will be realized, and the industry will see which models produce the greatest benefit for the patient population served. Table 1-2 highlights key characteristics summarized by Flareau and colleagues on each model.[39]

Table 1-2. Highlights of Potential ACO Models

Model	Highlights
IPA-directed ACO	Sets the independent practice association (IPA) or primary care physician group in a lead position for the ACO with specialty groups and hospitals in a subordinate role. This model brings the patient-centered medical home to a prominent position within the new ACO.
MSPG-directed ACO	Positions a multispecialty physician group (MSPG) to direct the ACO with a subordinate hospital. Physicians work with nonexclusive contracting rights, and the ACO partners with hospitals and ancillary services for clinical integration goals.
PHO-directed ACO	Establishes the physician-hospital organization (PHO) as the spearhead for the ACO that creates partnerships with physician practices serving as a collective risk-bearing organization. The PHO also negotiates contracts for the physician practices when they join the ACO.
IDN-directed ACO	The integrated delivery network (IDN) contracts exclusively or nonexclusively with physician groups. The IDN has control over hospital medical staff organizations, which could be under exclusive contracts to support beneficiaries needed for care under the ACO.
Private Insurance Payer–directed ACO	Private payers form a direct partnership with physicians that subcontract for hospital or other ancillary services.

These models do not constitute an exclusive list of potential configurations and, as ACOs evolve, there are certain to be new models that emerge across the industry. In fact, one of the key elements for public ACOs is agreeing to participate in the new Medicare Shared Savings Program. In a July 2012 press release from CMS, it was announced that 153 ACOs (including the 32 Pioneer ACOs and six

Physician Group Practice Transition Demonstration organizations) have entered into formal agreements with CMS from across the country to participate in the shared savings program.[40]

Medical Home

The patient-centered medical home (medical home) is another care delivery transformation model for the primary care sector that impacts ACOs development. First introduced in 1967 by the American Academy of Pediatrics, the "medical home is essentially the transformation of the practice of medicine, involving both cultural and workplace changes in the practice of family medicine."[41] There is however, a key difference between the medical home and ACO. In 2009, a report by the American Academy of Family Physicians Task Force, noted

> The Accountable Care Organization model mainly differs from the Joint Principles of the PCMH in that the medical home focuses on physician practice structure and processes improvements (e.g., electronic health recores, patient registries, same-day appointments, etc.) and not on accountability for cost and quality for a defined patient population.[42]

Limitations for ACOs: Limited Patient Accountability

Each ACO will be required to have 5,000 or more primary care Medicare patients, and only primary care patients count. Patients of a specialist who are not "signed on" with one of the ACO's primary care physicians (PCPs) will not be included as ACO patients for the 5,000 patient requirement or for financial reward purposes. If at the end of a year the ACO does not have enough patients, it has a 1-year grace period to correct this issue. If at the end of the grace period year the ACO's population has not reached at least 5,000, then the arrangement will be terminated and the ACO will not be eligible to share in savings for that year.

Although 5,000 patients generally is the minimum required to be in the program, ACOs will want to have more patients, because the minimum savings rate that an ACO must achieve to receive payments under the program is lower if an ACO has more patients.[43]

Limitations for ACOs: Open Network vs. Closed Network

ACOs are being formed under different structures but two forms are the open or collaborative network ACO model with nation-wide health information exchange using universal standards and the other is a closed or captive network ACO model using non-universal standards for exchanging health information within a proprietary domain. These two approaches or models leave out the "Computing in the Cloud" ACO model or what could be called the Accountable Care Network model (to be discussed in Chapter 11) where large scale health networks running globally under cloud-based services (e.g., Amazon Web Services, Google, or other service providers with large data centers and server farms), could bring down the total cost of computing for ACOs.

Limitations for ACOs: Data Sharing is Not Required

In a closed or captive ACO, data sharing is not necessary but a tremendous incentive to share information within a catchment or medical trading area (to be further discussed in chapters 3 and 11). The realities of ACOs, Meaningful Use, health information exchange, and health insurance exchanges require end users (clinicians and healthcare institutions) to value exchange of health information and data that is meaningful, easy to integrate into their own systems, and has the ability to be appropriately analyzed.

What these end users lack is the sophisticated ability to ask real questions about interoperability and standards. The ACO movement is getting larger hospital and physician organizations to talk with each other about the substantial sharing of data. The successful ones will quickly realize that sharing data with competitors is an absolute requirement for long-term success. Larger hospitals and physician organizations, those with more market shaping capability, will demand that vendors make information interoperable and shareable.

There are many other issues and topics to consider for ACOs, both public and private. Most importantly, will be the spectrum of health information technology issues that impact the functioning, efficiency, and development of ACOs. There are over 302 ACOs in development estimating to spend $500 million on health information technology in their first year.[44] Administration of these resources will require strong governance and project prioritization to enable stakeholder's use of new technologies to meet clinical transformation demands. Process design and effective training with new technology tools will also be essential to realize the full value for patients, providers and healthcare organizations alike.

Role of Health Information Technology

The health information technology revolution is underway, and with it comes a driving force for the advancement of healthcare delivery services, along with new capabilities to analyze, assess, predict, and solve problems for healthcare workers, patients, and stakeholders of the system. Accountable care organizations are embracing new technology applications and tools to meet the challenges set forth by

Figure 1-6. ACO Reference Model (ACORM)

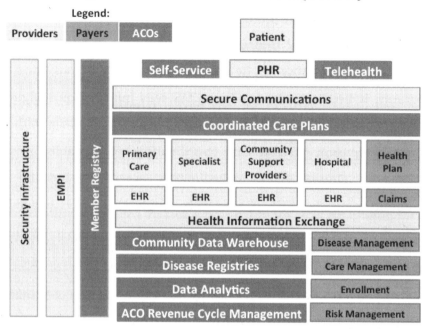

ACORM provides a conceptual framework for planning and implementing information technology elements in the ACO technological and organizational architecture. It is intended to provide health systems with a set of unprioritized elements for a Medicare ACO or other public or private ACO. Due to the early stage development of ACOs in 2012, quantifiable value for each ACORM element to an ACO is not yet possible to assess given the multitude of ACO configurations and each may have varying needs for different elements of ACORM. All of these elements may need to be addressed at different stages for each ACO depending on organizational and technology maturity. Many organizations will only need a subset of the elements referenced in ACORM to meet their needs in the near-term. The elements are arrayed in three groups defined in the legend: providers, payers, and ACOs. While there is certain to be overlap in the practical implementation of these elements, this grouping is based on an assortative relationship across the elements in regards to their most direct utility. Before discussing several of the elements, a number of overarching themes for ACORM should be noted:

➤ While much of the required information technology investment for ACOs overlaps with Meaningful Use, a new information technology strategic planning approach may be needed;

➤ Much of the technology called for is not readily available in the marketplace;

➤ Expect many health information technology products used by payers to be modified for use by providers;

➤ As the Medicare ACO and CMS Meaningful Use of EHRs program incentives increase to keep patients healthy and out of provider facilities, home health and telehealth technology innovation will accelerate;

➤ Privacy and security infrastructure will take on heightened importance and complexity;

➤ Key ACO information technology building blocks, such as HIEs, will quickly expand into new functionality areas; and

➤ While CMS called for end-to-end health information technology capabilities in the Medicare ACO start-up, many private insurance payer-directed ACOs can start with taking incremental steps in health information technology maturation.

ACORM Building Blocks

ACORM is comprised of several elements at various levels identified across the three groups. The "patient" is positioned at the top of the model, recognized as the single most important focal point for which all activities are directed. Underneath the patient are the first three elements of ACORM: personal health records, self-service tools, and telehealth. In the remainder of this section, a number of the elements of ACORM will be described and others, such as ACO revenue cycle management, health information exchange, EHRs, and data analytics, will all have dedicated chapters later in the book.

Personal Health Records

Personal responsibility on the part of the patient is a key component of the ACO concept, and the personal health record is designed to better equip patients to take ownership of their health. While personal health records are not required for patient accountability, they are the primary information technology–enabler for promoting patient accountability. Personal health records are often part of a patient portal or health information exchange, but they may also exist in the "cloud" (as in Microsoft's HealthVault or WebMD Health Record), as part of an enterprise electronic health record solution (as in Epic's MyChart), or as a custom Web site built by a health system. While personal health records are now part of the health information technology landscape, challenges remain concerning longitudinal data aggregation, security, and patient adoption.

Self-Service

Web-based self-service tools are those that allow patients to make appointments, pay bills, communicate with providers, and update information online and are often part of a patient portal. These tools can save patients time and money, increase patient satisfaction, increase patient commitment to the ACO's healthcare services and provider network, and increase the likelihood that patients will utilize the personal health record. As patients become more technology savvy, they are increasingly comfortable with these types of applications and are more likely to demand them.

Telehealth

Many interactions between patients and providers can be efficiently handled via e-mail or over the phone, but, until recently, providers have not been traditionally reimbursed for these interactions. Telehealth (also known as telemedicine) is improving accessibility through use of remote technology–enabled healthcare services for consumers through new channels for communications between patients, physicians, and care provider teams. In May 2011, CMS passed a final rule that streamlined physician and practitioner's credentialing for those who provide telemedicine services.[47] For consumers in areas where critical access hospitals (CAH) are their nearest locations to receive medical care, this regulatory change offers an example where lightening regulatory burdens can result in opportunities to expand services that improve patient satisfaction and outcomes where access to care is limited. As these technologies and their use become more broadly accepted, "e-visits" and other forms of telehealth services will be a fundamental component to controlling costs and improving productivity for public and private ACOs. In-home video conferencing is likely to become one of the most important avenues for patient-provider communication.

Secured Communications and Coordinated Care Plans

These two elements of ACORM represent key capabilities that help establish and maintain the relationships across physicians, community care providers, health plans, and patients in an ACO. With the advent of the Internet and digital technologies, there has been an increased drive for secured communications across multiple domains to provide access to needed information for appropriate stakeholders. As the use of social media continues to grow in the healthcare field (especially with consumer use of sites such as PatientsLikeMe, Sermo, CaringBridge, Facebook, and others) for exchanging healthcare information,[48] security features will continue to evolve to help enable increasingly safe knowledge sharing.

Coordinated care plans have historically represented networks of providers under contract to CMS to deliver care through an approved benefit package. These plans have been structured as preferred provider organizations (PPOs) , health maintenance organizations (HMOs) , and other structures within the managed care sector. As ACOs take shape in future years, the design and operation of these plans are likely to integrate with market dynamics and result in new mechanisms that are used to deliver care to the patients being served by the ACOs in each market. While secured communications provides a technology infrastructure element to connect physicians, community care providers, and patients, the coordinated care plans can provide the network or organizational structure for which patients access the physicians contracted to deliver the services they need from their ACO.

Electronic Health Records

EHRs are the basic building block in the ACO information technology infrastructure, as well as the centerpiece of the HITECH Act. The cost of implementing an EHR is decreasing while, at the same time, system acquisitions, implementations, and physician adoption is rapidly increasing thanks to HITECH incentives. Also, EHR vendors are beginning to add modules that have value for ACOs in meeting population health management objectives, such as health information exchanges, benchmarking tools, physician communications, and personal health records—all positive market developments for ACOs. Table 1-3 identifies a group of EHR vendor leaders in the market for both inpatient hospital-based systems and for outpatient primary or specialty care practice settings. The "ACO Enablers" are a general set of features that some of the industry leading EHR vendors endeavor to provide for their clients working in the establishment of ACOs.

Table 1-3. EHR Market Leaders

EHR Market Leaders	ACO Enablers
◆ Allscripts ◆ AthenaHealth ◆ Cerner ◆ eClinicalWorks ◆ Epic ◆ GE Centricity ◆ McKesson ◆ Meditech ◆ NextGen ◆ Siemens	◆ Discrete data capture ◆ Quality measure reporting ◆ Interoperability (bidirectionally) ◆ Referral workflow ◆ Performance dashboards

Incorporating disease management systems into an ACO's information technology infrastructure may improve this process greatly. Disease management specialists would be able to utilize granular, EHR data and drive alerts directly to the physician via the EHR or to the patient via the personal health record.

Care Management

Longitudinal care management has traditionally been the domain of payers using claims data as the primary data source. However, similar to disease management, ACOs will require a much more granular approach to care management, using EHR data. Some care management vendors have positioned their products for the provider space and some leading vendors are identified in Table 1-5.

Table 1-5. Care Management Leaders

Care Management Market Leaders
◆ Active Health Management
◆ Altruista Health
◆ Healthways
◆ ICA
◆ Matria
◆ Trizetto

Stage 2 of the Meaningful Use objective does include a requirement for documenting a care plan for transmission at transitions of care, which would make this functionality a necessary area of focus for health information technology vendors. Care coordinators and managers are likely to become central figures in the ACO model, using data from the

ACO's data warehouse to develop effective care plans. Care coordination may develop into a new specialty, with its own education, training, and certification requirements.

Risk Management

Actuarial services related to the ACO's financial risk management function are likely to be delivered by nonpayer third parties and will include handling all financial aspects of the ACO. Other financial services related to ACOs are likely to be bundled as well, including:

➢ Fund accounting and distribution

➢ Audit of attribution model

➢ Audit of shared savings payments

➢ Savings maximization models

The three vertically aligned elements on the left side of the model are technology elements that (*a*) require engagement for all patients or beneficiaries and (*b*) enable safeguarding mechanisms to protect the sanctity of a patient's protected health information.

Security Infrastructure

Privacy and security in healthcare is of increasing importance as the federal government steps up the surveillance, enforcement, and penalties around misuse of patient data. ACOs are and will be vulnerable to privacy and security breaches and face substantial challenges because of the large amount of data and large number of stakeholders (physicians, clinicians, and patients) involved. For example, consider an ACO with 100,000 beneficiaries; 1,000 physicians; 4,000 caregivers; and a number of vendor relationships. Providing system access to every stakeholder will require:

➢ An appropriate business associate agreement

➢ A "need to know"

➢ An audit trail

➢ Rules detecting unauthorized access

➢ Protection against download of patient data to a device that can be taken outside of the provider setting

This aspect of the information technology infrastructure will need to be carefully monitored and is likely to become an especially challenging aspect of ACOs. The importance of a strong security infrastructure cannot be understated, given the increasing number of data breaches occurring across the industry, costing an estimated $6.5 billion annually.[49] With the HITECH Act came additional Health Information Portability and Accountability Act (HIPAA) requirements that included "covered entities and business associates to account for disclosures of protected health information to carry out treatment, payment, and health care operations if such disclosures are through an electronic health record."[50]

Enterprise Master Patient Index (EMPI)

An EMPI provides a crosswalk to all of a patient's various identifiers (e.g., medical record numbers) housed in integrated and disparate systems of an ACO. Probabilistic matching (e.g., using date of birth, Social Security number, last name) is often used to make a positive match between patients in two systems when unambiguous identifiers are not available. Because ACOs need to carefully track patients across a number of care settings and providers, EMPIs are an important component of their information technology infrastructure. Key challenges include data governance (e.g., which entities can update core data), eliminating duplicates, and keeping the EMPI current.

Member Registry

Timely, accurate dissemination of patient enrollment data has been a challenge to payers for years, but ACOs must adopt this capability as a core competency. Meaningful ACO performance tracking will depend on such features as the ability to accurately track stop/start dates in real time. It may be possible to adapt current EMPI products on the market to hold registry indexes and fields.

This section provided a summary of many of the elements of ACORM. Enrollment is identified as another element, as it is essential to achieve beneficiary or patient volume levels necessary for healthcare administrators and physicians to plan for population level health management services to be provided by each ACO, public or private. Secondly, ACO revenue cycle management will be discussed in depth, as the topic of Chapter 9. Payment methodologies, regulatory issues, and information technology systems will be addressed in terms of impact and affect on ACO performance as a critical component of ACORM.

Setting the Stage

As the Institute of Medicine identified in 2001, there was a gap in the health information technology needs to meet the goals for improving the quality of care in America. Today, more than a decade later, this gap has been largely closed, but new challenges have emerged as the nation's infrastructure has evolved. With new systems have come unintended consequences and new complexities. While we have solved many problems, new issues have surfaced, brought about by technological solutions in the administrative, clinical, and regulatory domains. Figure 1-7 provides an illustration identifying the importance of health information technology in not only bridging the technology divide over time but, more importantly, serving as a driving force to help achieve the healthcare quality improvement goals set forth by the Institute of Medicine more than a decade ago, leading up to our current national quality strategy and the Three-Part Aim for ACOs established by CMS.

Figure 1-7. Bridging the Divide

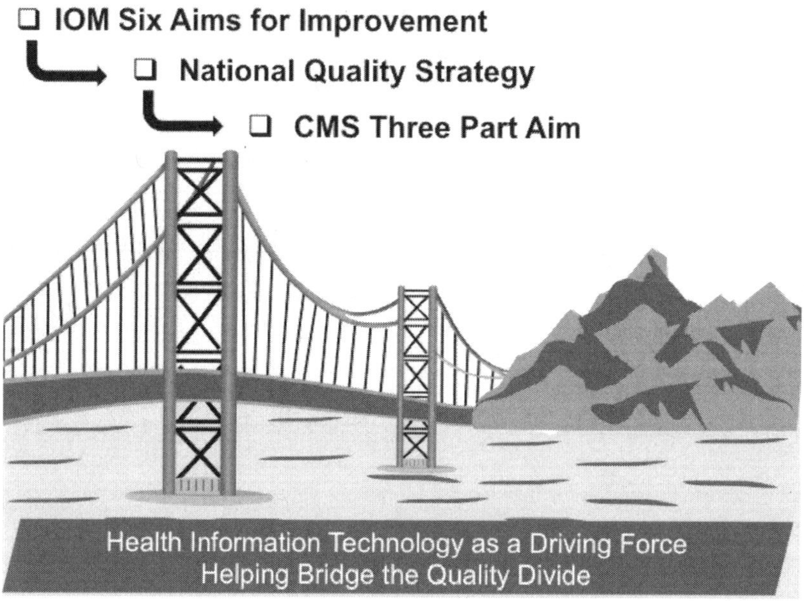

Without health information technology, many of the strides for improvement seen in the past decade would not have been possible. From "bench to bedside" is a phrase known to those in the field of translational medical research. Taking the developments of health information technology tools and applications from the labs, research centers, and pilot projects to getting them into mainstream healthcare services for the betterment of the patient populations being served is similar in its goal with this translational research objective, and the ultimate reward is improving health outcomes. Efforts of DHHS and many other private and public organizations have worked together to bring our nation's health system to this point in history. The need for working toward a nationwide health information network has never been greater as we realize the benefits that lie ahead in terms of improvement in the quality of care, access to care, reduction in medical errors, and reduced waste.

Remaining Chapters Orientation

Each chapter concludes with a section titled *Bridging the Divide*. Within these sections, final conclusions are presented along with a set of takeaways to serve as highlights from the chapter.

The factors influencing systemic change in healthcare (Figure 1-2) are also reflected upon throughout the text. The effects of the Baby Boomer population, system complexity, and the need for innovation have had a dramatic effect on the evolution of the US healthcare system over the last several decades, and the effects of these factors have equally fueled the advanced developments in the field of health information technology. To this end, welcome to *Accountable Care: Bridging the Health Information Technology Divide*, a work offered to provide new insights, detailed analysis, and defining points about the journey our nation has been on with many facets of health information

Chapter 2. Electronic Health Records for the Future of ACOs

Rick Jung and J.M. Bohn

We will make sure that every doctor's office and hospital in this country is using cutting-edge technology and electronic medical records so that we can cut red tape, prevent medical mistakes, and help save billions of dollars each year.[51]

President-elect Barack Obama

December 6, 2008

EHRs: Progress in Adoption

Across America a renaissance is occurring in healthcare with the implementation and adoption of electronic health records (EHRs) in both inpatient and ambulatory settings. For decades there was resistance across the industry to adopt these systems, but in recent years congressional support (as noted in Chapter 1) increased for a transition away from the paper-based culture of medical care to a modernized environment that makes safe and efficient use of electronic health record systems. In 2003, the Institute of Medicine released a report noting the need for "EHR system implementation and its continuing development is a critical element of the establishment of an IT infrastructure for health care."[52] These systems play a vital role in clinical care delivery, management, quality reporting, and administrative processes necessary to maintain electronic documentation of the protected information of a patient's medical diagnoses and treatments across care delivery settings. Since 2003, many initiatives have taken place at federal, state, and local levels to increase the acquisition and adoption of these systems to support the aims set forth by the Institute of Medicine in 2001 and the healthcare quality improvement goals across the United States.

Initiating this discussion on EHRs and their relevance to ACOs, it is important to distinguish between EHRs and electronic medical records (EMRs) .[53] EMRs are an electronic form of the paper medical chart for each patient. These systems are internal to a practice or hospital setting and provide:

➢ Electronic data tracking of longitudinal health records;

➢ Electronic monitoring of patient vital signs; and

➢ The clinical data repository, clinical decision support (CDS) , pharmacy order entry, clinical documentation applications, and warehousing of the patient's personal health data.[54]

EHRs provide the capabilities of the EMR but include interfacing and bidirectional data transfer with other organizations in the environment outside any given medical practice or hospital. Today, the industry is maturing rapidly with these technologies, and their capabilities are meeting the need for secured sharing of patients' health data within the rules of HIPAA.

Among many of their benefits, these systems serve as tools to assist physicians and caregivers in managing the complex aspects of patient health information. As ACOs are chartered with population health management, patient health information needs to be aggregated, compiled, and analyzed for various segments of a given population. The actions of ACOs, integrated delivery networks, and physician practices are to some extent driven by the needs of their patient population (e.g., provider organizations in Southern states with larger numbers of elderly and Baby Boomer patients will devote a higher percentage of services toward caring for this demographic segment). The evolution of EHR systems has involved development to enable the applications to manage the complexity of clinical workflows and integration with other clinical and administrative systems. The complex nature of healthcare operations is what has differentiated the development of EHRs from other industries' operational planning and management systems over the last several decades. The different degrees of interconnectedness that simultaneously exist with independent and autonomous authorities[55] within a healthcare organization as a complex system has extended the development cycle of these systems for decades, along with the need for meeting regulatory, confidentiality, and data sharing requirements.

What are some of the national trends that have driven us toward EHR adoption?

Most Americans have experienced an increase in the cost of health insurance premiums over the last few years that have surpassed cost-of-living increases. According to the Kaiser Family Foundation, average premiums for family coverage have increased 113% since 2001, while worker contributions have increased 131%.[56] Employer sponsored healthcare coverage is rapidly disappearing, and insurance companies have continued to increase prices. Federal government insurance plans (Medicare and Medicaid) comprised 31% of the payer mix in 2010, per an annual report by the US Census Bureau.[57] With the Baby Boomer generation just having begun to reach beneficiary age in 2011, this percentage is certain to increase over the coming decades. Supporting this trend is the Medicare Trust Fund's May 2011 Annual Report that indicated[58] the projected growth in funds required for hospital insurance and supplemental medical insurance as a percentage of GDP will continue to increase from its 2011 rate of 3.5+% to greater than 6% by 2050[59], translating into an even larger role in our nation's health insurance market in future years.

Given these trends, ACOs, along with clinical integration programs, are poised to help the industry reduce the rate of growth in healthcare cost and achieve greater levels of quality over time. Pioneer ACOs, as noted in Chapter 1, have been set up through CMS; by the third year, more than 50% of these provider organizations will have matured to the advanced Medicare ACO model. There is no question that the fee-for-service model is fading as the move toward more performance-based and value-conscious care delivery services, supported by advanced technological capabilities, are embraced. The remaining question is how quickly the transition has been and will continue to occur.

There is a multitude of surveys conducted annually, but the results from two national surveys provide some insights. The results of the 2011 annual National Ambulatory Medical Care Survey (NAMCS) by the National Center for Health Statistics (NCHS) shows the historical trend (Figure 2-1) since 2001 for the adoption of EHRs in the ambulatory setting across the United States.

Figure 2-3. HIMSS EMR Adoption Model

		2010 Final	2011 Final
Stage 7	Complete EMR; CCD transactions to share data; Data warehousing; Data continuity with ED, ambulatory, OP	1.0%	1.2%
Stage 6	Physician documentation (structured templates), full CDSS (variance & compliance), full R-PACS	3.2%	5.2%
Stage 5	Closed loop medication administration	4.5%	8.4%
Stage 4	CPOE, Clinical Decision Support (clinical protocols)	10.5%	13.2%
Stage 3	Nursing/clinical documentation (flow sheets), CDSS (error checking), PACS available outside Radiology	49.0%	44.9%
Stage 2	CDR, Controlled Medical Vocabulary, CDS, may have Document Imaging; HIE capable	14.6%	12.4%
Stage 1	Ancillaries – Lab, Rad, Pharmacy – All Installed	7.1%	5.7%
Stage 0	All Three Ancillaries Not Installed	10.1%	9.0%

©2011 HIMSS Analytics Data from HIMSS Analytics™ Database   N =   5,281 / 5,337

Each stage of the model represents the implementation of key elements of an EMR's capabilities. Three critical elements are: computerized physician order entry (CPOE) and CDS in place, followed by establishing closed loop medication administration. These elements not only showed some of the greatest increases in the percentage of hospitals that reached these stages, but have proven to be some of the most difficult in achieving safe and effective implementation. As industry adoption progresses, an increasing number of hospitals will move toward the Stage 7 level. In June 2012, HIMSS announced the launch of a similar model for the Ambulatory setting, A-EMRAM.[64] This new model will measure progress of ambulatory facilities integrated with a hospital or health system, as well as independent physician practices.

EHRs: Implementation and Effectiveness

In 2011, CMS issued its final rules for the first year of the Medicare ACO program and defined the Three-Part Aim[65] that serves as an overarching set of principles for Medicare ACOs and other new CMS programs:

➤ Better care for individuals
➤ Better health for populations
➤ Lower growth in expenditures

These final rules specified the requirement for EHRs as part of the CMS Meaningful Use of EHRs incentive program.[66] With this incentive program in place, ACO models throughout the public (Medicare and Medicaid) and private sectors are working to accelerate their acquisition and adoption of EHRs, as these systems will help healthcare providers achieve higher quality care at the population level, acquire the analytic capabilities to assume an increased share of clinical and financial risk, and have greater control over provider costs of delivering patient care. For ACOs, the implementation and effectiveness of their EHRs will be an integral part of their overall strategy. In fact, Davis and colleagues, in a 2012 article, identified a number of success factors as key to implementation and adoption of EMRs for ACOs.[67] These factors include:

➤ Executive cohesiveness around the vision for the system implementation,
➤ Having and maintaining a long-term partnership with vendors,
➤ Engage physician leaders early in the planning and implementation process,
➤ Establish a comprehensive governance structure,

> ➤ Focus on workflow standardization in clinical operations, and
> ➤ Track quantitative and qualitative benefits.

EHRs are one of the most costly and intricate systems to be implemented in any hospital or physician practice. For years, when there was greater resistance nationwide, these system implementations were perceived as just another "information technology implementation." Today, however, it is widely recognized that these systems bring about a comprehensive clinical transformation and the need for a deep understanding of all aspects of the organization's clinical and administrative operations. Workflow standardization is essential, as implementing an EHR drives the need for examining all the connection points, information exchanges, and transitions across an organization to ensure the most efficient transformation to future state operations possible.

In addition to the shared savings program and the HITECH Act, there are other initiatives driving the increased adoption of EHRs. The adoption of the patient-centered medical home model in recent years by primary care and specialty care providers has increased the necessity to implement and adopt EHR systems to meet goals for improving patient access to their records, continuity of care, and managing care and patient populations.[68] The DHHS Health Information Technology Regional Extension Centers (RECs) is another program funded under the HITECH Act that has been focused on supporting EHR system selection, implementation, training, and adoption for providers in small practices (e.g., those with 10 or fewer providers) and in rural communities. Over time, new programs will continue to emerge at federal, state, and local levels that will continue the national adoption of these systems.

Measure First, Manage Later

In almost all industries, the work being done by individuals and teams is measured to evaluate efficiency, effectiveness, revenue/loss impact, and overall value to customers and stakeholders. In the automotive industry, for example, the central computer (e.g., the enterprise resource planning system) keeps track of resources used, resources available, project schedules, and status on meeting production goals so that work is not duplicated and resources are not wasted. Healthcare services, for many years, lacked this centralized system for monitoring the quality and safety of care that patients are receiving in both inpatient and outpatient settings. The inability to measure and collect information makes it difficult to manage diseases and chronic conditions contributing to patients getting inappropriate and unnecessary care. Disparate systems, such as different EHRs from multiple vendors and multiple lab and imaging systems, have created requirements for patients to tell the same story over and over again, which has led to inaccuracies or incomplete patient health records. Having different and disconnected EHRs prevented physicians from having optimal and timely knowledge of the patient's condition and caused health systems to become taxed with redundant diagnostic procedures. The drive for increased interoperability, supported by common EHR and other health information technology data standards, will alleviate many of these challenges over time, as they are already being solved at local and regional levels working toward a nationwide health information network. However, the process is long, given the complexity of technologies, organizations, and other systems.

EHRs can provide measurable data for every patient, every disease state, and every point of interaction, enabling providers to manage the delivery of appropriate and necessary care. By measuring first, providers will be able to manage care more effectively for their patient population. In addition to collecting and measuring the data for the purpose of improving the quality of care, providers also must be prepared to use the data in the negotiation of contracts with payers as the industry continues its move toward models of pay-for-performance, value-based purchasing and accountable care.

As patients tend to stay with providers long-term, physician providers have the incentive to help manage their patients' health armed with the data that provides valuable insights to health outcomes and health status resulting from adherence or nonadherence to previously prescribed treatment plans. Enabling these relationships can take years, but if providers harness the potential of EHRs, they can devise and implement plans of care with their patients that result in better care at lower costs at the population level. Taking these steps then allows providers and their organizations to assume greater financial risk on the path to establishing an ACO utilizing the tools, such as EHRs, that will allow them to operate efficiently and effectively for the benefit of the patient populations they serve.

The continued emergence of new ACO configurations with clinical integration programs as part of the foundation are likely to arise from pilot projects across the country and out of CMS's Center for Medicare and Medicaid Innovation (CMMI) . Emergent models may embody new structures of owned/employed physicians and a diminishing percentage of fee-for-service arrangements, as the industry continues its movement toward pay-for-performance and value-based purchasing contractual arrangements. In these models, EHRs are and will be part of the core information technology infrastructure requirement for which physicians, hospitals, specialists, and other care providers and organizations will utilize to share data and deliver better care for their patient population.

The new revenue opportunities that are emerging through these new models have the potential to offset some of the substantial capital costs that come with significant organizational and clinical transformation initiatives. Strategic governance is crucial, as these implementations are multiyear programs that require significant capital investment and resources. Governance structures should include stakeholders from the C-level of the healthcare organization and the vendor to ensure alignment with strategic goals for effecting positive organizational change. This must also include measureable benefits realized for both quantitative and qualitative return on investment for the healthcare organization, its staff, the physician community, and most importantly the patients served through improved health outcomes at the population level.

New models of care delivery with integrated and interoperable EHRs will benefit patients with improved health outcomes and higher quality care at reduced cost and benefit employers with cost savings in reduced premiums for health insurance plans they offer to their employees. These issues are drivers in the maturation of public and private ACOs. As we learn from the lessons of the managed care era and embrace the role of EHRs as a tool to continue improving the quality of care delivered, we can better measure quality and cost of care to more effectively manage the health of the populations being served for decades to come.

From Volume to Value

It is estimated that about 30% of healthcare delivery in the United States today is either unnecessary or inappropriate.[69] Yet, if providers utilize EHRs and their underlying patient health data to make continuous improvements to prescribed treatment plans to effect changes in outcomes, higher quality healthcare can and will be achieved. It is important not just to provide an abundance of care for patients, but also to provide appropriate care. Not only will this result in increased value delivered to the patients, it will result in payments that are appropriate to the outcome of treatments. If, for example, an ACO chooses to assume the risk of contracting directly with a large employer, it will be able to offer a plan that eliminates costs of unnecessary care and keep administrative costs down so that premiums paid by the employer are reduced below rates they may be paying at the beginning of the contractual relationship. One of the keys to providing appropriate care and increasing the value in care delivered is to collect and measure the patient data contained in EHRs. Without appropriate analysis and determination of improvements to be made at the micro and macro level in caring for the health of the population, the value derived from EHRs is not maximized.

In this transition from a volume-driven care delivery system to one focused on value and performance-based compensation, independent physicians have fallen on hard times. The cottage industry they once knew is rapidly diminishing. Their information technology systems do not communicate with the systems of other practices and provider organizations; it is difficult to gain contracts with insurance payers; malpractice insurance is, in some cases, an exorbitant cost; and it is become increasingly difficult to meet financial obligations of the business for an independent practice. As noted in Figure 1-5, there are several potential organizational configurations for ACOs. Integrated delivery networks are one of the better-positioned entity structures to serve as the central point of command for ACOs, however. Physician consolidation under the integrated delivery network structure is increasing, led by hospitals who are often the parent entity of the integrated delivery network and have the resources and infrastructure to contract both exclusively and nonexclusively with a network of physicians in the geographic region that aggregates the needed referrals to amass patient volumes for care delivery through the integrated delivery network. While all the model configurations for ACOs are being piloted and tested, both publicly and privately, the move toward integrated delivery networks is being driven by its structural benefits in meeting resource supply needs, patient demands, and financial pressures. With the movement toward ACOs, the integrated delivery network is well positioned to implement the key design principles for ACOs[70] (e.g., improving accountability, increasing performance measurement, and reforming payment systems). Ultimately, this industry transition to a new era of healthcare provider organizational structures including the safe adoption of EHRs will lead to more cost effective controls and yield better outcomes for all patient population segments across our nation.

Standardized Care: Everybody Wins

EHRs contain patient health data that allows providers to track the outcomes of evidence-based medicine practices so they can evaluate what treatments work the best for given diseases and conditions. The notion of consistent care leading to patients experiencing improved health outcomes aligns with an ACO's mission and guiding principles. Consider the example of care for a diabetic patient population. An EHR allows the provider to track when patients are late getting a lab test, for example, and adhere to other standard-of-care protocols. Furthermore, the system can be set up to contact patients via their preferred method of communication (e.g., phone call, text, or e-mail) and, when patients get their lab work done, the results are automatically documented. Compliance benefits the patient, who is healthier, and the provider, who is rewarded through the shift to incentive-driven reimbursement models. In the results of one study of the care for a diabetic patient population, it was shown that a higher percentage of patients seen in EHR-driven practice settings achieved higher standards of care for diabetes treatment than did a percentage of patients seen at practices that were operating on paper-based patient records.[71] Examples such as this one provide evidence that with EHRs in place, quality of care can improve.

EHRs help drive standardization of care practices. As workflows are standardized across care delivery environments, standards of care can more adequately be reinforced, and measuring and comparing the outcomes of similar patient demographic groups becomes more relevant. As variability in processes is removed from the system of care in the way patients are treated, measurements become more meaningful, and it is easier to evaluate and determine best practices for integration into evidence-based medicine. Standardization of care occurs with the implementation and adoption of EHRs. Identifying and integrating best practices, such as evidence-based innovations, will afford healthcare organizations more opportunities to improve the quality and reduce the cost of care delivered.

The Evolution of EHRs

As any organization that has implemented an EHR knows, physician adoption has historically been a major obstacle. This trend is changing today with new federal incentive programs, but, over the last decade, resistance to change and adoption of EHRs was due in part to "inadequate capital, unclear ROI, maintenance costs, and inadequate IT staff."[72] These systems were viewed merely as a replacement of paper charts—an electronic file drawer—and not as a tool that would help manage the health of their patients or the business of their practice.

Today, however, the federal government, having recognized many of these issues that created barriers to adoption, launched programs to infuse funds that incentivize and support physician adoption of EHRs and help reduce barriers, both of which support accelerating the pace of adoption. Over the 3 years since the passage of the HITECH Act, the adoption of EHRs has been accompanied by new financial incentives (e.g., Meaningful Use, patient-centered medical home programs) tied to the implementation and adoption of EHRs and the improvement of population health outcomes. In an ACO, EHRs should evolve to better reflect how healthcare providers work and include functionality that will help them operate more efficiently. This is occurring throughout the industry with greater focus on clinical workflow redesign efforts that accompany the implementation of many EHRs in either initial set-up or in follow-up efforts.

Mobile Technologies

One of the limitations of some EHR systems is they have not been designed for application on mobile devices with a full set of features and functions that mimic the paper chart. EHRs need features and capabilities that are aligned with Meaningful Use, such as the ability to enter orders, e-prescribe, and view lab results. Physicians need access to tools of their choosing (e.g., iPhone and iPad versus desktop) to manage their patient population in the future ACO's multisite clinical care environment. Mobile devices are being adopted at an accelerated pace, so having EHR applications that can be used on these devices is essential to collect and provide the needed information at the point of care. The tools need to be simple, workflow oriented, and have the functionality that fits within the architecture of today's mobile technologies.

Consider the diabetes patient case mentioned earlier. When patients walk into their doctor's office, the physician needs to immediately know the following:

➢ Previous diagnosis of type 1 or 2 diabetes mellitus;

➢ Medication history;

➢ Patient lifestyle factors (e.g., weight management, diet, exercise, family history with diabetes, smoking status, alcohol use);

➢ Last five to seven lab results over the last five to seven quarters; and

➢ History of compliance or noncompliance with their treatment plan.

All of this information should be available at the physician's fingertips, along with an awareness of any new medications or interventions that may present better treatment options than those currently prescribed in the plan of care for the patient. Other than this essential information, does a physician need additional information? The answer is yes, but not at his or her fingertips. What complicates this scenario is that every diagnosis has different parameters in terms of the information the physician needs to know when the patient walks in the door. In fact, this is one of the challenges in designing EHRs that are lightweight—creating a user-friendly architecture that ensures optimal usability for the physician.

While being designed for mobile applications, EHRs need to store and present the provider with information needed to maintain efficient workflow and meet CMS Meaningful Use of EHRs criteria for Stages 1-3, so that the provider may capture financial incentives. Ensuring the capabilities are in place to meet these criteria is a system development priority that also allows physicians to track health outcomes of their patients. Mobile devices should be Web-based, as opposed to driven through a client server, so physicians can access EHRs remotely and have compatibility with a variety of systems. After Meaningful Use criteria have been met, ease of use is a final characteristic to be secured. The EHRs for ACOs should have a more workflow-oriented architecture, improved usability, and strong device connectivity to enable mobile use for physicians to improve efficiency and accelerate system adoption.

A New Solution: Best of Both Worlds

When you go to the automated teller machine to withdraw cash, make a deposit, or conduct other transactions, you do not need to go to your local bank; you can go to any automated teller machine at any bank and conduct the same transactions. Healthcare should have this same type of transparency, especially in the case of ACOs. Data needs to be simple to retrieve and accessible by *any* physician, so patients do not need to re-explain their health history every time they go to the doctor and risk inaccuracies or incomplete records being established.

Today, this type of communication does not always occur within integrated delivery networks, much less outside of them. Healthcare providers and organizations may always use different EHRs, given the wide array of EHR vendors in the market, and to make them compatible, they need effective, secure, and efficient health information exchange. Information needs to flow bidirectionally between specialists and primary care physicians to ensure that ACOs function properly and that the business needs of stakeholders are accommodated. Figure 2-4 presents a picture of an ACO Health Intelligence Hub.

Figure 2-4. ACO Health Intelligence Hubs

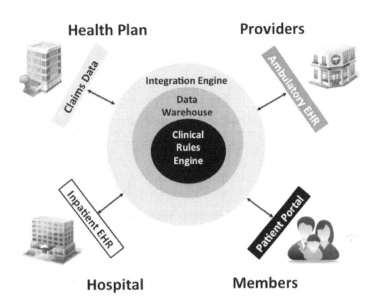

Four stakeholder groups (hospitals, members, health plans, and providers) are engaging and interacting with the EHR system through health information exchange that connects the multilevel technology architecture necessary to drive interconnectivity and efficient flow of information. EHRs and health information exchanges often are combined and offered by EHR vendors as they recognize the need for communication across sites and locations. However, it is unrealistic for a physician to implement a single technology platform from a single vendor, as they may care for patients at a variety of hospitals who may all be using different vendor systems. For an ACO, the challenge can be costly and must be evaluated with care, as EHR implementations are most often lengthy multiyear projects, and all physicians referring patients to the ACO's network will make significant capital investments to meet clinical integration goals, CMS Meaningful Use requirements, and to support necessary communication with other physicians and hospital sites across and outside the ACO.

A new solution is needed that ensures proper data flow, is Web-based, and can be installed on top of existing EHRs. A Web-based system ensures that physicians can easily connect to one another and avoid the challenges of the silo structure of stand-alone systems. Putting it all together, one model for EHRs in the context of ACOs can be referred to as:

WHEEL

- ➤ **W**orkflow-oriented;
- ➤ **H**IEs needed to ensure proper data flow;
- ➤ **E**fficient in terms of access to only the relevant data;
- ➤ **E**very provider can use it, because it is Web-based and is interoperable with different platforms; and
- ➤ **L**ightweight in terms of the physical device used to access it.

WHEEL is an example of another potential conceptual model to consider when establishing the EHR architecture.[73] It focuses on principles important to ACOs and ensuring secure and efficient communications for all physicians.

From Cost Center to Asset

As they stand today, EHRs are a huge cost center with a return on investment that, in the past, has largely been considered intangible and unclear.[74] However, analytics and performance metrics are improving as many executives have noted the importance of identifying return on investment (both quantitative and qualitative) from these multiyear and multimillion dollar projects. One example comes from Brigham and Women's Hospital (BWH) in Boston, Massachusetts. A 2006 article[75] noted that, between 1993 and 2002, [BWH] spent $11.8 million to develop, implement, and operate a computerized physician order entry (CPOE) system. Analysis of the project showed that, over the 10 years, BWH achieved gross savings of $28.5 million, net savings of $16.7 million, and net operating budget savings of $9.5 million. Key areas impacted that realized the savings were:

➢ Renal dosing guidance

➢ Nursing time utilization

➢ Specific drug guidance

➢ Adverse drug event prevention

Case Example: Sentara Healthcare ROI

Sentara Healthcare serves the southeastern region of Virginia and northeastern North Carolina and is comprised of more than 100 care-giving sites, including 10 acute care hospitals with more than 2,300 beds; 9 outpatient care facilities; 7 nursing centers; 3 assisted living centers; 9 advanced imaging centers; 3,700 physicians on staff; and 20,000 employees. Sentara Healthcare is among the very few organizations that have been awarded Stage 7 by HIMSS Analytics.

Sentara embarked on the implementation of eCare (comprised of Epic, other technologies, and workflow redesign) in February 2008. The total cost of ownership of the project totaled $237 million, so getting a return on that investment was critical.

As a result of their efforts with eCare, the following clinical improvements were realized and were primary drivers of the ultimate financial outcomes:

Case Example: Sentara Healthcare ROI (cont.)

- Computerized Provider Order Entry (CPOE). Nationally, post-implementation CPOE ranges from 25%-50%. Sentara Healthcare hospitals were achieving nearly 90% post-implementation CPOE.

- First Dose Medication Administration. The average time from physician order to medication administration (NOW orders) has been reduced by an average of 97.33 minutes, with turn-around times now running about 30 minutes.

- Sentara Healthcare estimates that 88,500 potential errors were prevented with the implementation of eCare's barcode scanning.

- Performance of Core Measures improved.

- Quality data collection was automated and reporting transitioned to Web-based reporting.

In addition to achieving clinical outcomes, document management and reduced transcription and supply expenses have improved, including:

- Scanning volume declined 38%.

- On-time performance is 98% (within 30 minutes).

- Pharmacy order scanning has been reduced by 94%.

- Same-day scanning and indexing of end procedure images was achieved.

- Clinicians enter more than 90% of progress notes into the system.

Medical group transcription and supply expenses were significantly reduced as a result of reimbursement improvements, reduced storage costs, medical records labor reductions, and malpractice claims and premium reductions.

Case Example: Sentara Healthcare ROI (cont.)

Sentara Healthcare's implementation began in February 2008 and quickly delivered financial benefits. As reported in the article "Making Music Out of Noise" (*JHIM*, Winter 2010), six hospitals had completed implementation by the end of 2009, and Sentara Healthcare was projecting nearly $16.6 million in annualized benefits. With seven hospitals using eCare as of the end of 2011, $50 million in benefits had been realized, far exceeding expectations. These financial benefits are attributed in large part to the following measures:

Benefit Derived From eCare	Financial Benefit in Dollars
Reduced Total Transcription Costs	3.0 million
Reduced Length of Stay/Reduced ADEs	14.7 million
Reduced Medical Records Supply Costs	2.1 million
Increase in Unit Efficiency/Retention of RNs	10.6 million
Increased Outpatient Procedures	9.1 million
Reduced Medical Records Positions	1.8 million
Reduced Optima (Health Plan) Costs	3.0 million

Other returns on investment may be nonfinancial or qualitative, such as experiencing a reduced average length of stay in a hospital emergency department setting as a result of implementing a CPOE system.[76] While challenges still exist with evaluating return on investment from EHRs that are important to stakeholders of each system implementation, it is possible to evaluate quantitative and qualitative benefits. Identification of variables, understanding cost factors, defining drivers of efficiency gains, and revenue stream increases can produce a clearer picture of the return on investment from the new clinical and administrative operating state that emerges with the implementation of EHRs.

Many physician groups and integrated delivery networks have spent excessive amounts of money on EHR systems, but they are still establishing the ability to share test results or other data among physicians and caregivers that extend beyond their existing organization or network. There are open-source offerings and other solutions that support these needs, but the choices of the past have been minimal. With the influence of CMS's Meaningful Use requirements, however, the options for having the capabilities in place to capture the necessary data and analytics ability to demonstrate clear return on investment are certain to become more robust and capable of meeting customer demands in the near future.

In ACOs, EHRs need to evolve so that the focus is on sharing data on health outcomes at the patient and the population level, rather than just collecting patient health data. One option is to link some element of physicians' compensation to this kind of data sharing, which ties in with the measure-first-manage-later concept discussed earlier.

In order for EHRs to work in this concept and fulfill their potential, the silo structure of today's platforms clearly needs to be reengineered. To be sustainable in an ACO, EHRs need to be interoperable, interconnected, and more compatible with platforms implemented by multiple vendors. This can be achieved by adhering to the Office of the National Coordinator's Permanent Certification Program for Health Information Technology[77], utilizing a regional health information exchange and planning for long-term participation in the nationwide health information network as it evolves to facilitate data transfer.

Future of the EHR

As the physician practice landscape continues to consolidate within integrated delivery networks and ACOs, health information technology solutions will evolve to support the emerging needs of these entities. Today's health information technology marketplace includes multiple discrete products and product categories (e.g., EHRs, health information exchange, analytics engines, patient portals, clinical decision support, computerized physician order entry, disease management, and revenue cycle management systems), all elements of the health information technology architecture needed to support successful ACOs.

Health information technology systems of the future will be unified, integrated solutions with the ability to manage the needs of tomorrow's integrated, data-driven delivery systems. Current EHRs will continue to be designed to address specific ACO needs for meeting and delivering information in accordance with the CMS Meaningful Use criteria. Over time, as design and testing costs are absorbed, future EHR product offerings will become more affordable under total cost of ownership considerations to help replace disparate legacy systems still in some provider organizations today.

Another fundamental shift for the core architecture of EHRs in the future will be the advancement of clinical decision support and reporting features that today are part of facility-based EHR systems. In the not too distant future, these features could well gravitate to the centralized ACO health intelligence hub. This movement will be driven by the shift away from physicians managing the patients in their panel to integrated care delivery systems managing patient populations across the complete care continuum.

In order to succeed with population health management, it will be critical to aggregate patient data to more effectively mine data and measure, evaluate, manage, and coordinate care more effectively across collaborating provider groups in the future ACO operating environment. We can expect to see the emergence of ACO health intelligence hubs or nerve centers operated by multidisciplinary teams of clinicians (e.g., health intelligence teams) , clinical support staff, and information technology data analysts. These health intelligence teams will collaborate to fulfill basic requirements such as care gap compliance. They will also leverage their clinical data assets to identify new patterns and protocols that can be applied to drive innovation in care delivery and to accelerate improvements in outcomes, efficiency, and cost control.

This transformation of health information technology architecture, systems, and the clinical workforce will have a major impact in the evolution of EHRs. Meeting the needs of physicians, caregivers, ancillary staff, and administrators will serve two basic purposes to note. First is to serve as a data entry system that feeds centralized ACO health intelligence hubs with the right data in the right format for population health management and analytic insights on performance. This will support operating and clinical quality measures required for the CMS Meaningful Use of EHRs program, the National Committee for Quality Assurance's (NCQA) Physician Practice Connections Patient-Centered Medical Home (PPC-PCMH™) program, Physician Quality Reporting Initiatives, and the Healthcare Effectiveness Data and Information Set

(HEDIS) requirements.[78] The other purpose is to serve as a thin client recipient of real-time data feeds from centralized ACO health intelligence hubs that use the WHEEL principle, noted previously, directing physicians on the precise care required for each patient they see, based on a synthesis of data and knowledge collected across the patients' care continuum. One of the goals for the future of EHRs in the ACO operating environment is the EHR in its current form may be displaced by more simple, but uniquely robust, applications, such as mobile Web-based devices tethered to the ACO health intelligence hubs that provide physicians with the right information, at the right time, to support their delivery of the best quality of care at the right place for lower costs. One case study of a progressive and dynamic physician practice that is on the forefront of advanced EMRs initiatives is Cornerstone Healthcare.

Case Example: EMR Advances at Cornerstone Healthcare

Cornerstone Healthcare, a High Point, North Carolina, based multispecialty physician group practice founded in 1995, has more than 200 physicians working across 15 locations throughout the central part of the state. In 2005, Cornerstone implemented Allscripts Touchworks™ EMR and, in 2009, upgraded to the Enterprise application. Cornerstone achieved the National Committee for Quality Assurance (NCQA) level 3 Patient-Centered Medical Home (PPC-PCMH™) certification in 2011 and is embracing the industry transition to accountable care–based service delivery, including participation in Cigna's Accountable Care Collaborative starting in 2012.[79] Knowing the challenges faced by the regional patient population, physician and technical leaders recognized the need for an analytic tool to strengthen outreach efforts with high-risk patients and a new tool to drive physician compliance in quality and performance metric reporting.

To strengthen outreach efforts, Humedica's MinedShare® data analytic tool was implemented in December 2010 as part of the American Medical Group Association's Anceta Collaborative. The application was integrated as part of the Patient Care Advocates program in March 2011 with Cornerstone's EMR to identify and contact high-risk diabetic patients with A1C over 9, BP>140/90, and/or LDL>130 who had not been seen in the office for 6 months. Through the spring of 2012, a 27.5% improvement had been seen in clinical parameters solely driven by this new outreach program and tool.

The second tool was an in-house add-on to the EMR to strengthen physician compliance with performance and quality metric reporting requirements. The tool went live with adult primary care physicians in mid 2011 and provided reminders for tests to be performed based on EBM guidelines and contractual performance metrics. With the increased requirements for physician quality reporting in the NCQA's PPC-PCMH™ program, CMS Meaningful Use of EHRs, and practice engagement in public and private ACO relationships, the need for physician quality and performance reporting has increased rapidly, driving the importance of such an analytical tool.

Challenges and Barriers for the Workforce

As EHRs evolve, one of the key issues to address is the workforce and the impact these systems have on it. There are generational issues at play when looking at the adaptability of the Baby Boomer generation versus Generation X and Generation Y in terms of physicians, nursing, and ancillary staff's adaptability to the rapidly changing world of healthcare with the continuous stream of new health information technology tools and applications they are confronted with on a daily basis.

The implementation of these systems brings about challenges and barriers of an educational, cultural, and technical perspective—all of which can have tremendous impact on efforts to improve the quality of care delivered and the potential for unintended consequences to be dealt with that can have negative impacts on workflow, quality of care, and overall cost of care. One overarching technical challenge for the industry is achieving interoperability, given the wide variety of EHR vendors in the health information technology market that ACOs must choose from in selecting a system to implement for and with their physicians, nurses, and ancillary staff.[80] While CMS Meaningful Use requirements will continue to drive interoperability progressing through Stages 2 and 3, the variability in vendor options and system features will continue to present numerous selection challenges for ACO leaders.

Unintended Consequences with EHRs and Computerized Provider Order Entry

Given the importance and promise of EHRs, a significant number of studies were conducted in the last decade regarding their impact and effects on quality of care. One study published in 2006 and 2007 by Ash, Campbell, Sittig, and colleagues identified nine types of unintended consequences related to use of computerized physician order entry.[81] Each of the consequences identified can have varying effects on the healthcare workforce and the quality of care delivered. Figure 2-5 illustrates the nine categories of unintended consequences.

Figure 2-5. Unintended Consequences[82]

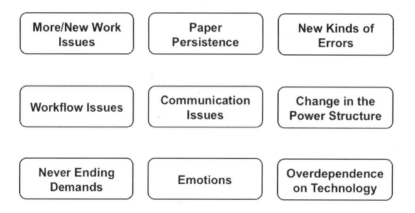

Each of these categories can impact the quality of care, occurrence of medical errors, and cost of care delivered in hospitals and physician practices alike. These unintended consequences have the potential to impact the progress of ACOs in their use and adoption of EHRs. One example to consider is workflow issues. Recognizing the occurrence of workflow gaps in transitioning from a paper-based medical record environment to the EHR-driven environment is essential in adoption of these technologies. In one study of a health system that analyzed its preparedness for meeting Stage 1 of the CMS Meaningful Use criteria, one of the central foci was on conducting an EHR workflow gap analysis that identified system improvements needed to bring the current (legacy) system up to needed standards to meet the criteria.[83]

Each of these unintended consequences is important, as they can affect the efficiency, effectiveness, and integration of EHRs in the inpatient and ambulatory settings throughout a system's life cycle, and they may reoccur with the implementation of new systems or system upgrades. All of these consequences occur within the sociotechnical dimensions described by Sittig and Singh in a 2010 paper regarding their impact on the complex adaptive healthcare systems.[84] Figure 2-6 illustrates the eight dimensions identified in their paper.

Figure 2-6. Sociotechnical Dimensions

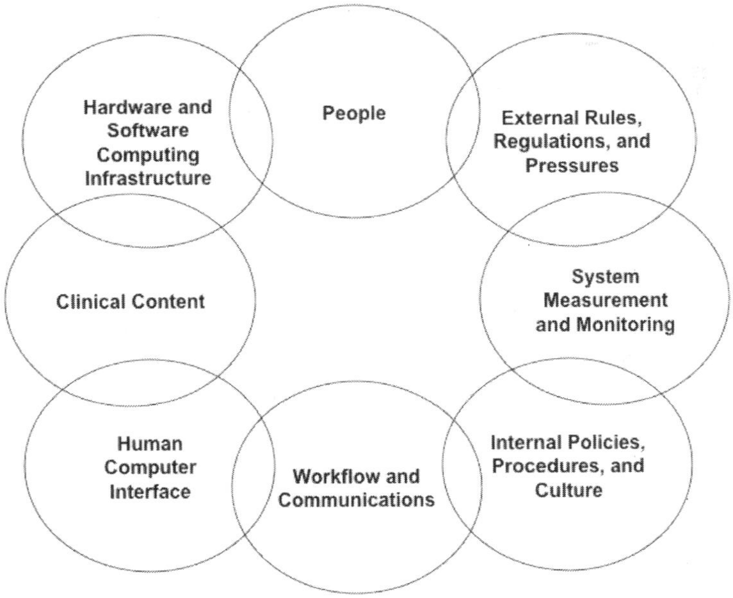

The importance of these factors (both the unintended consequences and the sociotechnical dimensions) is linked to the complex nature of these systems and, secondly, instituting plans to monitor the dimensions to mitigate the potential for harm to patients that comes with the occurrence of unintended consequences across these dimensions.

Impact on Physicians and Nurses

As EHRs are implemented, there are tremendous educational and cultural challenges that come with ensuring adoption of these systems. Physicians have extremely busy schedules and, in many situations, reimbursements for their services have been decremented year after year, driving an increasing number of them away from private practice and into employed situations under larger group practices or part of integrated delivery networks. For many, the issue of training on EHRs and other health information technology systems has been secondary to patient care. But, over the last decade, an increasing number of healthcare organizations have committed the resources to select and implement new EHR systems. With this multiyear system implementation and clinical transformation projects have come the increased need for additional investments in training to drive knowledge acquisition for physician and nursing staff to increase adoption, commitment, and adequacy of training.[85] However, EHR training is not just at initial installation; it becomes an element of the healthcare organization's culture, as the need for continuous learning with updates to applications, system upgrades, and new EHR systems continues to increase in importance ultimately to benefit the patient population served. Generational differences across the workforce have played a role in resistance to training, but, as the industry has moved forward with Meaningful Use of EHRs, the workforce is accelerating its adoption of these systems in clinical practices to improve the quality, safety, and cost of patient care.

Bridging the Divide

In Chapter 1, the ACORM model was introduced. One of the key building blocks to ACORM is the EHR. Many issues have been discussed, but one to consider is a high level strategy for successful implementation. There are many paths and ways to ensure successful adoption of these systems across the spectrum of care delivery settings. Sentara Healthcare and Banner Health noted one example of a successful strategy.[86] Coupled with the success factors for EHR implementation and adoption noted earlier in this chapter, a second set of tenets for successful EHR implementation and adoption from Sentara and Banner example includes:

➢ Establish mission and vision and understand the infrastructure,

➢ Ensure strong planning and execution of the work,

➢ Recognize that change is inevitable—prepare for and embrace it, and

➢ Ensure that strong and clear leadership is in place.

Collaborative leadership is critical, and engaging physician leaders as the spearhead for the ACO with a focus on driving teamwork and joint decision making across multidisciplinary boundaries leads to ACO maturity, achievement of shared savings goals, and accomplishing population health management and outcome objectives for an ACO's beneficiaries. The implications of organizational change management in EHR implementations are significant, as the changes to the healthcare organization's operations can affect the daily workflow activities of every physician, care provider, and other multidisciplinary worker in the system. Having a clear multistep process for helping stakeholders understand the changes underway, and those that are forthcoming, helps alleviate stress at individual and group levels, along with improving opportunities for EHR adoption.

Acknowledging and striving to apply the key tenets for successful EHR system implementations while working to mitigate risks and unintended consequences as they emerge will help strengthen our opportunities to improve the quality of patient care in ACOs as we reengineer the ecosystem of healthcare delivery in America.

Chapter 2: Takeaways

✓ Recognize the inherent complexity of EHR systems and how they serve as a foundational technology in an ACO's population health management objective.

✓ Know the distinction between EMR and EHR systems.

✓ Gain an understanding of return-on-investment measures for clinical and administrative measures evaluation and consider both quantitative and qualitative measures in developing a robust picture of the full ROI realized from any EHR system implementation.

✓ Consider the impact of bidirectional information flow through the ACO Health Intelligence Hub on all stakeholders when setting the communications framework for the broader ACO ecosystem.

✓ Consider the WHEEL conceptual model when establishing a new EHR architecture.

✓ Recognize the importance of monitoring for unintended consequences that may arise with EHR and CPOE implementations across the eight sociotechnical dimensions.

✓ Plan for the clinical workforce transformation and training needed to meet their needs.

✓ Development of mobile EHR applications should be a priority, ensuring they have a workflow-oriented architecture to enable mobile use by physicians.

✓ Understand EHR adoption trends and the barriers to physician adoption. Engage physicians early in implementation planning and for risk mitigation to enhance physician engagement.

[51] Remarks of President-elect Barack Obama. Radio Address on the Economy. December 6, 2008. Office of the President-Elect. Accessed online March 6, 2012, at http://change.gov/newsroom/entry/the_key_parts_of_the_jobs_plan/.

[52] Committee on Data Standards for Patient Safety. Institute of Medicine. *Key Capabilities of an Electronic Health Record System: Letter Report.* July 31, 2003. Washington, DC: National Academies Press.

[53] Garrett P, Seidman J. EMR vs. EHR—What is the Difference? *HealthIT Buzz.* January 4, 2011. Accessed online January 22, 2012, at http://www.healthit.gov/buzz-blog/electronic-health-and-medical-records/emr-vs-ehr-difference/.

[54] Flareau B, Bohn JM, Konschak C. Glossary and Acronyms. In: *Accountable Care Organizations: A Roadmap to Success.* 1st Ed. Virginia Beach, VA: Convurgent Publishing; 2011:208-209.

[55] Serrat O. Defining Complexity. In: *Understanding Complexity.* Knowledge Solutions. 2009 November. No. 6. Accessed online March 16, 2012, at http://knowledgesolutions.blogspot.com/2009/11/understanding-complexity.html.

[56] Kaiser Family Foundation and Health Research & Educational Trust. Employer health benefits 2011 summary of findings. September 27, 2011. Accessed November 25, 2011, online at http://ehbs.kff.org/pdf/8226.pdf.

[57] Income, Poverty, and Health Insurance Coverage in the United States: 2010. United States Census Bureau Annual Report. Table 10: Coverage by Type of Health Insurance: 2009 and 2010. p. 29. Accessed online January 20, 2012, at http://www.census.gov/prod/2011pubs/p60-239.pdf.

[58] Medicare Board of Trustees. Overview. In: *2011 Annual Report of the Boards of Trustees of the Federal Hospital Insurance and Federal Supplementary Medical Insurance Trust Funds*, p. 17. Accessed online September 21, 2011, at https://www.cms.gov/ReportsTrustFunds/downloads/tr2011.pdf.

[59] Bohn, JM. Introduction. In: *Your Next Steps in Healthcare Transformation.* Louisville, KY: Touchcast Press; 2011:4-5.

[60] Hsiao CJ, Hing E, Socey TC, Cai B. Electronic health record systems and intent to apply for Meaningful Use incentives among office-based physician practices: United States, 2001–2011. *NCHS Data Brief.* No 79. Hyattsville, MD: National Center for Health Statistics; 2011. Accessed online January 30, 2012, at http://www.cdc.gov/nchs/data/databriefs/db79.htm.

[61] Jones SS, Adams JL, Schneider EC, Ringel JS, McGlynn EA. Electronic health record adoption and quality improvement in US hospitals. *Am J Manag Care.* 2010 Dec;16(12 Suppl HIT):SP64-71.

[62] Jha AK, DesRoches CM, Campbell EG, et al. Use of electronic health records in U.S. hospitals. *N Engl J Med.* 2009;360(16):1628-1638.

[63] EMR Adoption Model[SM]. HIMSS Analytics. Accessed online January 23, 2012, at http://www.himssanalytics.org/hc_providers/emr_adoption.asp.

[64] HIMSS Analytics launches EMRAM for ambulatory practices. *Healthcare IT News*. June 6, 2012. Accessed online August 2, 2012, at http://www.healthcareitnews.com/news/himss-analytics-launches-emram-ambulatory-practices.

[65] Fed. Reg. Vol. 76, No. 212. November 2, 2011. I.(C). Overview of the Medicare Shared Savings Program. p. 67804.

[66] Fed. Reg. Vol. 76, No. 212. November 2, 2011. II.(B)5. Processes to Promote Evidence-Based Medicine, Patient Engagement, Reporting, Coordination of Care, and Demonstrating Patient-Centeredness. p. 67826.

[67] Davis CK, Stoots M, Bohn JM. Paving the Way for Accountable Care. Excellence in EMR Implementations. *JHIM*. 2012 Winter;26(1):38-45.

[68] National Committee for Quality Assurance fact sheet. NCQA's Patient-Centered Medical Home (PCMH) 2011. January 31, 2011. Accessed August 27, 2012 online at http://www.ncqa.org/tabid/675/Default.aspx.

[69] What are the Major Proposals to Contain Costs? In: *Background Brief: U.S. Healthcare Costs*. March 2010. Accessed November 25, 2011, online at http://www.kaiseredu.org/Issue-Modules/US-Health-Care-Costs/Background-Brief.aspx.

[70] Fisher ES, McClellan MB, Bertko J, et al. Fostering accountable health care: moving forward in Medicare. *Health Aff (Millwood)*. 2009;28(2):w219-w231.

[71] Cebul RD, Love TE, Jain AK, Hebert CJ. Electronic Health Records and Quality of Diabetes Care. *N Engl J Med*. 2011;365(9):825-833.

[72] Jha AK, DesRoches CM, Campbell EG, et al. Use of Electronic Health Records in U.S. Hospitals. *N Engl J Med*. 2009;360(16):1628-1638.

[73] WHEEL concept created and provided by co-author, Rick Jung. Spring 2012.

[74] Jha AK, 2009.

[75] Kaushal R, Jha AK, Franz C, Glasser J, Shetty KD, et al. Return on investment for a computerized physician order entry system. *J Am Med Infom Assoc*. 2007;14(4):415-423.

[76] Spalding SC, Mayer PH, Ginde AA, Lowenstein SR, Yaron M. Impact of computerized physician order entry on ED patient length of stay. *Am J Emerg Med*. 2011 Feb;29(2):207-11.

[77] Fed. Reg. Vol. 76, No. 5, January 7, 2011. I(B)(c)(2)(a) Initial Set of Standards, Implementation Specifications and Certification Criteria Interim and Final Rules.

[78] Flareau B, et. al. The Quality Continuum—Continuous Improvement. In: *Clinical Integration: A Roadmap to Accountable Care*. 2nd Ed. Virginia Beach, VA: Convergent Publishing; 2011:218.

[79] Cigna Works with Physicians to Bring Accountable Care to 65,000 More Individuals From Maine to Texas. Cigna Press Release, April 9, 2012. Accessed online April 22, 2012, at http://newsroom.cigna.com/article_display.cfm?article_id=1474.

[80] Blumenthal D. Wiring the Health System—Origins and Provisions of a New Federal Program. *N Engl J Med.* 2011; 365(24):2323-2329.

[81] Campbell EM, Sittig DF, Ash JS, Guappone KP, Dykstra RH. Types of unintended consequences related to computerized provider order entry. *J Am Med Inform Assoc.* 2006;13(5):547-56; Ash JS, Sittig DF, Poon EG, et al. The extent and importance of unintended consequences related to computerized provider order entry. *J Am Med Infom Assoc.* 2007;14(4):415-423.

[82] Ash JS, Sittig DF, Poon EG, et al. The extent and importance of unintended consequences related to computerized provider order entry. *J Am Med Infom Assoc.* 2007;14(4):415-423.

[83] Bowes WA. Assessing readiness for meeting Meaningful Use: Identifying electronic health record functionality and measuring levels of adoption. *AMIA Annu Symp Proc.* 2010 Nov 13;2010:66-70.

[84] Sittig DF, Singh H. A new sociotechnical model for studying health information technology in complex adaptive healthcare systems. *Arch Intern Med.* 2011 Jul 25;171(14):1281-1284.

[85] Adler KG. Successful EHR implementations: Attitude is everything. *Fam Pract Manag.* 2010 Nov-Dec;17(6):9-11; Morton ME, Wiedenbeck S. A Framework for Predicting EHR Adoption Attitudes: A Physician Survey. *Perspect Health Inf Manag.* 2009 Sep 16;6:1a.

[86] Bernd DL, Fine PS. Electronic Medical Records: A Path Forward. *Front Health Serv Manage.* 2011 Fall;28(1):3-13.

Chapter 3. Data Analytics and Business Intelligence

Chon Abraham, PhD, MBA

Most companies today have plenty of data. Conversely, creating intelligence and gleaning real insight from this data is what continues to elude organizations...research reveals a clear link between business performance and the use of analytics to drive fact based decision making.[87]

T. Davenport
2007

Introduction

Data analytics for healthcare organizations is evolving rapidly. As the technology revolution for the healthcare industry gains speed on a daily basis, more and more physician practices and hospitals are engaging vendors to provide support for analytic needs they have in managing their organizations. Historically, insurance payers have been a huge champion and user of analytics tools, due to the massive volume of data analysis done in health plan administration at the macro and micro level, but with the push for and adoption of EHRs across the healthcare industry, there is a rapidly increasing need for tools to support a broader group of stakeholders. Health systems regard their data sets from patient care records as assets to be safeguarded and maintained. Keeping within the rules of HIPAA, data can be used in statistical, quantitative, and retrospective analyses, along with use in predictive modeling and health outcomes research.

ACOs need strong business intelligence (BI) capabilities with their focus on managing health outcomes at the population level. Data analytics facilitates business intelligence and is critical to meeting organizational needs and goals in performance management, system level reporting, and data mining to support research, regulatory requirements, and operational needs. The current renaissance era of healthcare service delivery involving the formation of ACOs, both public and private, involves a shift to a pay-for-performance model in which the focus becomes one of quality of care, as opposed to quantity of care. Business intelligence tools will become essential to the capture, monitoring, and analysis of patient data in this paradigm shift to enhance clinical and organizational insights and efficiency.

Background on Data Analytics and Business Intelligence

Davenport suggests that organizations in all industries are perplexed with how to glean insight from the massive quantity of electronic data afforded to and by the firm operating in the digital age. As healthcare organizations become more digitized with the penetration of EHRs and other tools for electronic data storage, the next evolution in data management is making sense of that data and applying it in meaningful ways. ACOs will have to overcome this daunting task of gleaning insights from data amassed across the continuum of care that will be the crux of how its effectiveness is assessed. Thus, data analytics as a component of business intelligence will be of utmost importance to the utility of ACOs.

Business intelligence is a broad term that incorporates a broad category of applications and technologies for gathering, storing, analyzing, and providing access to data to help enterprise users make better business decisions. One of the keys to thriving in a competitive marketplace, as ACOs will quickly realize, is making sound business and clinical decisions based on accurate and current information, which takes more than intuition.[88] Data management, analysis, reporting, and query tools can help clinicians and business users wade through a sea of data to synthesize valuable information from it.[89]

The transforming of data into information that can provide knowledge for an organization is the formation of business intelligence. In essence, the transformation of data into insight does not happen without being deliberate in how the data is collected, stored, semantically cleaned, accessed, and reported.

So What Is Data for Business Intelligence?

The data for business intelligence pertains to raw, un-summarized, and unanalyzed facts that come from daily operations, transactions, or occurrences in the organizational environment.[90] EHRs are providing the foundational data for analysis. Business intelligence is regarded as the analysis of large amounts of data, which can be paired to provide information in a number of contexts for which healthcare is poised to benefit.[91] In addition to the above sources, third-party premium data from sources such as Microsoft's Azure™ Marketplace provides meaningful additional insights for both payers and providers.

And How Is Information Transformed for Business Intelligence?

Information evolves from data processed into a meaningful form. This insight as knowledge is related to knowing what information is required to answer a question, having functional knowledge of what the information means, and the forethought about how to apply it to solve problems. The rationale for transforming data into information and building knowledge addresses two domains (time and degree of innovation) that are imperative for ACOs to provide care across the continuum effectively. The pertinent dimensions addressed in business intelligence implementations are depicted in Table 3-1.[92]

Table 3-1. Questions Addressed by Business Intelligence

	Past	Present	Future
Information	What happened? (Technique: Reporting based on structured queries from standardization of transactional data)	What is happening now? (Technique: Alerts – based on semi-structured decision support elements)	What will happen? (Technique: Extrapolation – based on predictive analytics and forecasting techniques)
Insight	How and why did it happen? (Technique: Modeling, experimental design)	What's the next best action? (Technique: Prediction)	What is the best/worst that can happen? (Technique: Prediction, optimization, simulation)

With regard to how data is collected, ACOs are responsible for the care delivered across a continuum of care and will require streamlined processes to capture the necessary data. Pulling data from disparate systems that may only be accessible to physicians at facilities will need to change. With ACOs in particular, there is a necessity for establishing a data repository that enables transparency of clinical and administrative operations at each partner facility within the ACO. For example, Patient X could have received care at a number of different provider/ACO partner organizations in which each of the partners/organizations may retain their respective transactional data in the form of an EHR. Consolidating data from all of these repositories can be a challenge in terms of timeliness and readability, which is likely to impact physicians' ability to provide care with complete data. A data warehouse provides a means of consolidating this data based on a unique identifier for Patient X that is consistent across all information systems, enabling easier consolidation of information per patient. The data warehouse can also standardize the data for comparative analysis.

This data from the various transactional data repositories is extracted, transformed for standardization if needed, then loaded into a data warehouse and reconfigured into smaller data marts (i.e., smaller content-specific repositories).[93] These data marts will be accessed for content-specific querying by users needing reports, decision support capabilities for both clinical and operational issues, and predictive analysis for identifying patterns or forecasting. A critical element of the utility of the data marts in the data warehouse is the robustness of standardization of documentation procedures and the use of standard classification of disease and health problems codes. Figure 3-1 provides a depiction of typical data warehouse architecture with vendor software examples.

Figure 3-1. Typical Data Warehouse Architecture to Support Business Intelligence

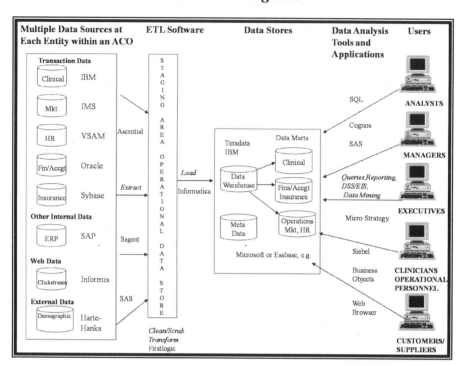

The critical functionality that all business intelligence systems share is the establishment of a logical, comprehensible interface between the human user and the data warehouse.[94] The flexibility of a dynamic business intelligence interface is to allow stakeholders of the organization (e.g., analysts, clinicians, managers, patients, suppliers, other organizational personnel) to access the data stores with proper permissions and analyze data on various levels (i.e., at the healthcare system, individual care environment, or patient level).[95]

Data Analytics Techniques for Business Intelligence

Data analytics in business intelligence can be accomplished via a variety of statistically oriented techniques. Several will be summarized here that aid in mining data for meaningful insights and identifying associative relationships.

Association Analysis

An association analysis "identifies affinities existing among the collection of items in a given set of records."[96] The association rules take the form of Set A $\Rightarrow$ Set B, or the criteria/indicators/occurrences such as medical ailments or a set of procedures in an order set (A) imply the criteria/indicators/occurrences are also present in Set B. To determine the strength of the association, the support and the confidence of each rule is determined. The support of a rule is the probability that the criteria/indicators/occurrences in the two sets occur together. This logic can be applied to a diagnosis if a patient presents with a set of symptoms that are analyzed as being associated with a disease and then the provider can be alerted of the likelihood of associated ailments. The greater the volume of data, the more accurate this technique is in determining associations. Thus, greater and timelier identification of diseases and effective regimens for patients within the ACO should be highly probable with the large volume of data that ACOs are expected to retain in a data warehouse.

Sequential Patterns

Identifying sequential patterns involves detecting "frequently occurring sequences or patterns from given records."[97] Using a sequence analysis is much like the association analysis but includes a time dimension. A sequence analysis is performed if a clinician wants to know the order in which a patient presents with certain ailments. In the case of patients seeing multiple providers, this information may be key in order to devise the most effective care regimen, which can then be compared by applying other business intelligence techniques to care regimens exacted by other clinicians within the ACO. This technique can also provide insights on what types of medical materials are used in sequence in the process of care across the ACO to aid in real-time inventory management and streamline supply distribution in the most economical way (i.e., not needing to maintain costly inventory).

Classifying and Clustering

Classifying involves separating "predefined classes...into mutually exclusive groups."[98] Classifications are done before an analysis is performed. For instance, this technique can be used to determine classifications of clinicians who perform similar disease practice regimens across the ACO or a group of patients who tend to receive a certain type of disease treatment that could be based on demographics or socioeconomic status, for example. The classification can give insight to differentiation of clinicians based on practice behaviors and treatment of patients according to factors other than purely the disease the patients have in common. Clustering is similar to classifying in that it involves separating the data into classes. Clustering identifies unknown classes, rather than predetermined classes, within the data. A clustering analysis also is referred to as unsupervised classification or segmenting.

Transparency provided by clustering and classifying can highlight inconsistencies or uniformity in clinician practices across an ACO. The classification technique can then be supplemented with other techniques, such as regression, to determine groups with the highest yet least effective costs of care associated with their practice regimen or clinical outcomes for patients in certain groups. Typically, in regression, the groupings are used as binary indicator variables. This type of insight can drive organizational policy such as best practices to mandate and compensation decisions.

Predictive Analysis

Prediction does what the name indicates. It predicts a "future value of a variable."[99] Predictive models must provide a rule to transform a measurement into a prediction and have a means of choosing useful inputs from a potentially vast number of candidates.[100] Predictive modeling is done using a variety of statistical techniques. Some commonly applied techniques are regression, neural networks, decision trees, and genetic algorithms.

Regression techniques model the associations between the input variables or the independent variables and the target variables or the dependent variables. Regression models are used to predict new cases, perform hypothesis tests, make inferences, and to model causal relationships. To perform a regression analysis, certain assumptions and diagnostics are performed in order to (1) determine if the data can be better represented by a linear or nonlinear regression function, (2) reveal if the data needs to be transformed to better fit the necessary assumptions, and (3) decide what variables should be included in the model. From a regression model, confidence intervals can be determined for the model parameters and for the prediction of new observations. An application of regression for ACOs may be the determination of a set of variables that contribute to cash flow (e.g., size of the ACO, patient case mix across the ACO, type of care environments, number of FTEs).

Neural networks are used to help solve complex problems, poorly understood issues for which large amounts of data have been collected, such as patient or population data in a data warehouse. Patterns in the data are discovered using neural networks that build models for each pattern and correct the model continuously. Essentially, data is entered into the model as training data for which the inputs (i.e., data plus their weights for predetermined impact on the outcome) produce a known set of outputs or conclusions. The business intelligence tool then assesses and determines, as artificial intelligence, the correct solution to apply. As the model is fed more data, each case is compared with the known outcome. If it differs, then a correction is calculated and applied to the nodes of the hidden processing layer to assess the change in the outcome every time, which is repeated until a correction value that is less than a specified threshold statistic is reached. In essence, the neural network uses rules that it learns through this process from the patterns in the data to construct a hidden layer of logic. Then, this hidden layer of logic processes inputs classifying them based on the experience of the model.[101] Figure 3-2 provides a graphic of this technique for assessing stroke disease, adapted from the work of Shanthi and colleagues.[102]

ACOs can apply this logic to determine the most effective regimens for care across service providers and to determine if different factors (i.e., different pairings/interactions of occurrences of variables that the model determines in the hidden layer) are more applicable in predicting outcomes based on certain facility or care environment characteristics.

Figure 3-2. Neural Network Example

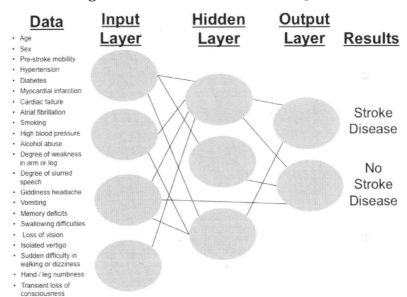

Decision trees with if-then logic allow data to be split into different groupings based on probabilities of an event occurring. Using decision trees, the branches can be traversed easily to reach conclusions about the probability of an event occurring. The simplicity of this method is often helpful when there are numerous significant known variables in contrast to hidden variables that are not initially known in neural networks.

Genetic algorithms are used to approximate a solution to optimization problems. They use concepts from biological evolution such as mutation, natural selection, and crossover. Genetic algorithms are often applied to scheduling problems or "optimization problems with many candidate variables."[103] This technique is typically applied to medical supply chain management problems to determine optimal replenishment plans, which can be a useful tool for ACOs, as well as independent healthcare organizations.

Data Visualization with Digital Dashboards

The purpose of data visualization is to present data to users from information systems in an easily comprehensible manner. Data visualization is the process of enabling users to better assess data in formats of graphics, charts, tables, maps, digital images, three-dimensional presentations, animations, and other digital technologies. This data typically is consolidated in a dashboard or snapshot that provides real-time views of key performance indicators.[104] Assessing these indicators as they apply to multiple partner engagement in an ACO will be an essential tool for ACO leadership to determine productivity and efficiency of ACO partners and their contributions to improving population health.

Healthcare oriented dashboards typically capture leading indicators of organizational productivity in relation to national standards for clinical and administrative areas of focus, such as chronic disease management, complication and mortality indices, length of stay, and readmissions rates, as well as revenue cycle management indicators. Dashboards can provide a quick means of displaying data to indicate the status of these indicators (e.g., meeting national standards or below expectations). This data is critical to clinicians and administrators who need to make timely decisions and are typically displayed on a dashboard to show correlations or causation between factors. Dashboards demonstrate these correlations and causations by incorporating drill-down capabilities for assessing why fluctuations in indicators occur over time.

An example of using dashboards for data visualization is with Deaconess Health System, a 500-bed acute care facility in Evansville, Indiana. This facility has improved clinical reporting by population demographics according to Greg Hindahl, MD, Chief Medical Information Officer (CMIO). Essentially, since implementing a dashboard platform more than 2 years ago, the facility improved its blood clot prevention compliance in its intensive care units from 79% to more than 90% in 6 months. "There is still significant fluctuation in the data from month to month, so this is a work in progress, but the dashboard helps to easily see these fluctuations and gives us an idea of where to focus attention for ongoing improvements," per Hindahl.[105]

Application of dashboards in the aforementioned capacities can enable benchmarking, especially as it relates to population health management initiatives, a primary focus for ACOs. Over time, a rich dataset could help administrators and clinicians understand their practices' trends as well as their populations.

Business intelligence tools are fertile ground for efforts such as value-based purchasing and ACO activities. If a clinician is going to be paid for quality, then he or she needs to understand the data. Business intelligence tools, including digital dashboards, can be a sound investment.[106]

Another example of the use of a dashboard is the Health and Productivity Dashboard (HPD) provided by HealthMedia Inc. , which has administrative implications for an ACO in the area of ACO employee healthcare cost management. The HPD captures leading indicators such as health status and professes confidence in health-related decision making that may be the cause of trailing indicators, such as employee absence days or reduced job performance or even likelihood of incident occurrence.[107] The basic concept for the dashboard in employee health management simply demonstrates that when data is presented in a clear and concise manner, administrators or business leaders are better equipped to understand the relationship of the multitude of complex issues such as health status, health conditions, occupation, compensation, absence, and on-the-job performance. The design provides a means to visualize correlations between poor health and employee productivity loss, as well as a means for benchmarking the various ACO partner organizations in terms of their respective employee productivity levels against comparison groups within the ACO. The primary functions of the HPD are as follows:

➤ Integrate data from a variety of sources,

➤ Filter the data according to rules of logic and analysis, and

➤ Automatically apply complex mathematical procedures.

ACO participants can be engaged over time to track their own changes, show the health status effect of these changes, and ultimately translate these changes into monetary terms for the ACO. Whether an independent healthcare organization, an ACO, or any self-sustaining business, not knowing the full cost of employee health puts decision makers at a disadvantage when estimating how much they are spending on the health of their workforce and how much they should be spending. Without this information, a decision maker's ability is limited to implementing effective health cost management strategies that target all aspects of the related cost, rather than the narrow conventional concerns; thus, dashboard technology such as HPD is extremely effective in helping meet these needs.[108]

Criteria for BI Tools and Vendor Solutions

Statistical data analysis techniques and tools such as dashboards are built into software supporting business intelligence tools. Vendor products vary greatly, but healthcare organizations, ACOs, and others must meet compliance requirements for the technical capabilities of the EHR modules enabling the data capture for business intelligence tool analysis in order to receive certification from national credentialing organizations. The NCQA launched its ACO accreditation program in the fall of 2011. While no specific business intelligence criteria were included, an underlying expectation was that all EHR modules of enterprise business intelligence solutions should conform to ONC-ATCB 2011/2012, Certification Commission for Health Information Technology (CCHIT) credentialing criteria. Tables 3-2 and 3-3 provide examples of requirements for enterprise business intelligence solution features and CMS Meaningful Use criteria associated with the credentialing requirements for a business intelligence solution.

Table 3-2. Key Features for Independent Software Vendors (ISVs) Regarding Business Intelligence[109]

100% Coverage of Meaningful Use Measures	Use BI-clinical to provide 100% coverage of quality and usage measures in the Meaningful Use guidelines. BI-Clinical also complies with the automated measure processing, calculation, and submission requirements of ONC
Scorecard and Benchmarking	Develop practice / physician scorecards, report against multiple reporting periods, compare and benchmark performance set and track goals for performance improvement
Clinical Decision Support	Create rules based on evidence-based guidelines, integrate BI-Clinical services with Point of Care UI (e.g., physician notes), create and track clinical alerts, and generate patient lists for proactively managing conditions
Quality Measure Monitoring	Provide additional pre-configured quality measures based on Joint Commission, PQRI and NQF specifications, customize measures based on supported vocabulary, track performance over time, manage data submissions
Usage Analytics	Track EHR usage (e-Prescribing, lab results, patient care summary, etc.), create scorecard and analytics views to monitor key performance indicators, create physician scorecards for actionable intelligence
Financial & Operational Measures	Provide complete financial and operational BI / Analytics (e.g., for PMS, HIS, RIS, etc.) fully integrated with clinical BI / Analytics

Table 3-3. Certified Meaningful Use Criteria[110]

BI-Clinical Framework 10.3 ONC-ATCB 2011/12 Certified Criteria		BI-Clinical Coverage
Calculate and submit clinical quality measures	170.304(j)	BI-Clinical measure processing framework has 100% coverage of clinical quality measures
Automated measure calculation	170.302(n)	BI- Clinical supports calculation & reporting on all usage measures
Clinical decision support	170.304(e)	BI-Clinical rules engine supports configuration of clinical rules to support clinical decision support
Patient reminders	170.304(d)	BI-Clinical measure processing framework can generate alerts & reminders for patient follow-ups
Generate patient lists	170.302(j)	BI-Clinical enables users to select, sort, retrieve, and generate lists of patients
Encryption when exchanging electronic health information	170.302(v)	BI-Clinical encrypts, decrypts and transmits health information as per Meaningful Use requirements
Audit log	170.302(r)	BI-Clinical has comprehensive audit data marts based on IHE ATNA to report on audit logs
All security criteria	170.302(o), 170.302(p), 170.302(q), 170.302(s) 170.302(t), 170.302(u)	BI-Clinical supports all security criteria under Meaningful Use Stage 1- access control, emergency access, automatic log-off, integrity, authentication, and general encryption

A Klas 2011 report[111] indicated that 64% of respondents plan on becoming an ACO by 2013, with 56% of them either using or moving toward one enterprise vendor for their business intelligence solution for ease of use and more robust reporting functionality targeted for use by clinicians and administrators alike. The primary criteria driving demand for business intelligence solutions are ease of use and analytical sophistication with reporting capabilities. "Providers recognize the need for advanced analytics and reporting capabilities, but complex and time-consuming systems turn many clients off. Customers say Dimensional Insight and Information Builders offer the best combination of usability and capability."[112]

The top five business intelligence vendor solutions in healthcare enable (1) data extraction from vast disparate data repositories, as opposed to just data warehouses; (2) use predictive analytics to evaluate revenue strategies for traditional as well as for ACO models; and (3) include and business intelligence mobile functionalities. However, "few providers have put them to use, with only 43%, 15%, and 12% of respondents adopting, respectively."[113] This suggests that the majority of healthcare providers are not yet adopting advanced business intelligence functionality. Table 3-4 summarizes some market leaders and information on their solutions provided in the Klas 2011 report.

Table 3-4. Vendor Business Intelligence Solutions

Vendor/Product	Description
Dimensional Insight (DI)	Top-rated vendor in the 2011 Klas report for the second year in a row. Dimensional Insight is a lower cost solution used mainly by small to midsize organizations for clinical and financial reporting. Flexibility is a key strength, along with pulling from disparate domains without a data warehouse.
Information Builder WebFOCUS	Easy-to-use and robust solution found mainly in midsize to large stand-alone hospitals. The WebFOCUS product is being used more for both clinical and financial reporting, having jumped from 6 to 10 enterprise customers. Cost, support, and system speed are strengths.
McKesson Horizon Business Insight (HBI)	Out-of-the-box BI solution from McKesson. Customers see dashboards and ability to reduce reporting burdens in versions 14 and 15 as two of the product's greatest strengths.
IBM Cognos 8	Highly customizable, sophisticated solution used mainly by integrated delivery networks (IDNs) and academic medical centers (AMCs) to meet varied and complex needs. Functionality is the main strength.
SAP XI Data Analytics	Solution designed for larger, more complex multi-facility IDNs and AMCs. Key strengths are the product's ability to meet virtually any reporting need and the product's sophisticated scheduler.

Another notable business intelligence vendor is Humedica. Humedica is referred to as a next-generation clinical informatics company that provides a number of aggregated services and data associated with business intelligence solutions to the healthcare industry. Through the use of its business intelligence solutions, Humedica incorporates nearly all of the aforementioned data analytics techniques to optimize models for assessing patient information across varied medical settings and time periods. Its solution generates a longitudinal and comprehensive view of patient care based on data from the Anceta Collaborative Data Warehouse, a shared data warehouse created by the American Medical Group Association, which tracks population health data and has disease-specific analytic models with comparative data that can be segmented by population segment and disease condition.

In one case, a healthcare system evaluating the conversion to an ACO model used Humedica's business intelligence application to assess the performance of various healthcare providers (as potential partners) in diabetes care.[114] Specifically, the potential partners were evaluated on the quality of care to diabetic patients demonstrated as a decrease in duplication of tests and patient hospital readmissions. This type of logic was also applied to assess the number of repeat claims and resultant revenue generation from third-party insurance providers. Mandates from the Affordable Care Act call for state insurance exchanges, revision of medical-loss ratios, and the expansion of healthcare insurance, among other initiatives, that can provide new opportunities to conduct analysis for partnership determination.[115] Thus, business intelligence solutions such as

Humedica's application enable providers to seek out and contract with healthcare partners and third-party insurance providers with scrutiny and confidence.[116]

Application of Data Analysis

Data analysis with business intelligence tools is considered to be of paramount importance for effective operations amongst 60% of US providers planning to become or join ACOs.[117] The Klas 2011 report also indicates that 16% of these organizations are actively employing predictive analytics with beneficial outcomes in the areas of medication administration safety, labor forecasting, financial impact modeling, and readmission rate predictions. Citiustech identified four areas for application of data analysis with business intelligence tools:[118]

➢ Clinical analytics,

➢ Regulatory reporting,

➢ Financial analytics, and

➢ Operational analytics akin to needs of an integrated healthcare system or ACO.

Each of these four areas is described below with examples provided from Duke University Health System and Sentara Healthcare.

Clinical Analytics involves comprehensive analysis and some quality reporting for clinical subject areas such as preventive care, immunization and patient safety, and population health management which are deemed to be key performance indicators for ACO management.[119] An example of business intelligence tool use for clinical analytics comes from Duke University Health System:

> The Duke University Health System (DUHS) combines the Duke University School of Medicine, the Duke University School of Nursing, the Duke Clinic, and associated hospitals into a system of research, clinical care, and education located across the state of North Carolina. A DUHS initiative entailed the use of an active Adverse Drug Event surveillance system built upon an integrated IT infrastructure servicing the entire healthcare system with decision support capabilities, coupled with process changes in care procedures. Alerts such as these are typically generated using predictive analytic techniques such as decision trees and neural networks that consider the patient's medication history, regimen, and medication data in the determination of a likely drug interaction or adverse event. Continuous monitoring of events across the healthcare system after implementing the intervention of the surveillance system and workflow process changes suggests a prevention of 157.8 potential cases of nosocomially acquired C difficile colitis per year in addition to a substantial decrease in costs to the healthcare system for hosting infected patients estimated at $578,968.[120] The success of this initiative spurred the development of other content-specific business intelligence initiatives that require analysis of safety data on medication safety, transfusion deviations, and patient falls.[121]

Regulatory Reporting is provided through the business intelligence tools by incorporating a set of measures for national ACO guidelines, including population health and cost measures, as part of a library based on recommendations by leading quality and regulatory organizations such as the Centers for Disease Control and Prevention (CDC), CMS, the American Medical Association (AMA), NCQA, and CMS's 2011 measures for the Physician Quality Reporting Initiative (PQRI). An example of the benefit for regulatory reporting is as follows from DUHS:

➢ DUHS used its data warehouse to provide a highly refined estimate of patients likely to need H1N1 vaccine in the wake of the pandemic H1N1 influenza outbreak.[122] Forecasting techniques were also used to estimate vaccine need according to CDC priority criteria allowing real-time reporting to state CDC officials concerning population statistics, based on patient clustering associated with ICD-9 codes, for expected vaccinations contributing to improved vaccine administration procedures for patient prioritizations. In essence, the business intelligence functionality enabled DUHS to create a list of high-risk patients within 24 hours of realization of the pandemic.[123]

Financial Analytics provides advance analytic tools for managing cost and revenue of each ACO partner in an integrated system, as well as providing analytics and insights for physician/facility-wide performance measurement. An example of a financial impact is as follows from DUHS:

➢ DUHS was projected to lose $2.1 million in the current fiscal year of the report, due to operational costs or lost revenue in its intensive care nursery. The expenses were associated with errors in (a) physician documentation, (b) medical record recoding potentially from recoding of notes for patient interventions or episodes in other care environments such as emergency rooms, (c) traditional revenue modeling, and (d) third-party payment management. DUHS utilized existing clinical and billing data in the data warehouse to develop a validated revenue model involving factorial statistics that presented expected payment for each patient. For example, they assessed potential candidates for process-level errors in which they determined the variability between actual and modeled revenues and were able to identify and correct charge-entry errors that impacted outlier payments. This approach eliminated the potential $2.1 million deficit and led to a profit of $400,000 within 4 months. The analysis also resulted in the correction and resubmission of previous accounts and returned more than $12 million in additional revenues and serves as the accepted model for future monitoring of charge captures across the entire network.[124]

Operational Analytics provides a comprehensive key performance indicators library for managing operational performance including throughput, productivity, and utilization subject areas. An example of operational analytics comes from Sentara Healthcare:

➢ Sentara Healthcare is a large integrated network operating in northern North Carolina and Virginia, with more than 100 care delivery sites, including 10 acute care hospitals with a total of 2,349 beds; 6 outpatient care campuses; 7 nursing centers; 3 assisted living centers; 8 advanced imaging centers; approximately 380 primary care and multispecialty physicians; and operates its own health plan, Optima Health, providing coverage to more than 430,000 members. Additionally, Sentara provides home health and hospice services, physical therapy and rehabilitation services, and offers patients access to their medical record information through Sentara MyChart as part of the Sentara eCare Health Network®.[125] Due in part to the volume and variety of services offered by Sentara, referrals management is an arduous task. Business intelligence tools help to identify challenges in meeting internal and external physician demands that were exacerbated by extensive wait times to contact central scheduling, post-posted appointments due to lack of pre-certifications, lost or incorrectly faxed scripts. These tools also helped determine models for efficient workload management and consolidation of revenue cycles for similar care environments across the integrated delivery network. Some notable outcomes reported in 2009 were a 69% increase in service level, 71% decrease in average speed of answer, and 149% growth in referrals for optical imaging (e.g., CTs and MRIs).[126]

ICD-10 and Business Intelligence

The United States is moving toward migration from ICD-9 to ICD-10 diagnosis codes. The current proposed rule from DHHS sets the conversion date nationwide to October 1, 2014[127], for this migration process, when all health claims would start being submitted and processed using ICD-10 diagnosis and procedure codes. The eventual change entails moving to the usage of a diagnosis code set of 14,000 to more than 140,000 unique codes (the data elements are described in further detail in Chapter 4). The drive for this expansion of the code set, which has already occurred in 25 countries outside the United States, will allow for greater specificity in disease/diagnosis classification, with up to seven alpha-numeric characters, and increase the granularity of the codes to more specifically account for ailments, injuries, and interventions. An example of a frequently used ICD-9 code is 883.0, which is for open wounds on fingers without mention of complication. The new ICD-10 provides 103 different codes that are the expansion of the ICD-9 code 883.0.

The first step in the process is to adopt the 5010 Electronic Data Interface standards that will begin in 2012. This will mandate an increase in the diagnosis field length to accommodate all the new codes. The American Health Information Management Association (AHIMA) provides a number of resources and references on the topic of ICD-10 and the future conversion.[128]

The potential benefit associated with using business intelligence in analysis of diagnosis codes is that, with the future increase in the granularity and specificity of the data, we will gain greater insight into relationships between diagnosis data, treatment regimen effectiveness, and trends across populations. The greater the granularity and specificity of the claims data with ICD-10 coding, the more likely we are to enable better predictive analysis with business intelligence. This is because there is a greater availability of predictor variables to enter into models for determining patterns in the data.

The ICD-10 migration will require healthcare organizations to update their health information technology systems, which should be a major consideration for ACO chief information officers in making information technology infrastructure modernization decisions. The software offerings currently being marketed not only seek to make the ICD-10 transition as seamless and as painless as possible, but also are proposing direct fiscal benefits in addition to the following:

- ➤ **Accurate and efficient coding**. Reduce time for proper code translations, increase employee productivity, and lower administrative costs.

- ➤ **Timely claims processing and payments**. Produce quicker turnaround on reimbursements, reduce denied claims, and improve cash flow.

- ➤ **Business intelligence dashboard**. Gain access to detailed real-time claims and reimbursement analytics to drive sound, profitable business decisions.

- ➤ **Early detection of denied claims**. Detect denied claims within minutes, instead of days, weeks, or even months, equipping your staff to resolve issues quickly, with less manual effort, and to ensure accurate and timely payment.

Bridging the Divide

New strategies are needed to meet the requirements put forth by the HITECH Act, Affordable Care Act, and long-term reimbursement implications for all healthcare reform initiatives. Organizations should make sure their business intelligence technologies support their patient and operational information needs and requirements in a wide range of areas. This includes the assessment of their quality and costs for both internal consumption and reporting purposes. Additionally, business intelligence can produce insights that show where shifting clinical responsibilities amongst clinicians (e.g., from a physician to nurse practitioner) can result in preserved quality of care and reduction in costs. It is important to look at and assess these different scenarios and approaches to deliver the necessary and most effective care. Predictive modeling as a type of data analytics in business intelligence can provide the mechanism for such assessments.[129] Use of data analytics in business intelligence solutions will surely be a major component of this effort, which has a direct impact or is associated with the following:[130]

➤ **Building awareness and establishing a clear vision**. There needs to be a shift from transaction-based to outcomes-driven payment.

➤ **Investing in a transformation infrastructure**. Test at the local level first. Currently, only one out of every four CEOs is leading the integration of the clinical, financial, legal, and advocacy decisions necessary for HITECH readiness.

➤ **Building clinical informatics expertise**. Need the ability to analyze aggregated data and manage new reimbursement protocols. This will lead to increased employment as new positions may be added, including those of medical informaticists, data mining experts, and clinical decision support analysts.

➤ **Invest in physician business services infrastructure**. Managed in separate business entities, these services include revenue management, human resource management, practice management, credentialing, EHR deployment and adoption support, and operations support.

➢ **Exploring a Medical Trading Area (MTA) Health Information Exchange**. Understand the distinct value proposition for HIE with your MTA (e.g., "the natural market" for which a healthcare organization operates) and the business case plus funding opportunities to enable its deployment.

➢ **Design an e-strategy for engaging patients**. Allow patients to have their own access and insights from business intelligence dashboards about performance of the clinicians, especially ACO partners. This provides patients and extended care providers suggested preventative care courses of action based on predictive analytics specific to the patient to both reduce risk of illness and improve health and wellness.

➢ **Develop a business intelligence strategy**. Complex reporting and collaboration between hospitals and physicians will be needed to examine information against the latest evidence to improve care for specific populations. This also lowers the overall costs for care around Potentially Preventable Events (PPEs), such as readmissions for at-risk patients and hospital-acquired conditions.

Providing the right tools and solutions to healthcare providers and payers to support effective clinical business intelligence strategy is critical, as discussed throughout this chapter. Here's one example of an industry leading solution utilizing the Business Intelligence tools from Microsoft®.

Case Example: Reducing Readmissions by Leveraging Microsoft®

Tools and Partners

As a leading industry provider of business intelligence tools and applications, Microsoft® provides many healthcare providers, insurers, and health IT vendors with development platforms and solutions such as Microsoft SQL Server®, PowerPivot® Fast Track Data Warehouse[131], and Parallel Data Warehouse for enterprise level BI with Excel® and SharePoint®. The solutions built on the Microsoft platform deliver data insights for healthcare organizations on information requirements for healthcare reform initiatives, quality improvement efforts, and clinical process monitoring to improve patient care. Many of the leading Health IT vendors utilize Microsoft for core applications and platforms to deliver advanced information needs for their healthcare clients.

In the ongoing need to reduce costs, improve outcomes, and enhance the patient experience, a large US based healthcare provider chose to focus on the top 17% of its most expensive types of readmissions to target and reduce readmissions using a predictive analytics solution developed on the Microsoft platform utilizing SQL Server. The strategy was to predict the population that would most likely be part of the top 17% of readmission types and build the plan to mitigate their risk and address the factors that would cause them to be readmitted. The strategy of predicting readmissions and eliminating the risk factors serves as a preventative tool that both improves the quality of care, reduces costs and provides a better patient experience. The overall ability to provide problem identification, data mining, trend analysis, and root cause analysis enabled the healthcare provider to better predict those patients with the greatest readmission potential by applying predictive analytics to the key drivers responsible for the particular readmission.

This innovative application runs on the Microsoft platform and is seamlessly integrated with Microsoft Excel, PowerPivot®, and SharePoint for easy access and use throughout the organization, providing hospital management with real-time business insights that allowed them to proactively improve follow-up/discharge procedures, which resulted in reduced risk potential for readmissions, improved quality patient outcomes, and a significant return on investment (ROI).

Case Example: Reducing Readmissions by Leveraging Microsoft® Tools and Partners (cont.)

The projected ROI is estimated to be 266% with a savings of $12 million from the top 17% of the most expensive types of readmissions system wide.

Collaborative solutions such as these in the healthcare business intelligence vendor community will continue to grow in importance and effectiveness for healthcare providers and insurers in the data-driven US and global healthcare markets.

Another strategy to consider is developing a productivity and performance plan to include standards for expected results, policy for penalizing ACO partner organizations who are performing below standard, and the use of data warehouses as a means to feed dashboards to help visualize key performance indicators for all ACO partners.

Reimbursements for healthcare organizations, ACOs, and others will become tied to their quality performance; thus, ACOs will be increasingly scrutinized for their productivity and performance.[132] Under the new performance-based or value-based purchasing paradigm, CMS will withhold 1% of all Medicare inpatient operation payments from nonqualifying hospitals starting in FY13.[133] The funds will be redistributed to hospitals based on performance-versus-care and patient satisfaction measures. ACOs need to understand the ramifications for lack of improvement or not meeting national performance expectations, as well as seeking technology as a means to help position themselves to be rewarded financially for demonstrating improvements in care.[134] Therefore, business intelligence should be at the forefront of strategic planning for ACO chief information officers and chief medical information officers, as it will become a necessity to understand the effectiveness of the complex systems that comprise their ACO operations. Thus, business intelligence is on the cusp of revolution—combining information, visualization techniques, social networking for some business contexts, and new models of collaboration.[135] This will be needed for optimized sustainability, increased adoption, and long-term growth of ACOs in the future.

Chapter 3: Takeaways

✓ ACOs will require strong business intelligence and data analytics capabilities to meet goals in performance reporting, data mining to support research, and operational analysis.

✓ Types of data analytics techniques include association analysis, sequential patterns, classifying and clustering, and predictive analysis.

✓ Neural networks are used to map patterns within data sets to help assess and determine both solutions and relationships.

✓ Four key questions addressed by business intelligence are:

   o   What happened in the past and why?

   o   What is happening in the present and why?

   o   How will future occurrences unfold?

   o   How do we empower others to make a better future?

✓ Data visualization involves presenting data to users from information systems in formats of graphics, charts, tables, maps, digital images, and three-dimensional presentations, to provide real-time views of key performance indicators.

✓ The expansion of International Classification of Disease codes to ICD-10 will bring about analysis of data sets with increased granularity and specificity to enable better predictive analysis with business intelligence.

✓ Business intelligence should be at the forefront of strategic planning for ACO chief information officers and chief medical information officers, as it will be a necessity to understand an ACO's operational effectiveness and efficiency in light of organizational and regulatory system complexities.

[87] Davenport T, Harris J. *Competing on Analytics: The New Science of Winning.* Boston, MA: Harvard Business School Press; 2007.

[88] Ericson J. Old Priorities, New Urgency. *Health Data Manag.* 2010 Oct;18(10):41-4.

[89] Glaser J. HITECH Lays the Foundation for More Ambitious Outcomes-Based Reimbursement. *Am J Manag Care.* 2010 Dec;16(12 Suppl HIT):SP19-23.

[90] Watson R. *Data Management: Databases and Organizations*, Fifth Edition. Hoboken, NJ: John Wiley & Sons, Inc; 2006.

[91] Glaser J, Stone J. Effective Use of Business Intelligence. *Healthc Financ Manage.* 2008 Feb;62(2):68-72; Fortin J, Zywiak W. Beyond Meaningful Use Getting Meaningful Value from IT. *Healthc Financ Manage.* 2010 Feb;64(2):54-59.

[92] Davenport T, Harris J, Morison R. *Analytics at Work: Smarter Decisions, Better Results.* Boston, MA: Harvard Business Press; 2010.

[93] Imhoff C, White C. Extending the Scope and Reach of Business Intelligence, Part 3. *Business Intelligence Network*, April 2010. Accessed online February 12, 2012, at http://www.b-eye-network.com/view/13358.

[94] Ferranti JM, Langman MK, Tanaka D, McCall J, Ahmad A. Bridging the Gap: Leveraging Business Intelligence Tools in Support of Patient Safety and Financial Effectiveness. *J Am Med Inform Assoc.* 2010 Mar-Apr;17(2):136-143.

[95] Ferranti, et. al. 2010.

[96] Watson R. 2006.

[97] Watson R. 2006.

[98] Watson R. 2006.

[99] Watson R. 2006.

[100] SAS Inc., *Business Analytics,* SAS Training Publication (2011).

[101] Laudon K, Laudon J. *Essentials of MIS,* 10th ed. Upper Saddle River, NJ: Prentice Hall; 2012; Shanthi D, Sahoo G, Saravanan N. Evolving Connection Weights of Artificial Neural Networks Using Genetic Algorithm with Application to the Prediction of Stroke Disease. *International Journal of Soft Computing.* 2009;4(2):95-102. Accessed online March 5, 2012, at http://www.medwelljournals.com/fulltext/?doi=ijscomp.2009.95.102.

[102] Shanthi D. 2009.

[103] Watson R. 2006.

[104] Nelson G. The Healthcare Performance Dashboard: Linking Strategy to Metrics. *SAS Global Forum 2010.* Accessed online February 10, 2012, at http://support.sas.com/resources/papers/proceedings10/167-2010.pdf.

[105] Byers J. Digital Dashboards Dig Deep. *CMIO Magazine*, October 2011. Accessed online February 11, 2012, at

http://www.cmio.net/index.php?option=com_articles&view=article&id=30138:digi
tal-dashboards-dig-deep.

[106] Riedel J. Using a Health and Productivity Dashboard: A Case Example. *Am J Health Promot*. 2007 Nov-Dec;22(2):1-10.

[107] Riedel J. 2007.

[108] Riedel J. 2007.

[109] Citiustech, Inc. Partner Integration Web page. Accessed March 1, 2012.

[110] Citiustech, Inc. Partner Integration Web page. Accessed March 1, 2012.

[111] Bird L. *Business Intelligence: Making Cents of Performance*. August 2011. Klas, Inc.

[112] Bird L. *Business Intelligence: Making Cents of Performance*. August 2011. Klas, Inc., p. 4.

[113] Bird L. *Business Intelligence: Making Cents of Performance*. August 2011. Klas, Inc., p. 3.

[114] Humedica Inc. SwedishAmerican Health System Selects Humedica MinedShare® for Its Clinical Analytic Solution and Joins Anceta Collaborative Data Warehouse. 2011. Accessed online March 4, 2012, at http://www.reuters.com/article/2011/06/27/idUS161189+27-Jun-2011+BW20110627.

[115] Glaser J. Strengthening Revenue Cycle Capabilities in an Era of Reform. *Healthc Financ Manage*. 2011 May;65(5):48-52.

[116] Humedica Inc. SwedishAmerican Health System Selects Humedica MinedShare® for Its Clinical Analytic Solution and Joins Anceta Collaborative Data Warehouse. 2011. Accessed online March 4, 2012 at http://www.reuters.com/article/2011/06/27/idUS161189+27-Jun-2011+BW20110627.

[117] Bird L. *Business Intelligence: Making Cents of Performance*. August 2011. Klas, Inc., p. 10.

[118] Citiustech, Inc. BI Clinical solution ambulatory Web page. Accessed March 4, 2012.

[119] Citiustech, Inc. BI Clinical solution ACOs & MCOs Web page. Accessed March 4, 2012.

[120] Ferranti, et. al. 2010.

[121] Ferranti, et. al. 2010.

[122] Ferranti, et. al. 2010.

[123] Ferranti, et. al. 2010.

[124] Ferranti, et. al. 2010.

[125] Sentara Healthcare Web site. Fast Facts. Accessed on March 4, 2012, at http://www.sentara.com/AboutSentara/Pages/FastFacts.aspx.

[126] Sentara Healthcare (internal document) "Referrals Management" 2009.

[127] Fed. Reg. Vol. 77, No. 74. April 17, 2012. I(A). Executive Summary and Background.

[128] American Health Information Management Association information on ICD-10. Accessed online February 11, 2012, at http://www.ahima.org/icd10/ and

http://www.ahima.org/icd10/resources.aspx.

[129] Glaser J. HITECH Lays the Foundation for More Ambitious Outcomes-Based Reimbursement. *Am J Manag Care*. 2010 Dec;16(12 Suppl HIT):SP19-23; Glaser J. 2011.

[130] Arlotte P. 7 Strategies for Improving HITECH Readiness. *Healthc Financ Manage*. 2010 Nov;64(11):90-94, 96.

[131] Capital and Coast District Health Board. Healthcare Agency Migrates from SAP to Microsoft and HP, Cuts BI Costs in Half. *Microsoft Corporation Case Study*. June 5, 2012. Accessed online August 8, 2012, at http://www.microsoft.com/casestudies/Case_Study_Detail.aspx?CaseStudyID=710000000816.

[132] Healthcare Financial Management Association. Strategies for Value-Based Health Care. *Healthc Financ Manage*. July 2011:1-8; Versel N. Hospitals use BI to Stanch Revenue Losses. *Informationweek*. August 3, 2011. Accessed online February 14, 2012, at http://www.informationweek.com/news/healthcare/policy/231300089.

[133] Glasser J. 2011.

[134] Glasser J. 2011.

[135] Nelson G. 2010.

Chapter 4. Interoperability and Standards

Chip Perkins, MBA

The "holy grail" of healthcare connectivity is a cornerstone for reaping the full benefits of eHealth. However, to fully realize this goal requires interoperability of such systems within health services organizations and jurisdictions, and across regions and countries.

Semantic Interoperability for Better Health and Safer Healthcare
SemanticHEALTHReport
January 2009

Introduction

Interoperable clinical data exchange is a key success factor in the business strategy of any ACO. The Three-Part Aim of CMS for ACOs is to improve America's healthcare system by reducing healthcare costs, improving outcomes, and providing patients with coordinated care. ACOs are intended to improve and drive higher levels of patient satisfaction and ensure that patients participate in the coordination of their own care. Coordinated care means that patients will get the right care at the right time without medical errors across the inpatient, outpatient, and home health care settings. Reimbursement and payments to providers will be made based on value and quality, not the fee-for-service model that is so deeply entrenched in our health system today.

Members of the computer savvy, Baby Boomer generation expect their care providers to use the latest in healthcare information technology innovation, provide better healthcare prevention and educational services, and to use technology to reduce the complexity of today's healthcare system in the United States. If we can use our ATM card across the globe to make cash withdrawals, why can't my cardiologist get electronic access to my latest lab test from my visit to the emergency room?

With today's disparate, complex health information technology systems and the aging Baby Boomer population, how will participating ACO physician members and patients share patient information needed to achieve better outcomes at a lower cost? The answer is in the ability of the ACO members to achieve significant levels of clinical and financial collaboration using sophisticated health information technology across inpatient, outpatient, and home care settings.

By focusing on the needs of patients and linking payments to outcomes, ACOs will help improve the health of individuals and communities and slow cost growth. Today, more than half of Medicare beneficiaries have five or more chronic conditions such as diabetes, arthritis, hypertension, and kidney disease. These patients often receive care from multiple physicians. A failure to coordinate care can often lead to patients not getting the care they need, receiving duplicative care, and being at an increased risk of suffering medical errors. On average, each year, one in seven Medicare patients admitted to a hospital has been subject to a harmful medical mistake in the course of care. Nearly one in five Medicare patients discharged from the hospital is readmitted within 30 days—a readmission many patients could have avoided if their care outside of the hospital had been aggressive and better coordinated. Improving coordination and communication among physicians and other providers and suppliers through ACOs will help improve the care Medicare beneficiaries receive, while also helping to lower costs. According to the analysis of the proposed regulation for ACOs, CMS could potentially save as much as $960 million over the first three years.[136]

ACOs will require organizations to build and demonstrate core competencies that improve care delivery, reduce costs, and improve quality. While there has been much discussion on the challenges an ACO will face from a financial and patient quality improvement perspective, less has been written on the absolute need of the underlying health information technology that is required to achieve the ACOs' goals. Physicians and hospital management have access to vast amounts of data, but much of the most basic patient data remains difficult to access by care providers. This chapter will focus on why effectively using health information technology for clinical data exchange (i.e., interoperability) and utilizing existing clinical terminologies is a foundational building block for an ACO to achieve its goals of improved health outcomes.

Background on ACOs

The College of American Pathologists (CAP) has published a comprehensive Accountable Care Toolkit[137] that is an educational resource on the transformational health reform regulations that emerged in 2010 and 2011.

As discussed in Chapter 1, in 2010, Congress initiated changes to the Medicare provider program through the Affordable Care Act, seeking to improve patient outcomes while lowering costs. One of the key initiatives of the Act is the creation of the Medicare Shared Savings program, which offers eligible healthcare providers, hospitals, and suppliers financial incentives to work together to improve the quality of care and reduce unnecessary costs for Medicare Fee For Service (FFS) patients by creating accountable care organizations. DHHS proposed the initial set of guidelines in March 2011 and issued its final guidelines in October 2011. The final rule includes 33 quality measures focused on patient experience, care coordination, patient safety, and preventive health.

The CAP ACO Toolkit identifies five basic tenets[138] of accountable care:

1. ACOs are legal entities serving a local Medicare population of 5,000 or more beneficiaries,

2. ACOs require physician engagement and leadership,

3. Clinical and anatomic laboratory services are critical components of these new care delivery systems,

4. New outcome reporting requirements for these organizations will be highly based on laboratory data, and

5. Physicians should assess local healthcare market and determine strategy/approach for engagement in ACOs.

The Interoperable EHR—A Prerequisite for ACOs

A fundamental business requirement of the ACO model is that all members of the care team and the patient have easy access to the patient's electronic medical record. EHRs provide care team members with improved opportunities for accessing patient information that can be used to enhance care and quality. Without easy access to the patient's health information, the care provider will find it more difficult to manage the patient's chronic disease, refer a patient to a specialist, review a lab result, or prescribe the simplest of medication. A patient's medical history, medical problem, and recent interaction with members of the care team must be accessible by all ACO members across all care settings. This fundamental objective of the ACO business model requires an integrated health information technology capability that allows the patient's clinical data to be freely exchanged, accessed, and understood by the care team—the interoperable EHR.

Inpatient care providers have historically struggled to exchange patient data across various institutional boundaries within a health system. The interfaces between inpatient EHRs and inpatient ancillary systems, such as laboratory, pharmacy, radiology, surgical, and emergency department, have often required interfaces that are expensive to maintain and support. Many hospitals still use one vendor to support the revenue cycle (patient access, scheduling, registration, and billing functions) and a second vendor to support their clinical order management, medication management, and clinical documentation. To add to the technology complexity, hospitals often rely on specialized vendor applications to support the Emergency Department, Surgical Services, and Intensive Care Unit departments. This "best of breed" strategy has created the need for organizations to develop custom interfaces to communicate messages between these disparate vendor systems. The interfaces require information technology support and are expensive for health systems to maintain. Over the past decade, many hospitals have moved their EHRs to a "one vendor" approach to leverage the integration provided by the single vendor platform and integrated electronic health record data base. Even vendors who claim to provide an integrated EHR solution, however, often use different technologies to bundle their solutions under one brand name.

There is also difficulty in exchanging data between inpatient and outpatient settings, which often use different electronic health record vendor solutions. Exchanging the most basic patient referral information between a primary care physician and the specialty physician in the outpatient setting is still sent by fax because information systems have not been connected. How many times have we read about gravely sick cancer patients who have to physically carry their paper chart or mammogram x-rays to the specialist inside the same healthcare system whose office might be right across the street? But despite these challenges, patients now have better tools and technology than ever before to participate in contributing to their own electronic health record by using health management portal solutions. As hospitals and providers achieve the proposed requirements for Stage 2 Meaningful Use, patients will be expected to have online access to their electronic health record and have the ability to update their information online. All these different healthcare stakeholders and health information technologies create significant challenges and complexity into the data exchange equation. And, finally, there is the limited amount of clinical data that is exchanged between the provider and payer for claims and billing purposes.

Standards for HIE

Chapter 5 will cover HIE in great detail; however, there are some critical points to note regarding standards for this domain of technology. Over recent years, we have seen the emergence of the HIEs at the community, regional, and state level whose goal is to facilitate the transmitting of patient data across various institutional settings. In order for ACOs and related coordinated care models to achieve their stated goals, a wide range of healthcare providers must be able to electronically access, exchange, and act on the patient's electronic medical record data to analyze variances, improve decision-making capabilities, and identify cost savings at the population health level, along with supporting treatment decisions to positively impact patient outcomes. HIEs are trying to fill that gap, acting as a community repository to aggregate and consolidate patient centric information. Many states have provided initial funding and grants to jumpstart the formation of HIEs. Due in part to the establishment of early interoperability and interface standards, many HIEs are now able to share basic provider directory information, diagnostic laboratory test results, prescription refill requests, and clinical consult requests with participating members. Coalitions of hospitals and physicians have joined together to create community HIEs focused on electronically connecting the medical community. As HIEs mature, interoperability of health data will expand and mature.

To accelerate the efficient use of health information technology and HIEs, the Office of the National Coordinator for Health Information Technology (ONC-HIT) established The National eHealth Collaborative (NeHC). NeHC is a public-private partnership that enables a secure and interoperable nationwide health information network to advance health and improve healthcare.[139] NeHC members include government agencies, health systems, health professionals, academic medicine, patient and consumer advocates, major payers and employers, nonprofits, technology providers, and others whose strategic goal is to promote the nationwide adoption of HIEs. Participating members have demonstrated initial success with the exchange of health information.

In 2009, the Social Security Administration (SSA) wanted to reduce the time required to review and approve disability claims. The SSA teamed with the NeHC and MedVirginia (a Virginia based HIE) to start electronically exchanging disability benefit claims information. The Veterans Health Administration, Department of Defense, and Kaiser Permanente have collaborated with members of the NeHC to exchange summary patient records for the Department of Defense (DOD) and Department of Veterans Affairs (VA) to create a virtual lifetime electronic record[140] for members of our Armed Services. These early pilot programs have demonstrated the importance of using data standards and the value of information exchange on a nationwide scale. If ACOs want to achieve this type of success, they will need to leverage similar technologies on a large scale.

To be discussed in Chapter 5 is the importance of the future of HIEs in connecting providers across public and private sectors. This is critical to achieving the Three-Part Aim for all CMS ACOs. As these initiatives evolve in the coming years, consistency in standards will be a key to ensuring that industry goals for interoperability are met.

Semantic Interoperability: Are Data Standards the Missing Link?

Having discussed the importance of clinical data exchange among care providers, for public or private payer ACOs to be operating and delivering the highest quality care to their maximum potential, patient data must be interoperable and available for health analytics analysis to improve decision making. The quality, accuracy, and applicability of the data are tremendously important for application across the care continuum. When diabetic patients monitor their blood sugar at home, the test result must be shared with their primary care provider and the rest of the care team. Uploading the blood sugar result to the primary care physician's electronic medical record system will not help other members of the care team unless the test result can be transmitted and shared across the ACO membership.

Participation in regional and state HIEs is growing, and the data is slowly starting to flow. Simply exchanging patient data, however, is not sufficient for interoperability. For the patient data to be actionable, the data needs to be semantically interoperable. Semantically interoperable simply means that the sending and receiving computer system can properly interpret the meaning of the data, which requires the use of standardized vocabularies. Figure 4-1 illustrates with a hub-and-spoke concept the need for semantic interoperability to support needed electronic communications across healthcare service provider stakeholders.

Figure 4-1. Interoperability

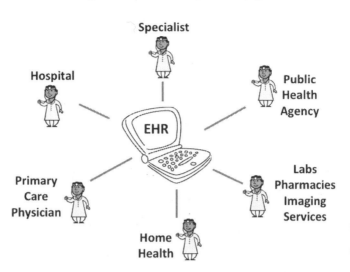

Each stakeholder has a need for various elements of data from the EHR. As systems continue to evolve, meeting the information needs of all the care delivery stakeholders will require achieving a high degree of interoperability.

How Are Standards Used?

Over the years, health information technology professionals have adopted many clinical standards and controlled vocabularies, but their lack of integration into EHR systems has lagged behind universal adoption and acceptance of the standards. In September 2011, the HIT Standards Committee's (HITSC) Clinical Quality Measures Workgroup (CQMWG) and Vocabulary Task Force (VTF) developed recommendations regarding the use of controlled vocabularies for the use in reporting quality measures required for Meaningful Use. The CQMWG and VTF both work on behalf of the National Coordinator for Health Information Technology. The groups jointly recommended the minimum set of vocabulary standards that would apply to each data element for the purpose of reporting 23 clinical quality measures to CMS.[141]

Controlled vocabularies such as SNOMED CT®, LOINC, RxNorm, UCUM, and CVX were identified as the recommended data element standards for reporting clinical quality measures and have been used to promote semantic interoperability and the exchange of consistent clinical information.

A brief description of each standard follows.

➢ SNOMED CT (Systematized Nomenclature of Medicine Clinical Terms) is a comprehensive clinical terminology, originally created by the College of American Pathologists (CAP) . In April 2007, the International Health Terminology Standards Development Organization (IHTSDO) , a nonprofit association with headquarters in Denmark, acquired the property rights. IHTSDO owns and distributes SNOMED versions internationally.

➢ LOINC, Logical Observation Identifiers Names and Codes, is a database and universal standard for identifying medical laboratory observations. LOINC applies universal code names and identifiers to medical terminology related to the electronic health record. The purpose is to assist in the electronic exchange and gathering of clinical results (such as laboratory tests, clinical observations, outcomes management, and research). The Regenstrief Institute, Inc., is the steward of LOINC.

➢ RxNorm provides normalized names for clinical drugs and links its names to many of the drug vocabularies commonly used in pharmacy management and drug interaction software, including those of First Databank, Micromedex, MediSpan, Gold Standard Alchemy, and Multum. By providing links between these vocabularies, RxNorm can mediate messages between systems not using the same software and vocabulary.

➤ UCUM, the Unified Code for Units of Measure, is a code system intended to include all units of measure being used contemporarily in international science, engineering, and business. The purpose is to facilitate unambiguous electronic communication of quantities together with their units.

➤ CVX/MVX—the CVX code is a numeric string that identifies the type of vaccine product used, and the MVX code is an alphabetic string that identifies the manufacturer of that vaccine. Taken together, the immunization can be resolved to a trade name (the proprietary name of the product).

For instance, the groups recommended that laboratory test information be standardized using LOINC for the test name and its results; SNOMED CT for applicable results values, such as microbiology organisms; and UCUM for units of measures.

On August 23, 2012, the ONC-HIT released the final CMS Meaningful Use Stage 2 rules. ONC-HIT also released a companion document, "Standards and Certification Criteria: 2014 Edition," as a guide for implementing standards to improve health data exchange. Many organizations and subject matter experts offer insights and opinions on new rules upon release, but a recognized industry leader, John D. Halamka, MD, MS, provides an excellent summary of these documents on his blog site, Life as a Healthcare CIO,[142] with links to the ONC documents.

The final Stage 2 rule specified HL7 2.5.1 as the transmission protocol for lab results, syndromic surveillance, reportable lab results, and immunizations.[143] For patient summary transactions, the Consolidated Clinical Document Architecture (CDA) is the only recommended standard. The National Council for Prescription Drug Programs is specified as the standard to exchange prescription information between entities. For clinical vocabularies, the companion rule to the final Stage 2 rule (Health Information Technology: Standards, Implementation Specifications, and Certification Criteria for Electronic Health Record Technology, 2014 Edition; Revisions to the Permanent Certification Program for Health Information Technology) identified vocabularies for key clinical content domains (Table 4-1).[144]

Table 4-1. Clinical Vocabularies Specified by Final Stage 2 Meaningful Use Companion Rule

Clinical Domain	Specified Vocabulary
Lab	LOINC (Ver 2.38)
Medications	RxNorm
Problem lists	SNOMED CT (International Release Jan 2012)
Discharge diagnosis	ICD-10 CM
Immunizations	CVX (Ver 08/15/11)
Demographics preferred language	ISO 639-1
Demographics preliminary cause of death	ICD-10 CM

Hospital laboratories and reference labs across the country have launched initiatives to map their local laboratory codes to LOINC, the universal language for laboratory reporting. The mapping allows the laboratory to send the patient results with the corresponding LOINC code that uniquely identifies the laboratory test and testing attributes. Mapping local laboratory terms to LOINC makes it possible to exchange laboratory results data between independent computer systems. This allows the receiving system to know exactly what type of laboratory test was performed without having to understand or translate the local test name or description. This mapping is critical to how the laboratory will interact with the ACOs' clinical teams and their disparate EMR systems and patient portals. Clinical data that has been enabled with terminologies such as LOINC support the development of data analytic tools, which can help to identify at-risk patients who require coordinated care.

One example of how hospital laboratories are starting to leverage LOINC codes is with the reporting of reportable laboratory results to public health agencies. Hospitals and laboratories currently use many nonstandard methods to report lab results to public health agencies. The Lab Interoperability Cooperative (LIC) is a grant-funded initiative to recruit, educate, and connect hospitals to their related public health agency by providing the necessary technical assistance to enable hospital labs to become meaningful users of certified EHR technology for submission of electronic data on reportable laboratory results to public health agencies.[145] The goal of the LIC is to provide services and education to hospital labs to help them implement the technologies necessary to enable automated submission of reportable lab results to public health agencies as defined by the Meaningful Use regulations.

Another well established clinical terminology that has been globally adopted to promote semantic interoperability is SNOMED CT®

International Release. The SNOMED CT core terminology provides a common language that enables a consistent way of indexing, storing, retrieving, and aggregating clinical data across specialties and sites of care. The International Health Terminology Standards Development Organization (IHTSDO) promotes the global adoption of SNOMED CT to ensure safe, precise, and effective exchange of clinical and health-related information. The IHTSDO maintains the SNOMED CT technical design, the core content architecture, the SNOMED CT core content (includes the concepts table, the descriptions table, the relationships table, a history table, and ICD mappings), and related technical documentation. SNOMED CT is considered to be the most comprehensive, multilingual clinical healthcare terminology in the world.

According to the IHTSDO Web site,[146] SNOMED CT aims to contribute to the improvement of patient care through underpinning the development of systems to accurately record healthcare encounters and to deliver decision support to healthcare providers. Ultimately, patients will benefit from the use of SNOMED CT to more clearly describe and accurately record their care, in building and facilitating better communication and interoperability in electronic health record exchange, and in creating systems that support healthcare decision making. SNOMED CT was originally created by the College of American Pathologists by combining SNOMED RT® and a computer-based nomenclature and classification known as Clinical Terms Version 3, formerly known as Read Codes Version 3, which was created on behalf of the UK Department of Health and is Crown copyright. SNOMED CT provides the core general terminology for the EHR and contains more than 311,000 active concepts with unique meanings and formal logic-based definitions organized into hierarchies. When implemented in software applications, SNOMED CT can be used to represent clinically relevant information consistently, reliably, and comprehensively as an integral part of producing electronic health records. SNOMED CT provides explicit links (cross maps) to health-related classifications and coding schemes that are in use around the world. This can include diagnosis classifications such as ICD-9-CM, ICD-O3, and ICD-10, as well as OPCS-4 classification of interventions. Additional cross maps are also under development or consideration. Cross maps facilitate reuse of SNOMED CT–encoded data for other purposes, such as reimbursement or statistical reporting. Use of SNOMED CT is free in IHTSDO Member Countries, including the United States. SNOMED CT is distributed in the United States by the National Library of Medicine (NLM).

The EHR problem list is an example of how SNOMED CT is being used to improve interoperability. A patient's "problem," or active diagnosis, is at the center of the information that drives clinical care practices and the overall care plan. Managing a patient's Problem List with structured, coded data is a critical function within an EHR. A Problem List based on structured data drives quality reporting, evidence-based care order sets and guidelines, computerized physician order entry, clinical decision support, and promote interoperability via the sharing of data across healthcare practices and other public reporting registries.

Problem List utility remains foundational to most critical EHR functionalities, American Recover and Reinvestment Act (ARRA) legislation, and CMS Meaningful Use requirements. This key focus has provided additional impetus toward structured and controlled use of a core Problem List. The CMS Final Rule for the Medicare Shared Savings Program has the following Stage 1 Meaningful Use requirement: "Maintain an up-to-date Problem List of current and active diagnoses based on ICD–9–CM or SNOMED CT." Healthcare delivery organizations are creating Problem List implementation strategies now with this understanding of the required SNOMED CT future state.

Many hospitals are now starting to update their EHRs to map the list of symptoms and conditions that are used on a Problem List to SNOMED CT, in addition to the ICD-9 CM/ICD-10 CM administrative billing code. To promote wider adoption of the SNOMED CT–enabled Problem List, the National Library of Medicine has released a Problem List Subset of SNOMED CT–encoded diagnosis terms based on datasets submitted by seven healthcare institutions: Beth Israel Deaconess Medical Center, Intermountain Healthcare, Kaiser Permanente, Mayo Clinic, Nebraska University Medical Center, Regenstrief Institute, and Hong Kong Hospital Authority. The purpose of the subset is to help healthcare provider organizations implement a standardized problem list to provide consistent care across patients. Adding the SNOMED CT identifier code to each patient diagnosis enables more Meaningful Use of EHRs to improve patient safety, healthcare quality, and health information exchange. In addition, enhanced standardization of data across the multiple health information systems allows multiple practitioners to provide more consistent care and improves the ACO's capability of clinical decision support and population health management.

Another source of clinician and patient-friendly terminology is the Convergent Medical Terminology (CMT). CMT was developed by Kaiser Permanente over many years for use within the Kaiser Permanente healthcare information systems and includes more than 75,000 terms and concepts. In September 2010, Kaiser Permanente, the IHTSDO, and DHHS jointly announced Kaiser Permanente's donation of its CMT content and related tooling to IHTSDO. Kaiser Permanente donated the terminology content that had been developed for its internal usage and a set of tools that is used to create and manage the terminology. CMT also includes mappings to classifications and standard vocabularies including SNOMED CT. The National Library of Medicine has now started to distribute the CMT content, which can be downloaded from the NLM Web site. CMT can be downloaded and incorporated into EHRs to help cross-reference clinical and patient-friendly terms used by physicians, patients, and other care providers.

In addition, recently, groups of EHR vendors and state governments have joined to reduce the barriers of sharing electronic health records by recommending a set of technical specifications to standardize connections between healthcare providers, health information exchanges, and other data-sharing partners.[147]

Data Governance

As providers and payers form ACOs and begin to build out their data exchange infrastructure, they will need an effective data governance strategy to manage the quality and integrity of the data used by the ACO and enforce data policies. Data governance is a set of business processes, procedures, and information technology tools that ensures important data is formally managed and controlled by the enterprise.

Data governance will ensure that data can be trusted and utilized by the organization in making strategic decisions and monitoring operating trends. Key individuals in the organization must be identified and be accountable to manage data as a strategic asset. Figure 4-2 provides a representative example of a typical data governance model that could be applied and engaged with many healthcare systems and vendors across the country.

Figure 4-2. Data Governance Model

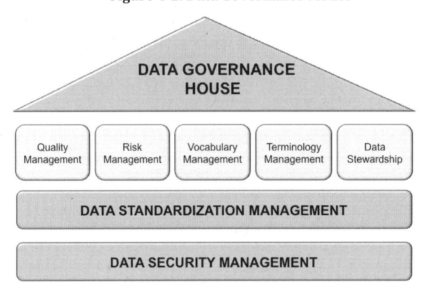

As the model illustrates, data security management and data standardization management serve as the foundation for the many other key elements and initiatives that fall under the data governance area. Formal data governance processes bring together existing policies, procedures, and tools that the organization uses to manage data. Some entities have defined a data governance model, such as the one represented above, to formally define stakeholders responsible for data quality management, data risk management, vocabulary management, terminology management, and data stewardship. In this model, an executive team meets regularly to discuss the enterprise strategy for data management, standardization of data, and use of industry terminology to promote interoperability. Some organizations identify a data czar, a senior executive, or a leader in clinical informatics who becomes the data steward for the organization. Healthcare providers and payers are using software tools to automate the incorporation of standard medical terminology and coding into healthcare software applications. As the adoption of clinical terminologies and standards becomes more widespread, this role will be one of critical importance in the ACO. One industry example of data governance comes from the Mayo Clinic.

Case Example: Mayo Clinic's Enterprise Data Trust[148]

An organization that has created a mature data governance model is the Mayo Clinic. The Mayo Clinic Enterprise Data Trust combines patient care, education, research, and administrative data from multiple systems to support information retrieval, business intelligence, and high level decision-making. Mayo created the Enterprise Data Governance (EDG) committee to treat Mayo's data as an enterprise asset. The EDG committee is comprised of 15 members, including the Executive Dean of Clinical Practice, Executive Dean for Education, Chief Information Officer, Chief Medical Information Officer, and Chief Planning Officer. The committee has a Vice Chair of Data Standards who leads the organization's efforts to standardize, model, and manage Mayo's vocabulary and metadata. The Mayo information technology department supports the committee's efforts with tools to manage the applications, vocabulary, and metadata activities. Mayo has teamed with Intermountain Healthcare and GE Healthcare to build a common vocabulary structure used throughout all Mayo applications. Mayo's long tradition of treating patient data as a strategic asset has evolved to a formal top-down data governance model to manage a cohesive Enterprise Data Trust.

EHR/HIE Interoperability Workgroup

Despite the industry's best efforts to simplify data exchange and connectivity standards, there is not one single set of standards used to exchange patient information between electronic health records and health information exchanges. The EHR/HIE Interoperability Workgroup[149] was founded to help standardize health data interoperability. The objective of the EHR/HIE Interoperability Workgroup is to define a single set of standardized, easy-to-implement connections to increase the adoption of EHRs and HIE services. The effort leveraged existing published standards for interoperability from the Office of the National Coordinator for Health Information Technology (ONC-HIT) . Ultimately, the specifications aim to remove impediments that make it difficult for EHRs to connect to HIEs, including technical specification differences, wait times for interface development, and high costs.[150]

The workgroup was originally formed by the New York eHealth Collaborative (NYeC) and is comprised of its federally designated counterparts in seven states (California, Colorado, Maryland, Massachusetts, New Jersey, New York, and Oregon) representing approximately 30% of the country's population. The eight EHR vendor members are Allscripts, eClinicalWorks, e-MDs, Greenway, McKesson Physician Practice Solutions, NextGen Healthcare, Sage Healthcare Division, and Siemens Healthcare. In addition, there are three HIE services vendors participating: Axolotl, InterSystems, and Medicity.

The first set of specifications from the EHR/HIE Interoperability Workgroup focuses on two Use cases and the detailed data and metadata specification for a compliant Continuity of Care Document.

The first Use case, Statewide Send and Receive Patient Record Exchange, describes how encrypted health information can be transmitted over the Internet. The second, the Statewide Patient Data Inquiry Service Use Case, describes the clinician's ability to query an HIE for relevant data on a specific patient.

The workgroup members collaborated to leverage existing HL7 standards, technical frameworks from IHE International, and HIE implementations to provide a fully detailed implementation specification. The implementation specifications were also aligned with Beacon community guidelines to be capable of gathering information required for reporting to ONC.

This type of collaboration between EHR vendors and state governments will advance the adoption of standards used for health information exchange and interoperability. As more and more collaborations are formed between vendors and government, these initiatives will reduce the technical and complex issues that limit the full adoption of interoperable EHRs.

As of 2012, 10 states and 26 vendors have signed on to the EHR/HIE Interoperability Workgroup to create standard data exchange specifications that will help simplify connectivity between EHRs and HIEs.[151]

Case Example: Care Connectivity Consortium

A recent example of an initiative to leverage standards-based health information technology is the Care Connectivity Consortium (CCC), formed in April 2011 by Geisinger Health System (Pennsylvania), Kaiser Permanente (California), Mayo Clinic (Minnesota), Intermountain Healthcare (Utah), and Group Health Cooperative (Washington). This consortium utilizes standards-based health information technology to share data about patients electronically. The goal of the consortium is to demonstrate better and safer care with better data availability. If a patient from one of the participating health systems gets ill while away from home and must receive healthcare in another system—or if any system sends patients to another—the care team at each participating health system will be able to access the patient's basic medical information (i.e., medications, allergies, and health conditions). The CCC participated in the HIMSS12 Interoperability Showcase and presented live demonstrations of the data exchange technology.[152]

Migration to ICD-10

As health systems in the United States are busy implementing EHRs, achieving Meaningful Use, and building links to HIEs, a major initiative is currently underway to update the antiquated ICD-9 clinical diagnostic and procedure classification code system that has been in place for three decades. Chapter 9 will address the topic of ICD-9 to 10 conversion in more detail related to the impact on revenue cycle management. The transition to the new version of ICD-10-CM and ICD-10-PCS was scheduled for nationwide conversion on October 1, 2013, to allow for better tracking of outcomes, severity of diseases, and provide much more detailed clinical diagnosis information that be used for health analytics. In April 2012, DHHS announced that the conversion date by which certain health care entities have to comply with the ICD-10 diagnosis and procedure code implementation would be postponed till October 2014.[153,154]

The CMS Fact Sheet[155] states that the adoption of the ICD-10 code sets is expected to:

> Support value-based purchasing and Medicare's antifraud and abuse activities by accurately defining services and providing specific diagnosis and treatment information;

> Support comprehensive reporting of quality data;

> Ensure more accurate payments for new procedures, fewer rejected claims, improved disease management, and harmonization of disease monitoring and reporting worldwide; and

> Allow the United States to compare its data with international data to track the incidence and spread of disease and treatment outcomes, because the United States is one of the few developed countries not using ICD-10.

The transition to ICD-10 is an expansive overhaul of the administrative coding system, and it will require much greater clinical documentation detail when coding diagnosis and inpatient hospital procedures and physician services. It significantly increases the number of codes from approximately 18,000 to more than 140,000. With the migration to ICD-10, hospitals will improve their capability to document clinical results using more structured templates that contain data coded to standard medical vocabulary, or they risk a significant decline in coding efficiency and increased claims denial rates. ICD-9 codes are currently interwoven throughout a number of legacy operational, financial, and clinical information systems, and they are pervasive in the entire revenue cycle. ICD-10-CM adoption will likely require significant updates to vendor applications, revised physician documentation work flow, retraining of employees, changes in reporting processes, and enhancement to third-party payer systems. Figure 4-3 illustrates the change and expansion in structure for diagnosis codes in the transition from ICD-9 to ICD-10.

Figure 4-3. ICD-9 vs. ICD-10 Data Elements Comparison

ICD-9 CM Diagnosis Codes	ICD-10 CM Diagnosis Codes
3-5 characters in length	3-7 characters in length
~ 14,000 codes	~ 69,000 codes
First digit may be alpha or numeric Digits 2-5 numeric	First digit is always alpha Digits 2-7 are alpha or numeric
Lacks detail and laterality	Very specific and has laterality

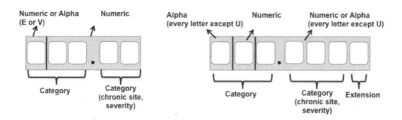

© 2012 College of American Pathologists

To assist in the translation process, CMS has published the General Equivalence Mappings (GEMs) , which is a tool that can be used as a starting point to convert data from ICD-9-CM to ICD-10-CM and PCS and vice versa. Mapping from ICD-10-CM and PCS codes back to ICD-9-CM codes is referred to as backward mapping. Mapping from ICD-9-CM codes to ICD-10-CM and PCS is referred to as forward mapping. Many of the ICD-9-CM codes do not map one-to-one to the new ICD-10-CM code. ICD-9-CM codes are three to five characters long, while ICD-10-CM codes are three to seven characters long. ICD-10 codes are very specific and include laterality. A common example that is often cited is that the one ICD-9-CM code for suturing an artery will translate into 195 possible ICD-10-CM codes that describe in greater detail the specific artery that is being sutured.

For another example, the ICD-9-CM code: 8659 Suture of Skin and Subcutaneous Tissue of Other Sites, translates into multiple ICD-10-CM codes, such as:

➢ ICD-10-CM: 0JQ10ZZ Repair Face Subcutaneous Tissue and Fascia, Open Approach

➢ ICD-10-CM: 0JQ13ZZ Repair Face Subcutaneous Tissue and Fascia, Percutaneous Approach

➢ ICD-10-CM: 0JQ40ZZ Repair Anterior Neck Subcutaneous Tissue and Fascia, Open Approach

➢ ICD-10-CM: 0JQ43ZZ Repair Anterior Neck Subcutaneous Tissue and Fascia, Percutaneous Approach

While the transition to ICD-10 will take significant effort and will likely be costly to most physician and healthcare systems, converting to ICD-10 will provide much better clinical diagnosis information. The improved coding detail can be used to improve clinical decision making and improve patient outcomes. Those organizations that do not take advantage of the transition to ICD-10-CM, and only take the mandatory compliance steps, risk the possibility of increased costs, lost coding productivity, and failure to realize the potential business value and return on investment.

Bridging the Divide

ACOs will result in a fundamental transformation of the healthcare delivery model, with a focus on quality outcomes and preventive care, and, over time, will move the healthcare delivery model further away from the current fee-for-service payment model. The need to access and share electronic health record information and medical knowledge will continue to grow rapidly as ACOs provide members with financial incentives to meet cost targets. As the population in the United States continues to age, and the Baby Boomers require more extensive and expensive healthcare, the healthcare industry will continue to be pressed to improve access to patient data, quality, and efficiency. The ACO providers will be incented to actively manage the care of chronic disease states that are expensive to treat and place higher emphasis on preventive medical care and patient-centered care. Health information technology and interoperable patient data exchange will be a strategic enabler that supports the growth of the ACO.

Meaningful Use Stage 1 provides the first step in moving a hospital and clinician office from a paper chart to an electronic record. Future stages of Meaningful Use will place additional emphasis on the ability for hospitals to electronically exchange patient data and leverage clinical terminologies and standards. Much of the electronic patient data that is being exchanged, however, is still unstructured and is not coded to standardized terminologies such as SNOMED and LOINC. The transformation will begin to gain momentum in Stage 2, when more data exchanges and increased use of controlled vocabularies are used to compute the core quality measures. The quality measures will be reported electronically. Stage 3 will push organizations to make more use of clinical decision support and to use health analytics and business intelligence to prospectively and retrospectively help ACO clinicians proactively manage their patients' health. Meaningful Use Stages 2 and 3 emphasize the use of more advanced and structured clinical data and functionality in the electronic medical record needed for longitudinal care planning, clinical decision support, and coordination of care and outcomes measurement.

As requirements evolve for Meaningful Use, further demands will be made upon clinical system vendors and providers to structure and standardize the vocabularies used in clinical documentation for questions, answers, patient treatments, and diagnostic results. To that end, the ONC Health IT Policy Committee, a public advisory body on health information technology to the ONC-HIT of the Department of Health and Human Services, submitted a set of vocabulary recommendations for the future code sets and clinical concepts (data elements) to be used in quality measures on September 9, 2011. While these are not explicitly recommended for use in other EHR functions, they establish a roadmap for semantic interoperability that must be considered in the development of applications and reporting strategies.

Given the changing reporting demands and electronic health record standards, and the need for a hybrid environment that utilizes multiple vocabularies and code sets, each ACO must establish the data governance processes needed to keep watch over the data dictionaries, terminologies, vocabularies, and data standards that will be implemented. Data governance is a discipline that ensures that enterprise data is formally managed. A successful enterprise data governance strategy will be a key requirement for sustaining the ACO.

Semantically interoperable EMRs are a strategic building block of healthcare technology required to support an ACO, and ACOs will utilize health information exchanges and patient registries as a foundation to communicate and exchange health information with participating members. The further adoption and use of healthcare terminology standards and controlled vocabularies will continue to break down the silos of patient information that exist today in hospitals, clinician offices, pharmacies, laboratories, and the community.

Chapter 4: Takeaways

✓ Interoperable clinical data exchange is a key success factor in the business strategy of an ACO.

✓ ACOs will need to deploy sophisticated health information technology solutions across inpatient, outpatient, and home care settings that provide seamless access to patient data.

✓ Semantic interoperability will improve the quality, accuracy, and applicability of patient data.

✓ The HIT Standards Committees (HITSC) Clinical Quality Measures Workgroup (CQMWG) and Vocabulary Task Force (VTF), under the direction of the Office of the National Coordinator for Health Information Technology, has developed recommendations regarding the use of controlled vocabularies for the use in reporting quality measures required for Meaningful Use. Subsequent phases of Meaningful Use regulations are expected to require additional use of clinical terminology and raise the bar for electronic reporting of core measures.

✓ ACOs will utilize health information exchanges (HIEs) and patient registries as a foundation to communicate and exchange health information with participating members. The further adoption and use of healthcare terminology standards and controlled vocabularies will continue to break down the silos of patient information that exist today in hospitals, clinician offices, pharmacies, laboratories, and the community.

[136] Department of Health and Human Services Press Release. Accountable Care Organizations: Improving Care Coordination for People with Medicare. March 31, 2011. Accessed online February 8, 2012, at http://www.hhs.gov/news/press/2011pres/03/20110331a.html.

[137] College of American Pathologists, Accountable Care Toolkits, Accountable Care Overview. Accessed online February 15, 2012, at http://www.cap.org/apps/docs/membership/transformation/new/toolkit_aco.html.

[138] College of American Pathologists, Accountable Care Toolkits, Accountable Care Overview, page 3. Accessed online March 4, 2012, at http://www.cap.org/apps/docs/membership/transformation/new/toolkit_aco.html.

[139] National eHealth Collaborative Web site. Accessed online February 25, 2012, at www.nationalehealth.org.

[140] Office of the Undersecretary of Defense, Personnel and Readiness [OUSD (P&R)]. Virtual Lifetime Electronic Record (VLER). Accessed online February 28, 2012, at www.prim.osd.mil/init/vler.html.

[141] Health IT Policy Committee, September 9, 2011, letter to Farzad Mostashari, MD, ScM, National Coordinator for Health Information Technology, Department of Health and Human Services.

[142] Halamka JD. Meaningful Use Stage 2 Rules Released. *Life As A Healthcare CIO*. August 23, 2012. Accessed online August 28, 2012, at

http://geekdoctor.blogspot.com/2012/08/meaningful-use-stage-2-rules-released.html; Halamka JD. More Meaningful Use Stage 2 Highlights. *Life As A Healthcare CIO*. August 24, 2012. Accessed online August 28, 2012, at http://geekdoctor.blogspot.com/2012/08/more-meaningful-use-stage-2-highlights.html.

[143] Centers for Medicare & Medicaid Services. 42 CFR Parts 412, 413, and 495. Medicare and Medicaid Programs; Electronic Health Record Incentive Program--Stage 2. Final Rule. August 23, 2012. (c) Public Health Objectives. p. 212.

[144] Department of Health and Human Services. 45 CFR Part 170. Health Information Technology: Standards, Implementation Specifications, and Certification Criteria for Electronic Health Record Technology, 2014 Edition; Revisions to the Permanent Certification Program for Health Information Technology. August 23, 2012. Accessed online August 26, 2012, at http://www.healthit.gov/policy-researchers-implementers/meaningful-use-stage-2-0.

[145] Lab Interoperability Cooperative Web site. Frequently Asked Questions. Accessed online February 24, 2012, at www.labinteroperabilitycoop.org/faq.htm.

[146] International Health Terminology Standards Development Organisation Web site. SNOMED CT® description. Accessed online February 26, 2012, at http://www.ihtsdo.org/snomed-ct.

[147] EHR/HIE Interoperability Workgroup Web site. Accessed online February 28, 2012, at http://www.interopwg.org/.

[148] Chute CG, Beck SA, Fisk TB, Mohr DN. The Enterprise Data Trust at Mayo Clinic: A semantically integrated warehouse of biomedical data. *J Am Med Inform Assoc.* 2010 Mar-Apr;17(2):131-135.

[149] EHR/HIE Interoperability Workgroup Web site Home page. Accessed online February 28, 2012, at http://www.interopwg.org/.

[150] EHR/HIE Interoperability Workgroup Web site About page. Accessed online February 28, 2012, at http://www.interopwg.org/about.html.

[151] EHR/HIE Interoperability Workgroup Press Release. 10 States Now Unified to Standardize Health Data Interoperability. February 20, 2012. Accessed online February 24, 2012, at http://interopwg.org/news/OFFICIAL-PR-10-States-Now-Unified-to-Standardize-Health-Data-Interoperability.html.

[152] Care Connectivity Consortium Celebrates Milestone at 2012 Annual HIMSS Conference Press Release. February 22, 2012. Accessed online February 25, 2012, at http://xnet.kp.org/newscenter/pressreleases/nat/2012/022212cccinteroperability.html.

[153] Fed. Reg. Vol. 77, No. 74. April 17, 2012. I(A). Executive Summary and Background.

[154] Department of Health and Human Services Press Release. HHS announces intent to delay ICD-10 compliance date. Accessed online February 24, 2012, at http://www.hhs.gov/news/press/2012pres/02/20120216a.html.

[155] Center for Medicare and Medicaid Services. ICD-10 Transition: An Introduction. April 2010. Accessed online February 18, 2012, at http://www.cms.gov/ICD10/Downloads/ICD10IntroFactSheet20100409.pdf.

Chapter 5. Health Information Exchange—Driving Connectivity

Greg Miller

...IT must play a central role in the redesign of the health care system if a substantial improvement in health care quality is to be achieved during the coming decade. [156]

Institute of Medicine
2001 Report. Crossing the Quality Chasm

The Institute of Medicine envisioned more than a decade ago that health information technology would be essential to eliminate medical errors and improve the quality of care delivered in the United States. Health information technology infrastructure for ACOs will help meet the continuously evolving requirements for higher quality and affordability by getting the right information to the right place at the right time. Section 3022 of the Affordable Care Act specifies that the Medicare ACO must have "clinical and administrative systems" and use "telehealth, remote patient monitoring, and other such enabling technologies" to report cost and quality measures, as well as coordinate patient care activities.[157] These same requirements will likely apply to Medicaid pediatric ACOs and private payer ACO models as well.

The availability and adoption of health information technology has grown rapidly over the past three decades. The need for these systems as prerequisites for healthcare and reimbursement reforms has increased interest in their adoption. Such other initiatives as EMR implementation incentives, the conversion to ICD-10 coding, and efforts to establish nationwide health information exchanges (HIEs) have reinforced the importance of technology in healthcare. For ACOs, health information technologies serve important functions of giving teams real-time access to patient records; stratification and identification of patients requiring treatment or intervention; collaboration and coordination across the continuum of care, monitoring and measuring quality and outcomes; and improving quality and affordability of both ambulatory and inpatient care.

With legislative and regulatory reforms accelerating ACO and clinical integration program development among hospitals and physician practices, ensuring interoperability among EMRs will support accurate and timely bilateral health information exchange between hospitals and office-based EMRs. Interoperability, in turn, will ensure the efficient coordination and continuity of care offered by any ACO.

Why Should IT Matter

It was reported in the *Archives of Internal Medicine* in January 2011 that

> ...poor communication between primary care physicians and specialists on referrals and consultations is an all-too-common problem that has real repercussions on patient care...It can lead to duplicate lab tests, repeat procedures, wasted time and resources, conflicting prescriptions, and potential harm to patients.[158]

That study proceeded to report that

> ...even though 69.3% of primary care physicians said they send specialists notification of a patient's history and the reason for the consultation all or most of the time, just 34.8% of specialists said they routinely receive such

information. Meanwhile, 80.6% of specialists say they send consultation results to the referring physician all or most of the time, but only 62.2% of primary care physicians say they ever get that information.[159]

The concept of sharing patient data and health information outside the four walls of a healthcare enterprise is anathema to many hospitals and health systems. It is driven by a multitude of factors, ranging from fiercely competitive markets to paranoia regarding data privacy and security. It is essential, however, to the management and operation of a successful ACO initiative that data be easily shared amongst all caregivers in a patient-centered, clinically integrated, coordinated care model in order to deliver care more efficiently and effectively and to ensure that all caregivers have the most up-to-date information about their patients at all times.

This level of patient-centered care coordination and collaboration among providers is the key to truly managing the health of individual patients and patient populations, and achieving improvements in quality and affordability is at the heart of the ACO model. Establishing an electronic exchange infrastructure is complex, however, not only because of the heterogeneous information systems spread across the care continuum—hospital information systems, ambulatory EHRs, and practice management systems—but also because many ACOs will span organizational boundaries beyond the walls of a single enterprise or entity. Because the ACO may be comprised of multiple organizations, establishing the electronic connections when the ACO does not "own" all the pieces and parts (e.g., hospitals, physician practices, imaging centers, reference labs) requires a flexible architecture for data exchange that can create a virtual integrated delivery network.

Virtualizing the Clinically Integrated Delivery Network

When asked by David Burda, the editor of *Modern Healthcare*, whether he would want to join an ACO if he were a new physician just starting out, Jay Crosson, the Permanente Medical Group senior adviser for health policy and former chair of the Medicare Payment Advisory Commission, answered, "I absolutely would."[160]

Why such a definitive response? Because Dr. Crosson experienced firsthand, during his work as a physician within the Kaiser Permanente system for more than 30 years, the value to both patient and provider when the hospital, physician, and payer are closely aligned with shared goals. Wherever a patient goes within the Kaiser system, be it a hospital or physician's office, each authorized provider—from nurses to primary care physicians to one or more specialists—has an overall understanding of the patient's history and health status based on his or her ability to review every interaction the patient has had with every member of the care team. This holistic and coherent approach—a 360-degree view—ensures that care is coordinated and congruent with the protocols and guidelines for that particular patient. In other words, the highest quality care is delivered at the lowest cost.

Kaiser Permanente has spent billions of dollars over many years on "bricks and mortar" infrastructure to achieve this level of coordination, including buildings, people, and health information technology. From an information technology perspective alone, Kaiser has spent billions on a hospital and ambulatory information system to ensure every physician across acute and ambulatory settings is using the same system; as a result, he or she has the most recently updated information about every patient.

There is no doubt that the integrated delivery network model as exemplified by Kaiser and such others as Intermountain Healthcare, Geisinger Health System, and Mayo Clinic, has achieved the greatest degree of success in improving care collaboration and reducing the cost of care. On the other hand, a model that requires a single or common ownership and substantial capital resources to build or purchase the infrastructure necessary to replicate an experience like Kaiser's is not realistic for nationwide or even regional ACO implementation, because a central goal of an ACO is to lower the cost of care, not increase it. Moreover, as ACOs take shape, many will be joint ventures that include participants and stakeholders who are not part of the same physical or legal organization—requiring a virtual network to accomplish their work. The expectation that every provider use the same information system is simply unrealistic, given human behavior, organizational dynamics, cost, and the nature of cross-organizational workflow; hence the value of new interoperability standards that will increasingly allow for information exchange at a lower cost of implementation.

Meanwhile, HIE vendors are working to assist providers in virtualizing healthcare records. This work is intended to help create the integrated delivery network experience and achieve the level of coherence experienced by Kaiser's providers without having to own all the pieces and parts and requiring everyone to be part of the same organization using the same information system. While data standards and interface development are complex, and while the currently available information is often limited, compared to single-source systems, it is the reality of healthcare today. Because of the current, episodic nature of an ACO's bundled payment and shared savings model, it presents complex issues of care coordination.

To successfully coordinate care on more than an episodic basis, distribute funds accurately, and improve quality as measured against benchmarks, community-wide coordination of patient information in a clinically integrated model is essential. HIE technology is the underlying connection of all stakeholders and participants in an ACO across organizational boundaries and disparate information systems, so that information can be shared community-wide and care coordination enabled. Participants require a range of connectivity in an ACO as illustrated in Figure 5-1. HIE technology can help meet and support those needs.

Figure 5-1. Spectrum of Connectivity for ACO Participants

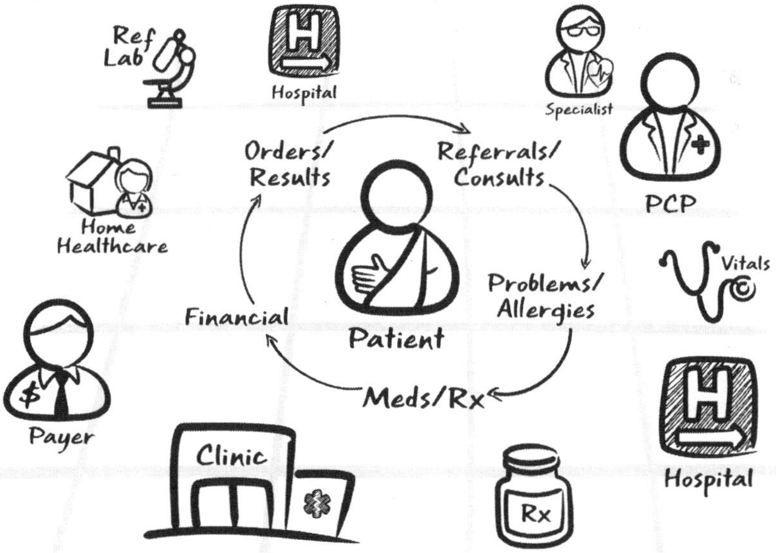

While we are specifically addressing the integrated delivery network type ACO, this spectrum of participants applies to each of the other four potential ACO models and the CIN defined in Chapter 1.

Defining HIE: Noun or Verb?

Before entering too deeply into the technology required to manage a successful ACO, it is important to define "health information exchange," because users of HIE often use the term in different contexts. HIE as a noun commonly refers to a third-party nonprofit organization formed to enable information sharing among multiple healthcare entities. Examples of this type of HIE are the regional health information organization and the health information organization. These entities and HIE are used interchangeably to refer to publicly funded initiatives serving either a local geographic region or a state. Some statewide initiatives, such as the Delaware Health Information Network, the Ohio Health Information Partnership, and the Colorado Regional Health Information Organization, are ARRA-qualified state-designated entities eligible to receive federal funds to support their operations. In the case of such regional initiatives as the Mississippi Coastal Health Information Exchange, there are a variety of funding mechanisms, both public and private, in place to support business operations. In addition to these HIE initiatives, many others are at various stages of formation and operation across the country.

Whether an HIE initiative is statewide or regional, its value in supporting an ACO and empowering comprehensive clinical integration hinges, to a great extent, on the quality and completeness of the data contributed by participating stakeholders. The resources of the federal State Health Information Exchange Cooperative Agreement Program are provided to designated state agencies and organizations that focus on engaging the right participants and allocate funds to create and strengthen infrastructure and capacity for health information exchange across and among healthcare providers in each state.

For a third-party HIE to support ACO operations fully, all providers—not only physicians and hospitals—participating in an ACO must also be participants in that HIE. This participation, however, is usually not the case. In a public regional or state HIE, the primary focus in the first few years is connecting hospitals and physician practices. In the future mature ACO model, *all* stakeholders involved in delivering care to a patient will be connected: hospitals and physician practices, as well as long-term care facilities, community health teams, nurse care managers, home health agencies, physical therapists, reference labs, imaging centers, and the like. It is, therefore, less likely that an HIE (in its noun form) will be able to fully support the information exchange needs of an ACO in the near term.

HIE as a verb commonly refers to the *activity* of exchanging health information across disparate information systems and multiple locations of care, both acute and ambulatory. The third-party HIE introduced above employs the verb usage of the term when it deploys HIE technology to enable the active sharing of information among its participants. Similarly, there are hundreds of local private information exchanges already in operation nationwide, sponsored by community hospitals, such as Hoag Hospital and El Camino Hospital in California, and health systems or integrated delivery networks, such as Intermountain Healthcare in Utah; BayCare Health System in Florida; and CHRISTUS Health, with care locations across seven states and

Mexico. Each of these self-funded private HIE organizations has deployed HIE technology to actively exchange health information to all members of the care team across acute and ambulatory care settings. In the private HIE setting, hospitals and health systems have a much stronger influence over stakeholder participation. As a result, the private HIE has a much higher likelihood of being able to support an ACO comprehensively by engaging all stakeholders beyond its hospitals and physician practices. This point can be illustrated (Figure 5-2) to show some of the various channels through which information must flow.

Figure 5-2. HIE as a Verb—Active HIE Among ACO Participants

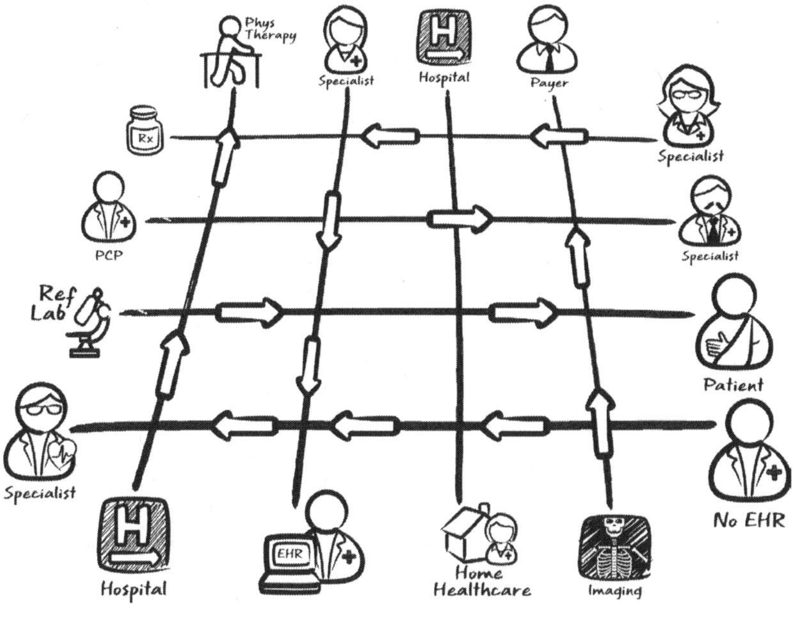

In the end, both the noun and verb forms of HIE are describing the same thing: the exchange of health information. The differences lie in the organizational structures, funding and sustainability mechanisms, goals of the entity, and stakeholder participation. The technology required for exchanging health information is essentially the same and, in either case, is necessary for the management of an ACO.

HIE Deployment Framework

Successful ACOs, clinically integrated networks, and other healthcare organizational transformation initiatives must possess an HIE infrastructure with specific competencies to support governance, operations, clinical quality measurement, financial goals, and objectives. In addition to the multiple underlying technologies required to manage an ACO, particularly those at the source that gather, store, assimilate, codify, or process data, several HIE-related technologies are also needed.

When it comes to deploying HIE capabilities, however, there is no one-size-fits-all model because, as discussed in Chapter 1, there are multiple configurations of ACO partnerships and ventures being formed in regional markets across the country. Therefore, an HIE deployment framework must be flexible, adaptable, scalable, and deployable in a model that adds capabilities incrementally to achieve the clinical integration objectives and goals of an ACO initiative. A flexible and incremental HIE deployment framework for ACOs, clinically integrated networks, and other initiatives can be depicted (Figure 5-3) as flowing through a number of levels.

Figure 5-3. Flexible and Incremental HIE Deployment Framework

Data Acquisition	• Data must be acquired from all clinical and administrative systems across acute and ambulatory care locations; From automated and non-automated practices
Data Exchange	• Electronic exchange of data across disparate systems and care locations
Data Aggregation	• Data from across the care continuum is aggregated. Terminology services are applied for semantic clarity and patient identity is matched
Risk Stratification	• Risk stratification to segment the population based on opportunity to impact clinical and financial performance
Analytics	• Advanced analytics to drill down and perform root cause analysis and build feedback loops for performance improvements and decision support
Clinical Integration	• Care coordination of populations – case management, disease management and wellness programs

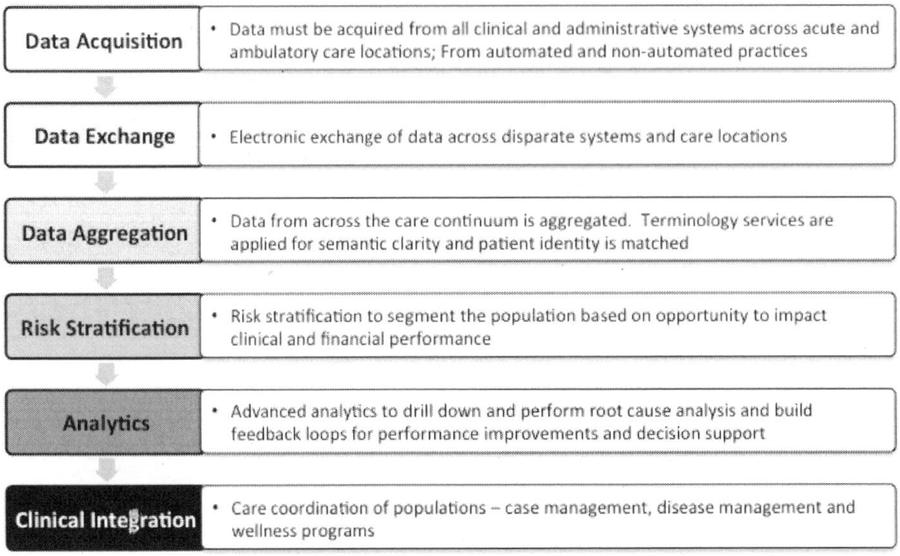

Nontraditional IT Competencies

The *New England Journal of Medicine* reported that the average Medicare patient sees seven different physicians in a given year, and patients with multiple chronic conditions may see up to 16 different physicians annually.[161] Due to the highly fragmented nature of our healthcare system today, most of these providers are not part of the same organization, making the coordination of care across providers time consuming and costly and increasing the opportunity for medical errors to occur.

As noted in the deployment framework in Figure 5-3, an ACO requires a sophisticated technology infrastructure at its foundation to facilitate its objectives of sharing health information among all stakeholders delivering care to a specific patient, in order to improve quality and reduce costs. The most essential feature of this infrastructure is the ability to share information and coordinate care across organizations in a virtual integrated delivery network-like infrastructure, also described earlier in this chapter. In fact, as Glaser and Salzberg noted in *Hospitals and Health Networks*, "While applications such as the EHR and the patient health record are important, data may be the most important ACO information technology asset."[162] We would suggest that what you do with the data, such as applying clinical intelligence and delivering at the point of care, is even more important.

Such traditional healthcare applications as EMRs, hospital information systems, emergency department information systems, office-based practice management systems, laboratory and radiology information systems, and patient administration applications are designed to record patient care information during an episode of care and are limited in scope to that care setting's organizational boundaries. While each discrete solution is important, many of these non–office-based technologies were not designed to provide output that could support the innovative coordination of care model needed for ACOs, which extends beyond the four walls of a hospital, an emergency department, an imaging center, or a lab.

To be successful, an ACO requires technology that can seamlessly integrate information and data across organizational boundaries spanning many discrete technologies, apply such clinical intelligence as advanced clinical decision support and analytics, and deliver knowledge at the point of care. Because the participants in the ACO likely will be affiliated with disparate organizations—and unlike Kaiser, not all will be using the same information system—support technology for the ACO will need to facilitate virtualization of the patient's record and make it available to the care team by connecting to disparate systems across multiple care locations and integrating data with local systems and technologies already in use. An illustration of the electronic virtual care team (Figure 5-4) shows the bilateral flow of patient information that is needed to facilitate effective HIE actions.

Figure 5-4. Electronic Virtual Care Teams

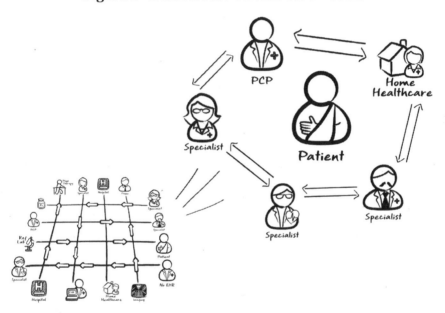

Section 3502 of the Affordable Care Act calls for the development and initiation of new community health teams to support medical homes (recognized as part of the foundation of ACOs). The efforts of these teams will be enabled by HIE capabilities that positively effect coordination of care and support the physicians and care teams delivering patient care in geographically dispersed locations throughout the regions they serve.

Supporting Every Provider of Care

While the HITECH Act is focused on enabling physicians to adopt EMRs, the reality is that many physicians still rely on paper records for patient care and use electronic data mainly for billing purposes. According to the CDC's 2009 National Ambulatory Medical Care Survey, only about 44% of physicians answering a survey reported using all or partial EMR systems (not including systems solely for billing) in their office-based practices. Of this 44%, about 21% reported having systems that met the criteria of a basic system, with only 6.3% having an extensive and fully functional electronic record system. This assessment means that more than half of all physicians in the United States still maintain paper-based practices. Within those practices, some physicians are comfortable using such electronic technology as e-mail and a Web browser, while others still prefer a paper chart and are reluctant to participate in HITECH incentives. Nevertheless, many of these same physicians will need to participate in an ACO model as these entities continue to expand in markets across the country. Educating these late-adopter physicians on the benefits and needs for health information technology adoption will be especially important as ACO start-ups get underway. This is particularly true because the Meaningful Use incentives, although going a long way toward encouraging adoption of EMR technology, will take years to reach critical mass.

The adoption of an EMR to record data electronically is only part of the equation. Data must be harvested from every care location, clinical intelligence applied, and knowledge exchanged with each member of the patient care team, which will likely be across a virtual integrated delivery network-like environment. This integration means that the HIE platform must support one-to-one, one-to-many, and many-to-many communications in a multidirectional, inbound and outbound active exchange framework. This data must be available to providers in their native workflow—as discrete data in the EMR, if it exists, or via a browser-based application in their practice. The EMR must be able to "outbound" data as discrete elements or in the form of a continuity-of-care document, so that it is consumable by other information systems in use across the care continuum. Similarly, in a non-automated care location, the browser-based application must not only display data, but enable the gathering and recording of data as an "EMR-lite," so that it can be exchanged with and accessed by other non-automated locations, as well as consumable in the form of a continuity-of-care document or as discrete elements by the heterogeneous information systems across acute and ambulatory care settings.

Many traditional HIEs are data aggregation platforms only, with a Web-portal application attached, so that participants can access information that has been centrally stored, in contrast to an active exchange infrastructure. The portal-based health information application (Figure 5-5) is fundamentally different from an active HIE.

Figure 5-5. HIE and the Portal-based Health Information Application

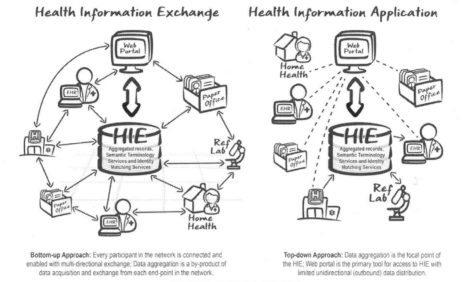

HIE vs. Health Information Application Comparison

Health Information Exchange

Health Information Application

Bottom-up Approach: Every participant in the network is connected and enabled with multi-directional exchange; Data aggregation is a by-product of data acquisition and exchange from each end-point in the network.

Top-down Approach: Data aggregation is the focal point of the HIE; Web portal is the primary tool for access to HIE with limited unidirectional (outbound) data distribution.

Multi-directional Exchange
Uni-directional Exchange
Access Only

One of the fundamental differences between the health information application and the active HIE is the effect on a provider's workflow. If a provider has adopted an EMR, the traditional portal-based HIE solution requires providers to work outside of their new workflow, which was specifically redesigned to support an EMR-based environment and electronic record keeping. Experience shows that if providers have gotten over the hurdle of adopting an EMR, then the most effective HIE solution is the multidirectional active exchange infrastructure model, which enables providers to stay in their native EMR-based workflow, while still enabling the active exchange of information—orders, results, consultations, and referrals—with other EMR-based providers, as well as with non-automated practices. The health information application model requires providers to exit their native EMR-based workflow and log onto a separate health information application portal-type solution, which is only for accessing the information. Most health information application-type solutions have the ability to export discrete data into EMRs, and, if so, it is only in a unidirectional model as displayed in figure 5-5.

So the fundamental difference between the portal-based health information application and the active HIE is that the health information application is an information access model and is not an active exchange—meaning that providers have to go "get" the information, as opposed to having information "pushed" to them in their native systems and workflow. This is a critical and important difference between the active HIE and a repository of data that has a meaningful impact on provider workflow and patient care.

To support clinical integration programs and ACOs, active exchange across organizational boundaries is required, with seamless integration into any EMR, while also enabling Web-based access to data for providers who are still in paper-based practices, and furthering the exchange with the ability to harvest data in each endpoint of the network. In this manner, the inbound-outbound, multidirectional active HIE model ensures data is synchronized across all caregivers.

While the number of HIE vendors is expanding, certification and interoperability requirements have conversely forced consolidation in the office-based EMR vendor market. Consequently, some physicians are finding themselves with unsupported products or outdated technologies that need replacement. Others work in markets where a handful of vendors predominate or in environments where local health systems are assisting with single or selected vendor implementations. While the idea of a single-vendor world is appealing, as mentioned earlier, it is not contemporary reality. Consequently, any sustainable ACO initiative likely will need to be interoperable with a number of different EMR/EHR solutions requiring health information exchange.

Of course, an ACO could be developed in the absence of such technologies; online registry reporting, for example, would quickly enable large groups of providers to populate a common Web-based system in which limited analytics could be run and from which improved care management might be delivered. We recognize this type of system as a starting point, however, and as not a sustainable state of operation—especially for newer models of care delivery requiring quality monitoring, rapid clinical process improvement, and financial performance measurement. As such, the technology needed to support an ACO would need to be vendor-agnostic and simultaneously support the workflow of the provider wherever he or she stands on the technology adoption curve from a paper-based environment to a fully automated practice.

Technology and Continuity of Care

One of the greatest challenges for physicians is being able to see what all the members of the patient's care team are doing, from visits to other practitioners and specialists to trips to emergency rooms and urgent care centers. The following case illustrates the complexities of a typical cross-provider care episode successfully facilitated under the active HIE deployment framework.

Mr. Johnson is a 59-year-old construction worker with a long history of diabetes. He has documented early retinopathy and hypertension, but no evidence of other end-organ changes from his chronic diabetes. He presents to his primary care physician, Dr. Clark, with fever, acute shortness of breath, and rales and wheezing in the left lower lobe. Dr. Clark diagnoses Mr. Johnson with acute pneumonia (confirmed on a chest x-ray) and admits him to Metro Community Hospital (MCH).

In the hospital, Mr. Johnson is newly diagnosed with renal disease (elevated serum creatinine, proteinuria, and mild acidosis). At discharge, he is placed in an intensive home care program for strict monitoring of sodium and protein intake, along with diabetes monitoring. He is discharged to the MCH home care agency to be seen by a visiting RN. His discharge medications include insulin, an oral antibiotic, and two new medications—a brand-name diuretic and a new ACE inhibitor for renal disease and hypertension.

During the visiting RN's third visit to Mr. Johnson, she becomes concerned by his rising blood pressure, weight gain, and general lethargy. She calls Dr. Clark to order new laboratory tests, which she then draws and delivers to the lab herself. The nurse questions Mr. Johnson, who insists he is compliant with his medication program.

Because MCH, the home care agency, Dr. Clark's practice, the local laboratory, and Bayside Pharmacy (which fills Mr. Johnson's prescriptions) all belong to an ACO, their clinical findings on Mr. Johnson are published in a common electronic community health record powered by HIE technology. This community health record features an innovative patient management dashboard displayed electronically to all authenticated members of Mr. Johnson's care team.

The home care nurse consults the dashboard and notices the list of medications from the MCH discharge summary does not reconcile with the list from Bayside Pharmacy. During further discussions with Mr. Johnson, she learns that he filled the two inexpensive generic prescriptions but not the expensive new diuretic and ACE inhibitor. With the recent decline in the construction business, Mr. Johnson's income has been severely reduced, and he admits he cannot afford to take the two medications for his renal disease.

The nurse also receives Mr. Johnson's recent laboratory test results via the dashboard. The results show a deterioration of renal function with increased serum creatinine levels and electrolytes, suggesting a recurrence of metabolic acidosis. She contacts Dr. Clark, who switches Mr. Johnson to an alternative generic medication for his renal disease. Dr. Clark then sends an electronic referral to a new nephrologist to see Mr. Johnson emergently so that he can receive more intensive evaluation of his worsening renal disease.

Because the visiting RN and Dr. Clark were part of an ACO with active HIE technology that supports high-quality care and efficient practice, they were able to intervene quickly with use of real-time and accurate patient health data to prevent another admission to the hospital. Without the collaborative capabilities provided by the technology framework and active exchange infrastructure, such a successful outcome would be in doubt and, at the very least, considerably less efficient and more expensive. Multiple bilateral connections can exist across organizations for the purposes of improving connectivity across the network of ACO participants, as illustrated in Figure 5-6.

Figure 5-6. A Virtual Integrated Delivery Network

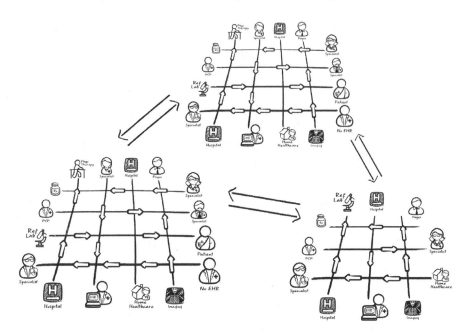

Health data exchange across boundaries leads to improvement in the quality and continuity-of-care information shared in a timely manner among the members of the virtual care team. It enables care collaboration across multiple providers and organizations and is critical for the ACO to achieve optimal levels of clinical integration and population health management, as well as the required quality and affordability improvements. Technological solutions needed to support such continuity of care and enhanced provider collaboration include:

➤ Data and workflow integration across disparate information systems and settings;

➤ A unified view of the patient across organizations and care locations;

➢ Real-time updates from participating entities and alerts of such updates to ensure timely care synchronization across all accountable parties;

➢ Clinical decision support, such as risk stratification to identify care opportunities, and clinical alerts to ensure adherence to care guidelines and protocols; and

➢ Aggregation of patient information to enable analysis and formulation of business intelligence on patient populations for the purpose of clinical quality monitoring, outcomes and performance measurement, and financial outcomes management.

Care Transition Technology Helps Avoid Penalties

In September 2012, CMS is instituting penalties for readmissions to the hospital that occur within 30 days after discharge, if those readmissions could have been avoided. These penalties, applied to Medicare inpatient payments, starts with a 1% withholding in 2012, but then continues to climb, reaching a 3% penalty in the year 2014. As Medicare inpatient volume represents a significant portion of the patient population for most US hospitals, the potential financial impact could be significant. As the US population continues to age and more people than ever become Medicare-eligible, the impact on hospitals and health systems nationwide could be disastrous.

To avoid readmissions, a combination of people, processes, and technology are needed to form a collaborative care model across the continuum. The core HIE capabilities described earlier in this chapter become the foundation for the technology to support the efforts to avoid readmissions and, thereby, avoid penalties. The HIE technology enables the secure exchange of information, so that care teams can monitor progress and proactively communicate a patient-centered, yet virtual care team. However, additional technology capabilities can expand the HIE platform to enable it to meet the needs of hospital systems, ACOs, patient-centered medical homes, medical groups, and other organizations as they strive to meet the complex needs of transitioning patients from acute care to ambulatory settings and then monitor their progress and care out in the community.

Technology to manage the transitions of care can be applied to any collaborative network of providers, such as an ACO, CIN, or PCMH, so they can better manage the flow of information and activity around patients. To manage the transitions of care effectively across a network of providers, the technology infrastructure must enable several key things:

➢ A secure network to exchange data;

➢ Interfaces to a wide range of EHRs, Practice Management Systems, and Hospital Information Systems;

➢ A patient-centric record;

➢ A comprehensive view of what care is being provided by all care team members; and

➢ Ways to communicate, notify, and alert providers proactively.

Technology to manage the transitions of care takes advantage of the HIE infrastructure, connecting to all endpoints of the network (i.e., hospitals, physician practices, long-term care facilities, labs, imaging centers, the patient) and acts like a hub for the network. Care coordinators can use the care transition technology to establish which providers comprise the patient's care team and automatically collect information about patients and activity from across the network in near real-time.

A care collaboration team can use the network hub in many useful ways, to help avoid readmissions to the hospital, such as:

➢ View clinical and administrative details about a particular patient;

➢ Real-time communication with all members of the care team to exchange notifications, alerts, requests, or other information;

➢ Identify gaps in care or other clinical needs and

➢ See what care is being provided by all members of the care team.

The care transition technology also helps members of a care team build a private exchange around a particular patient to share and disseminate data. A simple means of communicating intent using SBAR method (i.e., Situation, Background, Assessment, and Recommendation) enables a care team to establish a transitional care plan to be shared and updated as part of the system.

In addition, interacting with the patient is a critical function to help avoid readmissions. With care transition technology, you can proactively communicate, notify, alert, and manage patients' care, with the patients themselves being active participants. Patients can interact with their care team to access information, update content, and engage in other day-to-day interactions. These capabilities and data can also be extended to patient portals, patient health records, and other systems used by the patients.

The care transition technology enables the management of a group of patients such as the ACO members, patient-centered medical home patients, or recently discharged patients from the hospital. It provides a single view of activity, conditions, alerts, and other data points needed to manage the patient across the network. It enables the network to start managing the patient population immediately upon discharge and tracks referrals, orders, procedures, and patient compliance, while building up the quality of data for more advanced uses as the network matures.

With care transition functionality that leverages the HIE infrastructure, all members of a patient's care team are kept in sync across acute and ambulatory care settings. They are alerted to adverse events, complications, and changes in a patient's health status, so that hospitals and providers can proactively take action before a readmission occurs. Care transition technology can help hospitals avoid the CMS-imposed readmission penalties.

Semantics of Future Care

Readers familiar with the telephone game or sharing workplace water-cooler gossip have likely noted the often amusing outcomes of miscommunication. In healthcare, however, garbled communication can mean the difference between life and death. How is it possible, then, to share patient data across multiple physician practices, health systems, and allied health providers effectively and efficiently when their health information technology systems do not even speak the same language? Moreover, how do we make the underlying data actionable for managing the ACO?

The ability to create coherence between systems that do not speak the same language is an HIE function called semantic interoperability; it is vital to realizing the potential of sharing information across the continuum of care. Semantic interoperability establishes a seamless exchange of data between two or more systems or healthcare networks, ensuring that health data is not only understandable within its original context, but also capable of supporting clinical decision making, care collaboration, public health reporting, clinical research, health service management, and more.

From Logical Observation Identifiers, Names, and Codes to Systematized Nomenclature of Medicine (SNOMED), ICD-9, ICD-10, National Drug Codes, and Current Procedural Terminology (to name just a few), there is a multitude of code sets and terminologies requiring semantic interoperability in the contemporary ACO environment. Add the subtle nuances of clinician-friendly terminology and free text from physician dictation, and one begins to comprehend the semantic challenges of health information exchange.

Consider, for example, a simple description of an infected tympanic membrane as recorded in the chart of a patient with acute otitis media. Such terms as *erythematous*, *infected*, *inflamed*, or *reddened* all describe essentially the same clinical finding. To enable consistent data sharing across such variations in terminology and disparate code sets, an effective terminology services platform, incorporating a health ontology, is needed to meet sophisticated mapping process requirements and achieve the following results:

➤ A comprehensive health information schema that sorts through the fragmentation of multiple transactions related to the same event (e.g., prescription, refill, claim) and creates a single, optimized record of a person's health;

➤ A clear semantic understanding of the data. A health ontology organizes and filters information around concepts of clinical importance such as a disease state or a clinical specialty, rather than around the kind of test or the department in which a procedure was performed;

➤ A clear record of the person's healthcare events across the continuum of care over time; and

➤ A source of transformed information to exchange with third-party systems in formats native to such systems, regardless of the formats in which data was received.

The result: a unified view of the patient from multiple data contributors across the care continuum and heterogeneous information systems, enabling proactive decision support, trending, analytics, and empowering effective care.

In addition to resolving differences in terminology across the disparate data sources in the care continuum, a similar semantic problem exists with patient identity. A provider in the emergency department who is caring for a patient for the first time needs the most up-to-date information about that patient as a member of the ACO's patient population—particularly in cases in which the patient comes from outside the contracted payer patient population. This type of scenario poses a challenge. In each of the information systems at the endpoints of the network—hospital systems, ambulatory EMRs, practice management systems, and others—the patient has a unique medical record number. In situations in which the physicians or hospitals are using different systems (the far more likely scenario in most locations), data aggregation becomes a complex and limiting problem. Creating interfaces, developing common patient identity management systems, and doing so in a HIPAA-secure environment, are only a few of the challenges to aggregating relevant data on behalf of improved patient care.

Furthermore, in the silo-oriented US healthcare system, the multiple encounters are not linked via a unique common patient identifier across organizational boundaries and information systems. This problem does not exist in most developed countries with national health systems, because every patient has a single national medical record number, thereby linking together multiple care encounters related to an episode of illness. To effectively manage an ACO, it is essential for HIE technology to correlate, link, and assimilate multiple encounters, so that when a patient presents in the emergency department, the physician can quickly search for all historical data about that specific patient from any previous visit in any care location or from a provider who is a participating stakeholder in the ACO. Ensuring that "John Doe is John Doe" is extremely important as we seek to improve the quality of care and enhance patient safety in the United States. Figure 5-7 provides an illustration of this essential factor of semantic interoperability and patient identity management across organizations.

Figure 5-7. Semantic Interoperability and Identity Management Across Organizations and Systems

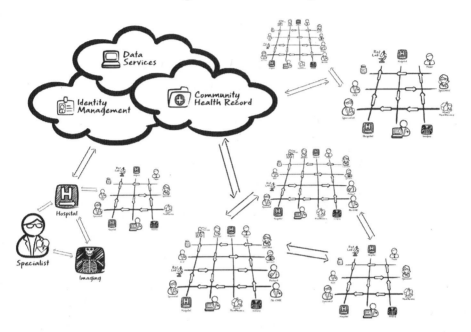

Because semantic interoperability facilitates collaboration, decision support, reporting, and detecting trends, meaningful uses of actionable data can result from effectively implementing an active HIE that accounts for both this language and patient identification issues. In light of this crucial requirement, ensuring that it is achieved for all ACOs will be critical to the success of healthcare delivery system transformation.

Case Example: A Health System HIE Enables Providers to Deliver High-Quality Care

A two-hospital health system in California has deployed HIE technology widely throughout the community it serves, connecting nearly 1,000 ambulatory providers, with and without EHRs. A free clinic in the community is connected to the Health System's HIE, and providers use an EHR in the practice. The Medical Director of the free clinic had a patient, a 55-year-old female, with a history of renal cell carcinoma of the left kidney. This patient came to see the Medical Director one day, complaining of persistent back pain for the past six months, after her previous nephrectomy.

After visiting with the patient, the Medical Director scheduled an MRI, using his EHR, for 3:15 pm that afternoon. The order was communicated and transmitted via the Health System's HIE infrastructure. At 3:43 pm the same day—less than 30 minutes after the MRI was performed—the MRI result appeared in the Medical Director's EHR. The test result was pushed in near real-time to the doctor, through the Health System's HIE infrastructure, and the data was integrated discreetly within the EHR.

Unfortunately, the test result showed a recurrence of cancer for the patient. While this was not good news, the Medical Director was able to talk with the patient immediately, while she was still in the clinic. The doctor was able to get the patient on a care plan far more quickly than was possible without the HIE in place, when he previously relied on "traditional" methods of result delivery—phone, fax, mail, and courier services.

While the patient was understandably upset by the news of the recurrent cancer, she felt more confident with her care team, due to the rapid response, and also did not suffer undue or prolonged stress, waiting for the test result to be produced and then for her to be notified. This process used to take up to 2 weeks before the Health System deployed HIE technology, but, with the HIE in place, the provider is more efficient, high-quality care is delivered, and patient satisfaction is enhanced.

Connecting the True "Last Mile"

While much of the attention of HIE is focused on establishing electronic connections between hospitals and physicians, the true "last mile" of connectivity is reaching the patients themselves. For an ACO to be maximally effective, it is essential for its patients to be active participants in managing their health. While generally classified under the category of patient engagement technologies, there are two primary solutions for connecting patients to the HIE: personal health records and patient portals.

Personal Health Records

The most basic tool for electronically exchanging information with patients is a secure messaging system in which the patients and their clinical team can dialog and share information. This provider-controlled system is highly desirable and a solid place in which to develop a patient-centric care model (discussed below under Patient Portals). Alternatively, there is the advent of the personal health record. The personal health record takes the relationship to a new place in which patients control and maintain an independent database of clinical information that they, the patients, consider appropriate. Think of the personal health record as a copy of the medical record that the patient or guardian maintains independently and, therefore, edits and manages over time. Personal health records usually offer electronic access to patient health information exchanged through the HIE, via a Web-based or mobile application.

There are many free and subscription-based personal health records available in the market today offered by vendors, payers, and providers.

While initially thought to be a panacea, only a small percentage of the American public has visited and created a personal health record, even when it is free, and less than half of those have returned to use it. Consequently, it is no surprise that Google recently announced it is leaving this market. That said, for some patients and guardians, the personal health record will offer a convenient and increasingly easy-to-use capability for tracking key information, such as prescriptions; managing chronic conditions; and using tools and content for managing one's health.

Patient Portals

Patient portals, unlike patient health records, are a way in which to enable the patient to converse securely with the healthcare team. This provider-controlled access tool may be sponsored by hospitals and/or physician practices in a tethered (containing information unique to that organization) or untethered form—in which case it contains multiple provider and organizational information. A patient portal offers a number of advantages over a personal health record, not the least of which is confidence by the healthcare team in the accuracy of the information it contains. Other technical advantages can include such features as Web-based, integrated voice reminders or mobile access to health information exchanged by the HIE, in a bidirectional exchange with their providers. In contrast, a personal health record is unidirectional. At the base level, patients with a patient portal have electronic access to critical information such as lab results, medications, allergies, and immunizations exchanged through the HIE. Like a personal health record, patients can present new information to their existing records exchanged via the HIE; however, the information would be seen and reviewed by the healthcare team and added on their behalf.

In addition, the portal has other more advanced capabilities, such as secure communication with providers, appointment scheduling, and electronic bill payment. Some patient portals go further to provide valuable content such as lifestyle, fitness, and nutritional coaching.

The most advanced patient portals have clinical decision support capabilities that monitor data exchanged via the HIE, constantly looking for information such as potential drug interactions or notifying the patient about treatment options that might be useful, based on their medical history. With outcomes-based reminders and alerts generated by the patient portal and leveraging data exchanged via the HIE, patients can take a more proactive role in managing their health.

Whether through a personal health record or a patient portal, empowering patients with electronic access to their health information aligns and engages patients with their providers and supports the ACO goals of improved outcomes at a lower cost. The topics of patient portals and personal health records are covered in depth in Chapter 8.

A Pragmatic HIE Strategy Delivers Results

Active HIE technology is central to achieving three factors for ACO success: stakeholder collaboration; an end-to-end care delivery network; and a strong technology infrastructure that brings together health records, patient populations, and clinical decision support.

Ensuring progress is, however, a challenge. A clear and logical HIE strategy can support effectively building and managing an ACO, yet many organizations do not know where to begin. One of the limiting factors to having independent physician groups band together as provider service organizations and forming ACOs in various markets is funding. Working together with other organizations that can assist in capitalizing the HIE development work is one way to climb across this barrier. In addition to the financial challenges, there are also operational and technical limitations. The most proven strategy for deploying HIE technology builds a solid exchange on a basic foundation. Additional functions can be layered according to specific needs and timelines, taking into consideration the workflow and technological maturity of the ACO's participants.[163]

An incremental bottom-up approach to deploying HIE is an effective way to produce both immediate and lasting value for the ACO. The bottom-up approach involves first connecting hospitals, physician practices, and such critical ancillary service providers as reference laboratories and imaging centers and liquefying transactions at a local level. This approach is in contrast to a traditional top-down regional health information organization approach to HIE that attempts to connect all possible stakeholders at once and aggregate all data simultaneously.

The first step is to engage physicians and other healthcare providers where care is delivered, connecting disparate information systems, and automating clinical messaging and workflow to create a solid and well-adopted HIE foundation. The HIE can then build upon that foundation and provide greater value over time by adding other functions and services. An important aspect of this first step is automating core healthcare transactions: ordering tests, referring patients among providers, and coordinating information among care teams. In accomplishing this critical step, the basic HIE connects core hospital systems (e.g., the laboratory, radiology, transcription, security, emergency department), EMRs, practice management systems, and other entities in such a way that information flows securely across the HIE infrastructure. Automating core transactions yields the following benefits:

➢ Creates immediate value for hospitals, physicians, and other providers—improved information quality and savings in time and money, leading to user satisfaction and high early-adoption rates;

➢ Enables a lower cost and more rapidly deployable approach than common methods of building an HIE, which require extensive and expensive infrastructure to accomplish the same goal;

➢ Establishes connections to all stakeholders participating in the ACO and fosters rapid coordination of care and collaboration; and

➢ As the level of connectivity across participants increases, and the HIE grows from the bottom up, its additional functions may include:

o Aggregating patient records and health information from all connected stakeholders to create a longitudinal record of care;

o Applying identity management services to ensure identification of a patient's correct longitudinal health record;

o Applying terminology services to ensure data is semantically correct across all data sources connected to the participants via HIE technology;

o Harvesting data from ambulatory care settings to establish registries and apply advanced clinical decision support, such as risk stratification, disease management, and population management tools for information retrieval, proactive, and personalized care management and analytics;

o Engaging patients through electronic connections via the HIE to personal health records or a patient portal, thereby, empowering patients to take a proactive role in managing their own health and helping clinicians achieve their outcomes performance metrics; and

o Deploying gateway services to exchange information with such external networks as the nationwide health information network, other HIEs, and public health agencies.

The bottom-up approach, which focuses first on system integration and exchange at a local level with local systems presently used by providers, has proven successful in a wide range of environments. It delivers significant value in a short time frame and at a lower cost than traditional "build it and they shall come" models of HIE deployment. Certainly, efforts to standardize and aggregate normalized data in a centralized manner are the ideal; however, they are also time-consuming and complex endeavors. Rather than compete with such systematic approaches, bottom-up HIE leverages those initiatives and will better position ACO development and management activities.

Thus, a good HIE strategy is based upon established standards while simultaneously ensuring flexibility and adaptability over time. The rapidly evolving contemporary environment does not adhere to any one specific standard or approach. Many methods are used, and even such common standards as HL7 come in several flavors. The HIE solution must be future-proof, complying with privacy, security, and communication standards, while still being open and adaptable to future standards as they evolve. The definitive component in the strategy is selecting technology that enables providers always to keep the patient in focus and empowers all authorized providers to actively participate, collaborate, and proactively coordinate care.

The pragmatic approach to delivering immediate and sustainable results for HIE initiatives is depicted in Figure 5-8.

Figure 5-8. Pragmatic HIE Model

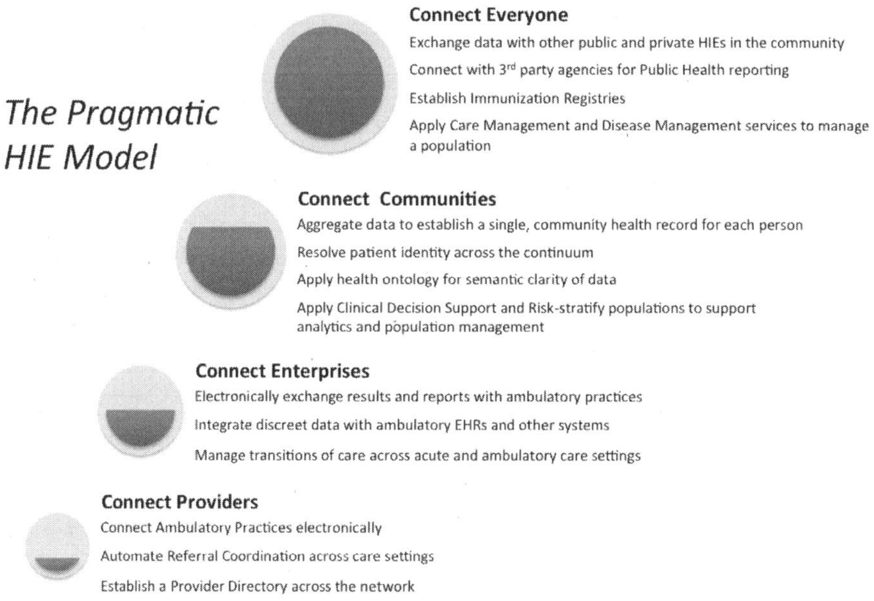

The Pragmatic HIE Model

Connect Everyone
Exchange data with other public and private HIEs in the community
Connect with 3rd party agencies for Public Health reporting
Establish Immunization Registries
Apply Care Management and Disease Management services to manage a population

Connect Communities
Aggregate data to establish a single, community health record for each person
Resolve patient identity across the continuum
Apply health ontology for semantic clarity of data
Apply Clinical Decision Support and Risk-stratify populations to support analytics and population management

Connect Enterprises
Electronically exchange results and reports with ambulatory practices
Integrate discreet data with ambulatory EHRs and other systems
Manage transitions of care across acute and ambulatory care settings

Connect Providers
Connect Ambulatory Practices electronically
Automate Referral Coordination across care settings
Establish a Provider Directory across the network

The Road to Interoperability and Data Exchange

The road to establish an HIE deployment framework starts with engaging physicians from the ACO in process design, to ensure their buy-in and help identify information they need to support population health management. As HIE efforts mature, establishment of an oversight committee focused on all elements of HIE will be important to provide leadership and guidance to cross-functional implementation teams and to set strategic objectives for long-term success of the ACO's HIE initiative.

The last element of our roadmap concerns strategic benefits realized for the ACO at the community level. Implementation of effective, active HIE will accelerate the ACO's ability to support requirements for data needed by physicians and other clinicians in population health advanced clinical decision support, population stratification, patient care identification, disease and care management, quality monitoring, and performance measurement. Ultimately, each ACO's roadmap will vary to some degree, depending on the participants involved and the model being implemented.

Clinical Data Reporting Systems

As EMRs and information exchange systems mature and come into being, a critical and parallel discussion needs to center around clinical data reporting systems. These systems provide the business intelligence for which the ACO needs to operate. They are an essential component of what was missing in the 1980s to support physician hospital organizations that largely failed. Understanding population health management and truly managing down to the provider and patient level with clinical and financial data will be necessary for successful health systems to manage clinical and financial risk. Modeling software that begins to identify how best to manage populations of patients continues to be developed and is expected to be a major area of focus in the coming years.

With many vendors competing in the clinical data reporting systems market space, there are numerous factors to consider when picking a system to aid in data reporting down to the physician level, such as:

➢ Whether or not the system can accept discrete data,

➢ Whether or not the vendor has experience with the source systems,

➢ Whether a registry is available, and

➢ Whether or not the reporting components can be modified by the end-user organization or whether they require code changes.

All of this and more should be taken into consideration for these important vendor selection and system acquisition decisions. Many large systems are looking at implementing full data warehouses. While the nature of this is beyond the scope of this book, many clinical data reporting systems may be eclipsed by more mature reporting systems over time. If this is the local tactical approach, then the ACO will have to weigh the value of the short-term reporting system in the context of realizing its cost and relative shelf life. In all cases, some type of clinical data reporting system will be necessary and likely need to be implemented well before health information exchange is fully matured. As such, the ACO leadership will need to define a limited number of metrics from which to start as the new organization is built and the competencies and technologies become increasingly available.

Bridging the Divide

Many topics have been discussed, culminating in the pragmatic HIE model, and numerous healthcare organizations across the country are advancing the national agenda for moving toward a nationwide health information network (NwHIN) . The NwHIN is not a physical network that runs on government servers, nor is it a large network that stores patient records. It is a set of standards, services, and policies that enable secure health information exchange over the Internet. For several years, establishing regional health information organizations (RHIOs) was a central part of the plan for enabling the NwHIN.[164] In light of business model and funding challenges experienced by many RHIOs, the ONC-HIT engaged a change in national strategy for enabling NwHIN. Today, the initiative is led by federal agencies (the Veterans Administration, Department of Defense, Social Security Administration, and Centers for Disease Control, among others) and private organizations to exchange electronic health information securely. These organizations have collectively helped develop NwHIN standards, services, and policies for sending and retrieving electronic health information to support patient care, streamline benefit claims, and improve public health tracking.[165]

Two issues to note regarding the continued evolution of NwHIN are the future roles of RHIOs and the establishment of a national level governance structure to support NwHIN. Over the years, RHIOs have been established through public and private efforts in communities and states across the nation, and their role continues to be evaluated.[166] Secondly, a national level governance framework that will involve public-private organization engagement will be needed in some form and is currently under debate for the direction of how it will be organized.[167]

Achieving semantic interoperability will ensure strong collaboration and important uses of patients' health information. Addressing the regulatory changes that will continue to come from CMS and ONC-HIT will be of paramount importance in reducing barriers to enabling virtual care teams through the HIE deployment framework.

Chapter 5: Takeaways

✓ ACOs depend on the ability to share and act on information about specific patients and population groups through peer-to-peer and peer-to-patient communications in a highly secure network. Physicians, clinical care teams, hospitals, and health systems involved in delivering care to a patient need a complete picture of a patient's past care and current needs in order to more effectively deliver high-quality, safe, cost-effective care.

✓ Collaboration and coordination of care among physicians and other healthcare providers across acute and ambulatory settings is a cornerstone to achieving effective management of an ACO. An ACO cannot operate effectively or efficiently without the meaningful exchange of health information across all providers and all care settings.

✓ Virtualizing the integrated delivery network is the fastest and most cost-effective method to connect providers and foster care coordination and collaboration amongst providers. Advances made in technology are making the virtual integrated delivery network model possible by bridging information, systems, services, and people to create a coherent collaborative care model, which enhances provider workflow and eliminates the variation of care coordination in manual environments. Two related points include:

Chapter 5: Takeaways (cont.)

o Collaborative care keeps the patient in focus at all times, connecting cloud services; brick-and-mortar clinical, administrative, and financial systems; and local applications, such as clinical decision support systems and EMRs, with the community of people who care for the patient.

o These advances enable organizations, affiliated providers, and other allied caregivers who work together but are not part of the same entity to collaborate on a platform and create a high level of coordinated care for individuals and populations of patients.

✓ Care transition technology leverages the HIE infrastructure and keeps all members of a patient's care team in sync across the continuum of care, and team members are alerted to adverse events, complications, and changes in a patient's status. With care transition technology, hospitals and providers can proactively take action, before a readmission occurs. Care transition technology will help hospitals avoid the CMS-imposed readmission penalties.

✓ Clinical decision support and analytic tools for both hospital and ambulatory settings are critical components of effective care management, enabling proactive management, identification of gaps in care, and enabling timely intervention by providers.

✓ As an HIE deployment matures, a robust set of acute and ambulatory data will be derived from across the care continuum. As the field of analytics evolves, along with advances in modeling and simulation capabilities, new tools will enhance monitoring, measurement, and alerting capabilities for total population and patient-level health management.

Chapter 5: Takeaways (cont.)

✓ The most effective approach to deploying HIE technology is one that is pragmatic and starts by engaging and connecting providers in a way that quickly and meaningfully enhances their workflow. The next step is to electronically connect the providers to enterprises (e.g., hospitals) and enable discreet data integration with ambulatory EMRs and other systems in place across the care continuum. Two related points include:

o With all points of the network connected electronically, a virtual IDN and virtual care teams begin to emerge. As clinical events occur across the care continuum, producing volumes of data, this data can be aggregated, patient identity resolved, and a health ontology applied, to create a semantically coherent single best record for the patient across care teams and across the community of care.

o An HIE that incorporates advanced clinical decision support capabilities enables proactive care management and identification of gaps in care. Robust analytic and business intelligence solutions will turn the aggregated data into meaningful and actionable information for effective ACO management.

[156] Institute of Medicine, Committee on Quality of Health Care in America. Using Health Information Technology. In: *Crossing the Quality Chasm: A New Health System for the 21st Century*. Washington, DC: National Academies Press; 2001:164.

[157] H.R. 3590, Patient Protection and Affordable Care Act, §3022(b)(2)(F) and (G). Requirements for ACOs (2010).

[158] O'Malley AS, Reschovsky JD. Referral and Consultation Communication Between Primary Care and Specialist Physicians: Finding Common Ground. *Arch Intern Med*. 2011 Jan 10;171(1):56–65.

[159] O'Malley AS, 2011.

[160] Video interview: Former MedPAC chairman Jay Crosson on ACOs. *Modern Healthcare*. August 9, 2010. Accessed online July 20, 2011, at http://www.modernhealthcare.com/article/20100809/VIDEO/308099999.

[161] Partnership for Solutions. *Chronic Conditions: Making the Case for Ongoing Care*. September 2004. Introduction, p. 3. Accessed online March 23, 2012, at http://partnershipforsolutions.org/DMS/files/chronicbook2004.pdf.

[162] Glaser J, Salzberg C. Information technology for accountable care organizations. *Hospitals and Health Networks*. September 2010. Accessed online July 23, 2011, at http://www.hhnmag.com/hhnmag_app/jsp/articledisplay.jsp?dcrpath=HHNMAG/Article/data/09SEP2010/090610HHN_Weekly_Glaser2&domain=HHNMAG.

[163] Agency for Healthcare Research and Quality, National Resource Center for Health Information Technology. Webinar. May 14, 2010. Building and maintaining a sustainable health information exchange (HIE): Experience from diverse care settings.

[164] Coiera E. Building a National Health IT system from the Middle Out. *J Am Med Inform Assoc*. 2009 May-June;16(3):271-273.

[165] The Role of the Direct Project and NwHIN Exchange in HIE Platforms. Accessed online July 17, 2012, at http://www.medicity.com/whitepapers-briefs.html.

[166] Lenert L, Sundwall D, Lenert ME. Shifts in the architecture of the nationwide health information network. *J Am Med Inform Assoc*. 2012 Jul 1;19(4):498-502.

[167] Terry K. Health IT Groups Criticize Information Exchange Regulation Plan. *Information Week*. July 5, 2012. Accessed online July 18, 2012, at http://www.informationweek.com/news/healthcare/interoperability/240003218.

Chapter 6. The Paradigm Shift for Quality Care

Cynthia Davis, MHSA, RN, FACHE

Given the rise of chronic conditions and the rapid aging of the population, there has never been a more urgent need to improve quality and reduce costs through the optimal use of technology.[168]

Louis Burns
CEO, Intel-GE CareInnovations

Introduction

A multitude of forces is converging upon our healthcare system—its physicians, nursing workforce, ancillary, and administrative professionals who strive to provide the highest quality of care possible to the patients they serve. Yet, as we see on a regular basis, even today with so much effort going into improving quality of care, errors still occur, mistakes still happen, and resources are wasted. Preventable adverse events resulting in medical errors were estimated by the Institute of Medicine in 1999 to be the cause of as many as 98,000 deaths in US hospitals.[169] A more recent study, published in the *New England Journal of Medicine* in 2010, on the quality of care in a group of one state's hospitals provided evidence that, with all the efforts and resources being invested, medical errors were still occurring at an alarming rate.[170] However, efforts to effect positive change and quality improvement have increased greatly over the last two decades. Methodologies such as Six Sigma, Lean Thinking, and organizational change management techniques have been implemented and engaged to reduce errors, waste, and inefficiency, and, ultimately, improve quality. While there are examples of positive impacts, more needs to be done, and this is one of the key objectives for health information technologies.

In the US healthcare system today, health information technologies are playing a key role in efforts to improve the quality of care across the nation. Electronic health records (EHRs), health information exchange, changes to medical coding languages, and new clinical decision support tools are just a fragment of the tools and applications being implemented throughout health systems and physician practices alike. Measuring and evaluating the impact of these new technologies on clinical quality outcomes can take months to years to evaluate and provide conclusive evidence for or against the position of how much these systems help improve quality of care.

Momentum across the nation for adoption of EHRs and other health information technologies provides new opportunities for measurement and evaluation of the impact of these systems on quality of care. Return on our investments from these efforts can come in the form of financial gains but, more importantly, in the improvement of health outcomes and clinical process improvements. In a 2011 article by Hoffman and Podgurski, comparative effective research (CER) outlines an important approach for the evolution of clinical quality improvement. The solution posed by the authors involved applying CER methodology to develop a "personalized comparison of treatment effectiveness (PCTE)" program, drawing from an EHR's database of de-identified patient health information and records. The primary objective would involve comparing similar patient groups (whenever possible) to identify the best treatment options for a given patient's cohort.[171]

The implementation of a PCTE program allows physicians the opportunity to request results of a study conducted through data mining of their EHR's database, including statistical analysis, "and the results of well-regarded prior studies of the treatments in question, especially randomized controlled trials."[172]

Significant potential exists for the development of such an approach to clinical quality improvement. The promising future of business intelligence and data analytics tools in the capturing, monitoring, and analysis of patient data can serve as a strong enabler for meaningful and accountable quality improvement. However, a program such as PCTE will require clinical oversight to ensure excellence in the quality of processes, study design, and needed monitoring, given the sensitivity of electronic patient health information. Table 6-1 provides a summary of additional points to support a PCTE program.

Table 6-1. Points for Consideration With Establishing a PCTE[173]

PCTE Establishment Points
EHR records need to include a representative patient population for the cohort being studied.
Recognize that the accuracy and completeness of an EHR's data set is a top priority, as it will enhance the validity of results from data mining efforts in each study.[174]
Consider establishing internal compliance programs focused on patient follow-up and data entry to drive quality and integrity of study results.
Acknowledge that, in the case of rare diseases and conditions that a physician may encounter, suitable or appropriate study groups of de-identified electronic patient health information may not exist or be available.

Operationalizing a PCTE program requires the first step of having a robust EHR system in place. As organizations are continuously seeking new methods of improving the quality of clinical care, the PCTE model will serve as a future potential initiative to be explored for improving the health of the populations served.

The complexity of the US healthcare system with the networks and processes that exist between payers, providers, and patients also contributes to the challenges with measuring the impact of new technological innovations on quality of care. New technologies are reducing barriers, but, in some cases, also produce unintended consequences and have the capacity to effect e-iatrogenic events, those that bring about "patient harm caused at least in part by the application of health information technology."[175]

The healthcare industry is continuing to move forward rapidly with adoption of new technologies to support quality care. Innovation is a recognized key to growth, and quantum leaps in improving care delivery in America may best be achieved through new models of care, such as ACOs supported by the integration of new applications, tools, and systems that enable healthcare workers with advanced capabilities to improve outcomes at the micro and macro levels within the patient populations they serve.

With this introduction as a backdrop, this chapter will address myriad issues ranging from (a) a national quality strategy that influences the efforts of technology developers and care delivery organizations alike, (b) the influence of organizational leadership on quality of care and the structure of organizations delivering care, (c) measures of quality, and (d) a summary of technologies supporting quality initiatives. An awareness of the transformation underway from the fragmented and decentralized system of the past to the learning environment that captures lessons learned, measures the impact of innovations, and incorporates new technologies is needed for a complex adaptive system such as the US healthcare industry to advance and evolve.

What objectives can be achieved in this journey of improving the quality of care delivered in America?

➤ Improved efficiency

➤ Reduced waste

➤ Decreased rates of preventable adverse events

➤ Faster adoption of technologies by physicians and caregivers

➤ Improved health outcomes for patients

Achieving these objectives is part of the nation's goals to improve the quality of care for its citizens and for all those who come here in search of the best healthcare services available. With the aging of the Baby Boomer population, the increased need for improving the quality of care delivered to this generation is bringing about a paradigm shift in focus on the quality of care throughout the nation. Physicians, nurses, and ancillary professionals are focused on this journey and, for ACOs, the quality mission is simple: establish a patient-centric environment that is driven by performance and value, delivered to the patients served.

Transition to Value-driven Care

For much of the 20th century, healthcare services in America were characterized as being volume-driven and considered a fee-for-service-based industry. Evolving through a focus on individual patients and treatment of chronic diseases and conditions, it was a system known to have systemic problems with overuse of services and misalignment between services paid for and the quality of care received by the patient population. As the nation moved into the 21st century and had seen the rapid growth of managed care companies, it was apparent that change was needed once again. Along with recommendations from the Institute of Medicine and other organizations, a movement started toward value-based care delivery.[176] As Porter and Teisberg noted in *Redefining Health Care* in 2006, "A seminal shift in mind-set has occurred, and cost reduction is today no longer the dominant focus of reform. Safety, error reduction, and (to a lesser extent) quality of care have finally been brought into the mainstream of health care reform."[177]

In the midst of this shift, the nation is moving toward a system that is focused on quality of care with an incentive structure that rewards for acceptance and management of financial and clinical risk with a new focus on caring for patients at the population level. The evolution of health information technologies, and especially those that bring capabilities for predictive modeling, intelligent clinical decision support, and patient health records management would enable physicians and provider organizations with new tools to support making this transition. Figure 6-1 illustrates some highlights of this transition.

Figure 6-1. Transition From Volume-Driven Care to Quality/Value-Driven Care Environment

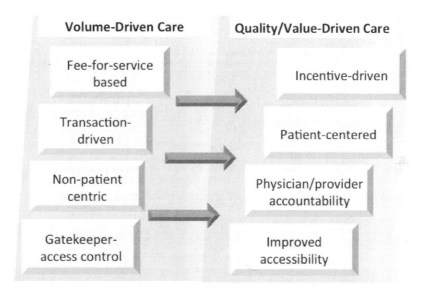

This transition has included instilling accountability with the physician and provider jointly. As the managed care era established a "gatekeeper" model for determining patient access to healthcare services, in the value-driven care era, expanded access, improved coordination of care, and increased affordability of care have all been key drivers. The concept of patient-centered care has become a focal point for all systems, processes, and technologies. The accelerated adoption of the patient-centered medical home model in primary and specialty care practices during the past decade required meeting a number of quality measures and incorporating the use of electronic health records and other health information technologies for performance measurement reporting. An important strategy for the future of new technologies is more emphasis in new design and redesign to strengthen "patient-provider relationships, communications, access, and patients engagement in their own care"[178] capabilities of new applications and tools. ACOs, both public and private, are addressing these issues in their technology roadmaps to support their shifts to population health management, meet CMS Meaningful Use requirements, and various clinical and administrative reporting requirements.

Leadership to Improve Quality

Organizational transformation is occurring in virtually every healthcare organization across America. Sweeping reforms at the federal level are driving policy change; new joint ventures; large-scale workforce training initiatives; and decisions for acquisition, procurement, and implementation of new health information technologies that most often take years to fully adopt and sometimes hundreds of millions of dollars in capital funding depending on the magnitude, scope, and complexity of the project.

As the focus of this book is on health information technologies for healthcare organizations, managing the cultural transition that occurs with system implementations is critical to maintaining high quality of care. Transitions can bring a disruption to clinical workflows, changes in the power structure of clinical operations, introduction of new digital communications, and availability of new data and insights. The changes that come with new systems, such as EHRs and computerized provider order entry systems, can infiltrate every level of an organization. In light of this fact, leadership starting from the board level is a critical success factor. Jiang and colleagues provided a synopsis of the results of a 2006 survey (3,898 hospitals with 562 hospital chief executive officers responding) regarding board of directors' involvement in quality initiatives.[179] Results from the survey responses included:

➢ 81% noted their governing boards established strategic goals for quality improvement,

➢ 61% said their hospitals maintain a board committee that focuses on quality issues,

➢ 88% feel their board is just as responsible for patient care quality as they are for financial stewardship of their organizations, and

➢ 75% stated that "most to all" board meetings have a quality improvement related topic on their agenda.

The board quality committee plays a crucial role in healthcare organizations. Results of the survey indicated that the presence of such committees was associated with strengthening the overall oversight function of the hospital's board of directors and decreased mortality rates for heart attack, congestive heart failure, pneumonia, stroke, hip fracture, and gastrointestinal bleeding.[180] Part of the importance of these senior executive committees is to model and demonstrate the culture they want for their organizations. This can be viewed as one of the most important roles for healthcare leaders in today's transformational times in the healthcare industry.

Another issue to consider is how to get boards of directors to engage in quality activities for their healthcare organizations to help improve health outcomes for the populations served by ACOs, both public and private. Joshi and colleagues identified four strategies (Figure 6-2) to strengthen the level of engagement of boards of directors in the quality initiatives and mission of healthcare organizations.

Figure 6-2. Strategies for Strengthening Board Engagement in Quality[181]

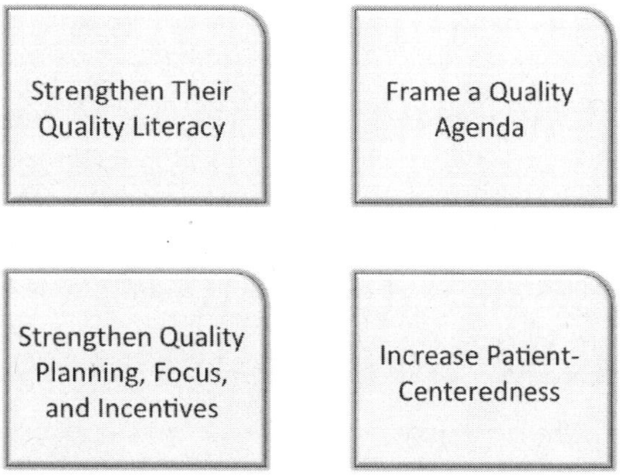

Strengthen Their Quality Literacy	Frame a Quality Agenda
Strengthen Quality Planning, Focus, and Incentives	Increase Patient-Centeredness

First and foremost is patient-centeredness. As the central focus for every hospital, ACO, physician, and care provider is the patient, those planning board meetings should consider integrating reference stories to illustrate the direct impact that quality improvement activities are having toward enriching the lives of the patients being served. Ensuring involvement of representatives from the patient population can also help demonstrate improvements being made for the board. Second is to increase the quality literacy for board members, Joshi and colleagues suggested a number of actions. Increasing attendance at quality conferences, holding quality strategy retreats for the board, and providing quality education opportunities all can contribute to improving the degree of quality knowledge possessed by board members. Third, to frame a quality agenda, efforts should be made to ensure that meaningful dialogue takes place between the chair of the board and the senior hospital officer(s) regarding quality progress and impediments to it, in addition to ensuring that adequate time on board meetings is allotted to address quality improvement issues. Fourth, a vision for improving quality of care and patient outcomes is needed and should be based on key measures of clinical outcomes. In addition, the hospital's quality plan should be in alignment with the overall hospital/health system strategic plan, and the board should review and understand key clinical quality measures, with incentives for board members connected to specific quality metrics to help drive engagement.

Evaluating Progress

One of the keys to evaluating progress in the healthcare environment and for the benefit of patients in their health outcomes is remembering the foundational structure given to the industry by Avedis Donabedian, MD. Dr. Donabedian, who is widely considered the father of healthcare quality management, defined a framework of three dimensions to assess healthcare quality: structure, process, and outcomes.[182]

Figure 6-3 illustrates Donabedian's three dimensions, which still embody much of what is done in healthcare today.

Figure 6-3. Donabedian Quality Framework

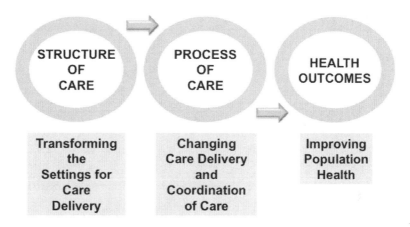

Applying Donabedian's quality framework to better understand the implications associated with health information technology system implementations across the three dimensions can lead to a number of questions for physicians and the healthcare workforce.

➢ **Structure**: Do we have the right health information technologies to fit our model of care delivery?

➢ **Process**: Are our health information technologies integrated with our clinical and administrative processes? Do we effectively use our systems to evaluate improvement in the processes of care delivered? Do our systems integrate with evidence-based medicine practices that drive improvement in effective clinical decision-making?

➢ **Outcome**: Are our technologies patient-centric?

These are just a few possible questions that organizations can ask in applying one of the foundational models for healthcare quality management in developing and assessing measures of quality and impact on each of the three dimensions of healthcare quality.

The Front Line of Care and a Focus on Patient Safety

In managing change and driving for quality improvement at the front line of care, our nation's nursing and ancillary workforce must be involved in not only ensuring effectiveness of organizational change, but also evaluating efforts to improve patient safety and health outcomes for the patients served. With a focus on patient safety, the Donabedian quality framework provides a model relationship to manage changes in the structure of care that effect changes in the processes of care delivery. Understanding and applying this model is critical not only for healthcare leaders but also for those on the front line of care delivery.

While Dr. Donabedian's original model was introduced in 1966 in his seminal paper, *Evaluating the Quality of Medical Care,*[183] Coyle and Battles introduced an improvement to the methodology in 1999. They introduced the notion of including "antecedents of medical care" in the model as additional factors that impact patient safety.[184] Antecedents were described by Coyle and Battles as patient and environmental risk factors that, when taken into account in the evaluation of quality measures, would provide additional insights into the correlations and linkages between changes in structure and clinical processes that affect measures of patient health outcomes. Patient factors were said to include "genetics, socio-demographics, health habits, beliefs and attitudes, and preferences," while environmental factors could include the "patients' cultural, social, political, personal, and physical characteristics." As ACOs and other healthcare provider organizations move forward in seeking new ways to improve the quality of care, consideration for these factors should be given in evaluations of the transformation of the structure of care that delivery settings are having on the clinical processes and their impacts on the healthcare workforce focused on improving patient safety and health outcomes on the front line of care.

CMS's Transition to Value-Based Care Model

CMS has been on a path to transitioning to more value-based purchasing programs as a basis for all services it pays physicians and providers for in caring for their beneficiary population. The CMS Value-Based Purchasing Roadmap[185] issued in 2009 delineated new priorities that included:

➢ Transition to incentive-based payment mechanisms based on the value of care delivered;

➢ Changing the structure of care delivery with growth and expansion of ACOs;

➢ Drive toward accountability for financial performance and clinical outcomes being held by both physician and provider organizations for the beneficiary populations and communities they serve; and

➢ Increased use of electronic health records to improve coordination and collaboration by physicians and provider organizations, along with increased use of personal health records to strengthen consumer engagement in monitoring and tracking the quality of care received. Patients beliefs, values, and cultural norms impact consumer engagement in their care delivery process.

As part of this overall strategy, CMS launched the eRx Incentive Program, the Physician Quality Reporting Initiative (PQRI), and the Medicare Shared Savings Program (e.g., Medicare ACO), the latter two of which are performance-driven based on evaluations against specified performance measures and benchmarks. As these programs are focused on the Medicare beneficiary population, they will provide stronger insights on the healthcare system's performance in meeting the needs of the Baby Boomer population in the coming decades. Other performance measurement programs, such as the Healthcare Effectiveness Data and Information Set (HEDIS), serve as key reporting requirements for private payer health plans. Determining the best ways to harmonize these different performance measures to ensure more efficient quality reporting for physicians and provider organizations is a priority for the industry.

Quality Measures

Appendix B provides a list of the 33 final quality measures released by CMS in December 2011 for the Medicare ACO program. The pay-for-performance program for these measures is being phased in over a 3-year period. In the first year, payments will be based on reporting of all 33 quality measures. In year two, pay for performance applies based on 25 of the measures (plus pay for reporting applies to 8 measures), and, in year three, pay-for-performance is based on 32 of the measures.[186] With the new capabilities of EHRs and other health information technologies, there will be new opportunities to achieve greater harmony among the required ACO measures, Meaningful Use of EHRs measures (to be addressed in Chapter 7), PQRI measures, and other programs.

To support the industry movement toward ACO establishment in the public and private sectors, the NCQA established an ACO accreditation program with three levels (Table 6-2) and 40 measures of clinical and cost quality evaluation.

Table 6-2. Three Levels for NCQA ACO Accreditation[187]

Level	Description
1	Healthcare provider organizations that have started ACO formation but not yet reached full ACO capability maintaining status for 2 years
2	Entities that demonstrate a broad range of ACO capabilities maintaining status for 3 years
3	Level 2 organizations that demonstrate strong performance or improvement in measures across the triple aim for 3 years

The National Quality Forum (NQF), the recognized industry-leading organization that approves and endorses healthcare quality measures, issued its 2010 report, *Guidance for Measure Harmonization*. In it, the NQF, noted a number of key principles (Table 6-3) to be taken into consideration in planning for the harmonization of future quality measures.

Table 6-3. Principles for Quality Measures Harmonization[188]

Principles
Harmonization should not slow innovation of measure development and use.
The issue of harmonization should ideally be addressed before a measure is sent to the NQF.
Quality measures should be based on best available measure concepts.
Notional harmonization should occur before harmonization of technical specifications for a new measure.
Harmonization should eliminate unintended differences among related measures.
If it is decided not to harmonize a measure, the value of different notional and technical specifications for the measure must outweigh the encumbrance imposed.
Measure harmonization efforts should support establishing standard definitions and specifications.

In addition to these issues, the health IT related safety measures area remains relatively weak across the industry. Regarding this issue, a 2011 report by the Institute of Medicine recommended to DHHS that measures evaluating health IT impact on patient safety should be developed jointly between the public and private sectors and make reporting on such measures a mandatory and annual requirement.[189]

All of these issues drive home the importance of quality measures, especially as provider organizations, physicians, and payers transition to operating within ACO structures. Evaluating performance of the organization is one aspect of performance measurement that healthcare leaders must attend to, as it enables the learning health system to continue improving and maturing.

Aligning With Physicians to Improve Quality

In the process of evaluating organizational performance, it is critical to get physicians engaged in quality and safety planning initiatives. The Medicare ACOs and private sector ACOs are to focus on improving the quality of care for the beneficiary population served as a whole. The physicians partnering with provider organizations in each ACO have an obligation to engage in the mission to improve the quality and safety of patient care. However, variation in care practices, resulting in variation in quality of care delivered still exists. Technologies that aid in the diffusion of information to physicians helps reduce variation but occasionally messages can be mixed or lost, all of which can hinder progress in the shift from a volume-driven system of care to a quality- and value-driven system of care.

Without physician engagement, these challenges and others cannot be overcome. As Porter and Teisberg noted in *Redefining Health Care*, "The only truly effective way to address value in health care is to reward ends, or results, rather than means, such as process steps."[190] Rewarding for "ends or results" is about achieving better patient health outcomes and improving patient safety in the new era of accountable care for the US healthcare system.

The Institute for Healthcare Improvement, one of the leading nonprofit organizations in healthcare today, focuses on research and innovation related efforts to drive knowledge and adoption of best practices. In a 2007 white paper, *Engaging Physicians in a Shared Quality Agenda*, they introduced a six-step framework for engaging physicians in quality and safety initiatives.[191] Three of these steps are:

➢ **Solidify mutual purpose**. The "mutual purpose" is geared toward identifying the higher level objectives to be focused on by the healthcare organization and its physician partners. These can be clinical, administrative, or infrastructure related, but it is essential that the objectives be of significance to drive engagement.

➤ **Apply improvement methods**. One key step to solidifying physician engagement is ensuring that viable quality improvement methodologies are put to use. Standardization of practices and making effective and efficient use of data and approaches to ensure best use of physicians' time are critical to the success of applying quality improvement methodologies to help engage key physicians.

➤ **Employ an engaging style**. Physicians undergo a unique and lengthy journey in their training for their profession. Those operating and trained in the US healthcare system are recognized for their "high analytic academic achievement, ability to delay gratification, diligence, perseverance, self-abnegation… and willingness to undergo a very prolonged apprenticeship"[192] in addition to placing value on scientific medical evidence and having a higher level of power that comes with their responsibility for the delivery of quality care to their patients. Considering this background, key strategies should be employed that include engaging physicians early in the process, ensuring meaningful communications and messages are delivered often, and identifying early adopters among physicians to engage as champions.[193]

Ensuring the engagement of the physician community in defining and implementing quality initiatives is critically important. Their involvement from the board level to the front line of care will help ensure that the full perspective of all those involved in the delivery of patient care services is accounted for and that commitment is attained for the benefit of each ACO's patient population.

Scorecards

In the development of executive scorecards to track such quality opportunities and indicators, what are some of the keys to defining them?

➢ Engage the board and stakeholders;

➢ Understand your variation and how you compare nationally;

➢ Measure the right things at the right times and over multiple years;

➢ Ensure measures are valid, reliable, and understandable; and

➢ Provide timely insights that afford Board, C-level healthcare executives, and stakeholders the opportunity to initiate proactive efforts to continually improve quality.

ACOs, physician practices, clinically integrated networks, and other provider organizations may select measures of success based on a highest priority set of measures that are regularly reported to external organizations. These may include CMS in regards to Meaningful Use of EHRs, eRx Initiative, PQRI, Medicare Shared Savings, and the NCQA's HEDIS measures or those required for patient-centered medical home and ACO accreditation.

Automation and continued implementation and adoption of EHRs will continue to bring new opportunities to improve quality reporting, bringing stronger insights for the C-level healthcare executive, giving way to real-time assessment efforts across the continuum of care settings to continually improve population health management efforts in working toward achieving CMS's Three-Part Aim for ACOs. One area for improvement identified for healthcare organizations and ACOs across the country is the need to reduce hospital readmissions. In 2011, IHI provided a summary of interventions to reduce hospital readmissions[194] based on best practices. A few of these interventions are:

➢ Patient and healthcare worker education on self-care issues for the patient following discharge,

➢ Strong management and communication of changes in medication regimens, and

> ➤ Ensuring timely post–acute care follow-up by the care provider team.

As these types of interventions and others are instituted within an ACO's beneficiary population, the care delivery team can monitor the effects on population level health outcomes. These effects and changes can then be reported periodically through executive scorecards and other assessment tools to provide feedback to all stakeholders in the system.

Implications for Patient Safety

Health information technologies are being used to transform the way care is delivered across all care delivery settings in the US healthcare system. As information technologies are developed, piloted, and implemented, lessons are learned about their effects, both direct and indirect, on the patients being cared for daily.

Complexity, as we have discussed throughout this book, is an underlying factor that is driving challenges and the need for change throughout the healthcare industry. While interconnectedness exists across organizations and stakeholders, there exists both linear and nonlinear relationships that impact the industry's ability to achieve quality and cost goals. Standardization of clinical practices and workflow in patient care operations is one effort that is focused on reducing variation. The implementation of EHRs creates across multiple care delivery settings a platform for these efforts, but most systems require some degree of design tailoring to fit any one healthcare provider's or ACO's operating environment. While research on specific technologies such as EHRs, computerized physician order entry, clinical decision support, and barcode medication administration systems has been done and is ongoing to evaluate their impact on improving the quality of care, one new initiative on a national level that is focused on patient safety is the Partnership for Patients, a $500 million initiative out of the Center for Medicare and Medicaid Innovation.[195]

A national initiative was launched in April 2011 by DHHS to bring together hospitals, employers, health plans, physicians, care providers, and state and federal agencies with a focus of achieving two goals by the end of 2013: reducing harm done to patients (e.g., decrease preventable hospital-acquired infections by 40%) and reducing hospital readmissions by 20%.[196] Twenty-six organizations were contracted competitively through the establishment of regional Hospital Engagement Networks, a $218 million program to participate in the Partnership for Patients initiative. In less than its first year, more than 6,500 partners have joined the partnership, including more than 3,000 hospitals with 2,345 physician, nursing, and pharmacy organizations alone.[197] Ten areas of focus for the Partnership are identified in Table 6-4.

Table 6-4. Focus Areas for Partnership for Patients

Focus Areas
Adverse drug events
Catheter-associated urinary tract infections
Central line–associated blood stream infections
Injuries from falls and immobility
Obstetrical adverse events
Pressure ulcers
Surgical site infections
Venous thromboembolism
Ventilator-associated pneumonia
Preventable readmissions

Achievement of these goals will take a comprehensive focus on improvements through proper implementation and adoption of technologies, training and educational programs, applying lessons learned from other organizations, and reporting on performance measures to evaluate progress. Much the same as the approach and philosophy for ACOs, the program is intended to drive quality improvement and change in the way we deliver care in the transition from a volume-driven system to one driven by value and performance working toward achievement of the Three-Part Aim: better care for individuals, better health for populations, and lower growth in expenditures.

Technologies and Safety

As healthcare organizations large and small move forward with implementation of EHRs, barcode medication administration, computerized physician order entry, clinical decision support systems, electronic medication administration reconciliation systems, and other health information technologies, there are many obstacles that can arise and lead to preventable adverse events and medical errors.

Workarounds with barcode medication administration systems are an example of an obstacle to healthcare worker adoption that can lead to preventable adverse events, as shown in the results of a study of barcode medication administration systems in use at five hospitals.[198] Medication errors can occur in the prescribing of medications and in the administration process[199] across inpatient, ambulatory, long-term care, and home care settings. Patient harm resulting from health information technology applications can include dosing errors, illness detection failures, and delayed or inappropriate treatments resulting from inadequate human-computer interactions and/or loss of data.[200]

As the number of EHR systems adopted across the United States increases, the need for greater attention to human factors and system usability characteristics will continue to increase. Usability of health information technologies, and especially EHRs, involves both the physical attributes of the devices that house the applications and the usability of the data contained within the system. Usability testing evaluates a system's functionality, effectiveness, and efficiency. These factors are critical to the issue of patient safety because dysfunctional, ineffective systems that have flaws in computer-user interfacing may be causes of preventable adverse events and other unintended consequences that affect the healthcare workforce and directly or indirectly lead to patient harm.

In one case, an example of a heuristics evaluation was conducted with physician end users of an EHR system in an academic oncology care setting. Questions covered efficiency, flexibility, and accessibility of the system, and feedback identified issues such as problems with data visibility, appropriate matching of data, memory support (e.g., providing users with needed information to minimize cognitive processing requirements), minimalist views (having appropriate amounts and types of information on the screen at any given time), and flexibility in use of data.[201] This type of information will be needed by provider organizations, physician practices, and care delivery settings across the nation in the coming years to ensure that the systems we implement are most effective in optimizing the advancement of care delivery processes.

Bridging the Divide

Health information technologies bring great promise for improving the quality of care delivered, but with them comes a number of challenges that are being dealt with daily throughout the US healthcare system. Patient safety is the single most important goal for every healthcare organization. The complexity of the healthcare system at the micro and macro level invokes a requirement for intense focus on continuing development of performance measures that provide insights to clinical quality, cost, and efficiency of patient-centric operations. Future measures should also provide more insight to health information technology safety issues, as called for in recommendations by the Institute of Medicine in its 2011 report, *Health IT and Patient Safety: Building Safer Systems for Better Care.*[202]

The periodic results from evaluating measures from programs such as the three stages of CMS's Meaningful Use of EHRs program over the coming years will support continued improvement in care coordination, data capture and sharing, clinical processes, and, ultimately, better patient health outcomes.

As ACOs, clinically integrated networks, and other healthcare delivery organizations evolve, attention to the spectrum of these quality issues should be at the top of the priority list for healthcare executives seeking to improve the quality of care in the communities they serve.

Chapter 6: Takeaways

✓ Healthcare organizations are mired with interdependencies. Elements of each complex system that influence quality of care delivered.

✓ Recognize the importance of the transition from the volume-driven care environment to the quality- and value-driven care delivery environment.

✓ Boards, physicians, nurses, and other healthcare leaders need regular assessments of quality indicators that provide both the quantitative and qualitative pulse of the ACO in its economic impact in the community, effect on improving population health, and progress in improving operational efficiency and effectiveness.

✓ Leadership is key to supporting a front line worker approach to organizational transformation.

✓ Consider the Donabedian Quality Framework (i.e., structure, process, and outcomes) when evaluating impact of technological changes that will have a systemic effect on a healthcare organization, its workforce, and its patients.

✓ Health information technologies (EHRs in particular) hold great promise for improving quality of care, but attention must be given to monitor for their influence on unintended consequences, preventable adverse events, and other patient safety related impacts.

✓ Keep the patient experience the focus of the efforts.

[168] Intel's Louis Burns to Give Keynote on Healthcare at World Congress on Information Technology 2006; Intel Assumes Global Impact Program Sponsorship. *Business Wire Press Release*. April 2006. Accessed online March 25, 2012, at http://www.businesswire.com/news/home/20060403005383/en/Intels-Louis-Burns-Give-Keynote-Healthcare-World.

[169] Committee on Quality of Care in America. Institute of Medicine. Chapter 2: Errors in Health Care: A Leading Cause of Death and Injury. In: *To Err is Human. Building a Safer Health System.* Washington, DC: National Academy Press; 1999: 26.

[170] Landrigan CP, Parry GJ, Catherine B. Bones CB, Andrew D. Hackbarth AD, et al. Temporal Trends in Rates of Patient Harm Resulting from Medical Care. *N Engl J Med* 2010;363(22):2124-2134.

[171] Hoffman S, Podgurski A. Improving health care outcomes through personalized comparisons of treatment effectiveness based on electronic health records. *J Law Med Ethics*. 2011 Fall;39(3):425-436.

[172] Hoffman, et al. 2011.

[173] Hoffman, et al. 2011.

[174] Terry AL, Chevendra V, Thind A, Stewart M, Marshall JN, Cejic S. Using Your Electronic Medical Record for Research: A Primer for Avoiding Pitfalls. *Family Practice*. 2010;27(1):121-126.

[175] Weiner JP, Kfuri T, Chan K, Fowles JB. E-Iatrogenesis: The Most Critical Unintended Consequence of CPOE and other HIT. *J Am Med Inform Assoc.* 2007;14(3):387-388.

[176] Committee on Quality of Health Care in America. Institute of Medicine. Executive Summary: Recommendations 9 and 10. In: *Crossing the Quality Chasm. A New Health System for the 21st Century*. Washington, DC: National Academies Press; 2001:17-18.

[177] Porter ME, Teisberg EO. Quality and Pay for Performance. In: *Redefining Health Care. Creating Value-Based Competition on Results.* Boston, MA: Harvard Business School Press; 2006:85.

[178] Leventhal T, Taliaferro JP, Wong K, Hughes C, Mun S. The patient-centered medical home and health information technology. *Telemed J E Health*. 2012 Mar;18(2):145-149. E-pub 2012 Feb 3.

[179] Jiang HJ, Lockee C, Bass K, Fraser I. Board engagement in quality: Findings of a survey of hospital and system leaders. *J Healthc Manag*. 2008 Mar-Apr;53(2):121-34; discussion 135.

[180] Jiang, et al. 2008.

[181] Joshi MS, Hines SC. Getting the board on board: Engaging hospital boards in quality and patient safety. *Jt Comm J Qual Patient Saf.* 2006 Apr;32(4):179-187.

[182] Stanford University. Closing the Quality Gap: A Critical Analysis of Quality Improvement Strategies. *AHRQ Technical Review Number 9. Chapter 5. Conceptual Frameworks and Their Application to Evaluating Care Coordination Interventions*, Section 5b. Methodological Approach, Model 2: Donabedian's Quality Framework. June 2007. Accessed online October 2, 2011, at: http://www.ncbi.nlm.nih.gov/bookshelf/br.fcgi?book=hstechrev&part=A25445.

[183] Donabedian A. Evaluating the Quality of Medical Care. *Milbank Quarterly*. 2005;83(4):691-729. Reprinted from *Milbank Memorial Fund Quarterly*. 1966;44(3):166-203.

[184] Coyle YM, Battles JB. Using antecedents of medical care to develop valid quality of care measures. *Int J Qual Health Care*. 1999 Feb;11(1):5-12.

[185] Centers for Medicare and Medicaid Services (CMS). Introduction. In: *Roadmap for Implementing Value Driven Healthcare in the Traditional Medicare Fee-for-Service Program.* Baltimore, MD: CMS; 2009:1-3.

[186] Centers for Medicare and Medicaid Services. Quality Performance Scoring. In: *Accountable Care Organization 2012 Program Analysis: Quality Performance Standards Narrative Measure Specifications Final Report.* December 12, 2011; p. 7. Accessed online March 27, 2012, at http://www.cms.gov/SharedSavingsProgram/downloads/ACO_QualityMeasures.pdf.

[187] National Committee on Quality Assurance. NCQA Accountable Care Organization Accreditation brochure. Accessed online March 29, 2012, at http://www.ncqa.org/LinkClick.aspx?fileticket=Mv2IW8SCCvI%3d&tabid=1312.

[188] National Quality Forum (NQF). *Guidance for Measure Harmonization: A Consensus Report.* Washington, DC: NQF; 2010:5.

[189] Committee on Patient Safety and Health Information Technology. Institute of Medicine. Summary and Recommendations 1-8. In: *Health IT and Patient Safety: Building Safer Systems for Better Care.* Washington, DC: National Academy Press; 2011:5-14.

[190] Porter M, Tiesberg EO. How Reform Went Wrong. In: *Redefining Health Care. Creating Value-based Competition Results.* Boston, MA: Harvard Business School Press; 2006:88.

[191] Reinertsen JL, Gosfield AG, Rupp W, Whittington JW. *Engaging Physicians in a Shared Quality Agenda.* IHI Innovation Series white paper. Cambridge, Massachusetts: Institute for Healthcare Improvement; 2007. Accessed online April 23, 2012, at http://www.ihi.org/knowledge/Pages/IHIWhitePapers/EngagingPhysiciansWhitePaper.aspx.

[192] Terrell GE, Bohn JM. State of Affairs. In: *MD 2.0: Physician Leadership for the Information Age.* Tampa, FL: American College of Physician Executives; 2012:10.

[193] Davis KD, Stoots M, Bohn JM. Paving the Way for Accountable Care—Excellence in EMR Implementations. *J Healthc Inf Manag.* Winter 2012;26(1).

[194] Schall M, Coleman E, Rutherford P, Taylor J. *How-to Guide: Improving Transitions from the Hospital to the Clinical Office Practice to Reduce Avoidable Rehospitalizations.* Cambridge, MA: Institute for Healthcare Improvement; June 2011. Accessed online April 26, 2012, at http://www.ihi.org/knowledge/Pages/Tools/HowtoGuideImprovingTransitionsfromHospitalto HomeHealthCareReduceAvoidableHospitalizations.aspx.

[195] Center for Medicare and Medicaid Innovation. Partnership for Patients Program. Accessed online March 25, 2012, at http://www.innovations.cms.gov/initiatives/Partnership-for-Patients/index.html.

[196] US Agency for Healthcare Research and Quality. Patient Safety and Health Information Technology E-Newsletter. May 9, 2011, Issue #68. *Partnership for Patients Aims to Improve Care and Lower Costs.* Accessed online March 25, 2012, at http://www.ahrq.gov/news/ptsnews/ptsnews68.htm#HIT; Department for Health and Human Services. *Partnership for Patients: Better Care, Lower Costs. Making Care Safer.* Accessed online March 25, 2012, at http://www.healthcare.gov/compare/partnership-for-patients/safety/index.html.

[197] Centers for Medicare and Medicaid Services. *Fact Sheet: Hospital Engagement Networks: Connecting Hospitals to Improve Care.* December 14, 2011. Accessed online March 26, 2012, at http://www.cms.gov/apps/media/press/factsheet.asp?Counter=4219&intNumPerPage=10&che ckDate=&checkKey=&srchType=1&numDays=3500&srchOpt=0&srchData=&keywordType=All& chkNewsType=6&intPage=&showAll=&pYear=&year=&desc=&cboOrder=date.

[198] Koppel R, Wetterneck T, Telles JL, Karsh BT. Workarounds to Barcode Medication Administration Systems: Their Occurrences, Causes, and Threats to Patient Safety. *J Am Med Inform Assoc.* 2008;15(4):408-423.

[199] Committee on Identifying and Preventing Medication Errors. Institute of Medicine. Incidence of Medication Errors. In: *Preventing Medication Errors: Quality Chasm Series.* Washington, DC: National Academy Press; 2007:109.

[200] Committee on Patient Safety and Health Information Technology. Institute of Medicine. Intersection of Patient Safety and Health IT. In: *Health IT and Patient Safety: Building Safer Systems for Better Care.* Washington, DC: National Academy Press; 2011:22.

[201] Corrao NJ, Robinson AG, Swiernik MA, Naeim A. Importance of testing for usability when selecting and implementing an electronic health or medical record system. *J Oncol Pract.* 2010 May;6(3):120-124.

[202] Committee on Patient Safety and Health Information Technology. Institute of Medicine. Summary, Recommendations 1-3 and 10. In: *Health IT and Patient Safety: Building Safer Systems for Better Care.* Washington, DC: National Academy Press; 2011:5-14.

Chapter 7. Meaningful Use

Mary Staley Sirois, MBA, PT

The value of an idea lies in the using of it.

Thomas Edison
American Inventor and Businessman
(1847-1931)

Chapter 2 provided detail of the state of the industry with regard to the pursuit of implementation and adoption of EHRs. The introduction to the industry of these systems started in the late 1960s, but their adoption was slow for several decades. Over the years, studies of the benefits from EHRs have led the healthcare community to realize the need to work on accelerating adoption of these systems. EHRs are part of the global development of the health information technology landscape that are and will continue to enable transformational changes for ACOs and other care delivery organizations in the 21st century.

Momentum has been gained industry-wide through better information about the benefits of using EHRs and, secondly, from the financial incentive support programs established by the federal government to aid eligible professionals, eligible hospitals, and critical access hospitals in their pursuit of acquiring, implementing, and embracing within their culture the use of EHRs.[203] In 2009, President Obama signed the HITECH Act into law as part of the ARRA. The HITECH Act introduced eight programs (Table 7-1) for healthcare workforce training; research related to electronic health records and health information technology use; and advancement of academic curricula focused on health information technology issues that, over time, are intended to support the development of the nation's healthcare infrastructure and workforce in transitioning to "meaningful users" of EHR systems.

Table 7-1. HITECH Programs[204]

Program Title	Grant Description
Beacon Community Program	Program for communities to strengthen their HIT infrastructure and HIE capabilities
State Health Information Exchange Cooperative Agreement Program	Support to states or state designated entities in establishing HIE capability
Health Information Technology Extension Program	Establishes HIT regional extension centers for technical assistance, guidance, and best practices to accelerate healthcare providers' efforts to become meaningful users of EHRs
Strategic Health IT Advanced Research Projects (SHARP) Program	Grant program to fund research on breakthrough advances in: security of HIT, patient-centered cognitive support, healthcare application and network platform architectures, and secondary use of EHR data
Community College Consortia to Educate HIT Professionals Program	Seeks to accelerate HIT education and training programs at community colleges or expand existing HIT college training programs
Curriculum Development Centers Program	Grants to college institutions for HIT curriculum development
Program of Assistance for University-Based Training	Increases the number of professionals qualified to work in a specific HIT role that requires university-level training
Competency Examination for Individuals Completing Non-Degree Training Program	Supports development of initial administration of a set of HIT competency exams for colleges

Since they were initiated in 2009, each of these programs has contributed to funding efforts to improve our healthcare workforce and advance new translational ideas to further the US healthcare system's ability to make better use of EHR technologies. To this end, an increasing number of provider organizations (e.g., integrated delivery networks, hospitals, physician practices, academic medical centers, and public health facilities) have been implementing EHRs in recent years, as these systems are part of the infrastructure needed in the topography for establishing the nationwide health information network originally called for by President George Bush in 2004[205] and reinforced by President-elect Barack Obama in 2008.[206] In light of the importance of these issues, this chapter is dedicated to presenting a detailed description of the new CMS Meaningful Use of EHRs program and its importance to ACOs, other healthcare provider organizations, and healthcare professionals.

Meaningful Use Overview

Over the last decade, the healthcare industry has accelerated efforts to catch up with other major industries in its implementation, adoption, and use of information technologies in order to modernize its use of such tools and applications, as has been the case in other major industries for many years. With the support of federal incentives, this pace will continue as the industry is focused on improving the quality of care delivered through the efficient and effective adoption of health information technologies. However, much work needs to be done, as quality has not always been shown to improve in some cases to date.[207] A key to improving the industry's quality of care delivered is through achieving Meaningful Use of EHRs. ARRA specified three main components for a new Meaningful Use of Certified EHR Technologies Program:[208]

➢ The use of a certified EHR in a meaningful manner, to include electronic prescribing;

➢ Demonstration of electronic exchange of health information to improve quality of healthcare; and

➢ Submission of information on clinical quality and other measures in a form specified by DHHS for specified reporting periods.

Following the release of this legislation, work commenced on developing the underpinning rules for what would be CMS's three-stage Meaningful Use of EHRs program: a multiyear initiative (Figure 7-1) that will impact ACOs, other provider organizations, and healthcare professionals in their education, training, and use of health information technologies for years to come.

Figure 7-1. Three Stages of Meaningful Use

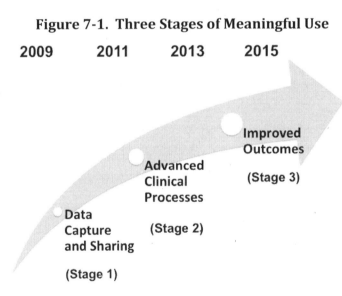

The Meaningful Use Program stipulated that, starting in 2011, eligible professionals, hospitals, and critical access hospitals would start to receive financial incentives for demonstrating and attesting to Stage

1 requirements. The July 2012 update from CMS on June 2012 statistics regarding registrations and payments made to eligible professionals and hospitals to date (cumulative for 2011 and 2012 through June) in Stage 1 included:[209]

> Total Medicare-eligible professionals paid to date 62,177 ($1.1 billion);

> Total Medicaid-eligible professionals paid to date 46,136 ($963 million);

> Total eligible hospitals paid to date 3,388 ($3.9 billion),

  o 764 of these hospitals (92 of which were critical access hospitals) have received both Medicare and Medicaid payments; and

> Total Medicare Advantage Organizations paid for 11,117 eligible professionals ($189 million).

The incentive program is broken into two divisions offered separately under a Medicare Meaningful Use Program and a Medicaid Meaningful Use Program, with details provided in this chapter. Incentive payments for the Medicare program will be paid through 2016, and payments for the Medicaid program through 2021.[210] Medicare payment adjustments will commence in 2015 for those eligible professionals, hospitals, and critical access hospitals that fail to demonstrate their ability to meet Meaningful Use requirements.[211]

ARRA reinforced the Office of the National Coordinator for Health Information Technology (ONC-HIT) and expanded its resources and responsibilities.[212] Falling under the purview of the Department of Health and Human Services, the ONC-HIT is chartered with activities "consistent with the development of a nationwide health information technology infrastructure that allows for the electronic use and exchange of information."[213] Furthermore, the ONC-HIT was granted authority for the following duties[214] that support its serving as a national oversight body:

➢ Review and determine endorsement of standards, implementation specifications, and certification criteria for electronic exchange and use of health information technology;

➢ Review federal health information technology investments to ensure progress is being made toward goals;

➢ Coordinate federal health information technology policy;

➢ Be responsible for updating of the federal health information technology strategic plan;

➢ Maintain a Web site for the ONC-HIT;

➢ Maintain or recognize voluntary certifications for health information technologies;

➢ Prepare reports on implementation of programs, lessons learned, and impact assessments on a national level of health information technologies with respect to communities with health disparities;

➢ Evaluate benefits and costs of electronic use and exchange of health information technologies;

➢ Make annual estimates of resources needed to reach the goal of utilization of an electronic health record on a national level; and

➢ Establish a governance mechanism for the nationwide health information network.

The scope of these duties provides strategic guidance and oversight for health information technology industry stakeholders to help advance efforts to work toward a nationwide health information network. As part of this effort, the ONC-HIT noted three key benefits for providers and patients in the use of EHRs:

➢ "Complete and accurate information,

➢ Better access to information,

➢ Patient empowerment."[215]

In addition to these benefits, the ONC-HIT notes three reasons for using EHRs over paper-based systems: improves information availability at the right time and right place to improve care decisions and coordination, improves care follow-up, and strengthens convenience factors related to information availability. The final rule for the Medicare Shared Savings Program in its first year performance-reporting period calls for participating providers to meet Meaningful Use of EHRs requirements. This is one of the 33 quality performance measures; therefore, those ACO providers who qualify as meaningful users of EHRs will have the opportunity to boost performance scores over those performing at the same level of clinical quality but not considered meaningful users. The final Medicare Shared Savings Program rule notes the use of survey-based measures, claims, and administrative data measures and the GPRO Web interface for the quality data reporting (see Appendix B).

System complexity related to health information technologies and the systemic effects of the aging population have contributed to the heightened awareness and need for the Meaningful Use of EHRs program, along with the need for a national and coordinated effort toward payment and delivery reform. With establishment of an ACO, the complexities associated with getting the needed health information technology infrastructure in place are offset by the benefits of having data that can be utilized across aligned stakeholder organizations for providing effective and efficient quality care in a manner that ensures patient satisfaction and engagement.

Incentive Eligibility and Payments

ARRA defined eligibility for professionals and hospitals for both the Medicare incentives and Medicaid incentives. At the heart of the Meaningful Use and ACO rules is the caregiver or caregiving organization. Coordination of electronic health record use across each ACO and other provider organizations will improve the ability of the ACO to collect, report, and share information needed to ensure quality of care. The following list provides a summary on the eligibility requirements and criteria for eligible professionals, eligible hospitals, and critical access hospitals.[216]

Eligible Professionals Requirements for both Medicare and Medicaid Incentives

➢ Payments for eligible professionals are per individual practitioner;

➢ Eligible professionals who work in a practice setting may qualify for an incentive payment if they successfully demonstrate Meaningful Use of certified EHR technology;

➢ Eligible professionals are only eligible for one incentive payment per year, regardless of the number of practices or locations where they provide services;

- Hospital-based eligible professionals cannot receive incentive payments. Professionals are considered hospital-based if 90% or more of their services are performed in a hospital inpatient (Place Of Service code 21) or emergency room (Place Of Service code 23) setting; and

- If professionals are eligible for both programs, they must choose between participating in one or the other but may switch once before 2015 (after receiving an initial payment).

Professionals Eligible for Medicare Incentives

Professionals eligible for Medicare incentives include:

- Doctor of medicine or osteopathy

- Doctor of dental surgery or dental medicine

- Doctor of podiatry

Professionals Eligible for Medicaid Incentives

Professionals eligible for Medicaid incentives include:

- Physicians (doctors of medicine or osteopathy)

- Nurse practitioner

- Certified nurse-midwife

- Dentist

- Physician assistant who furnishes services in a federally qualified health center (FQHC) or a rural health clinic (RHC) led by a physician assistant

For the Medicaid incentives, the eligible professional must meet one of these criteria:

➢ Minimum 30% Medicaid patient volume (not counting patients from the Children's Health Insurance Program),

➢ Minimum 20% Medicaid patient volume and is a pediatrician (not counting patients from the Children's Health Insurance Program), or

➢ Predominantly practices in an FQHC or RHC with a minimum 30% patient volume attributable to needy individuals.

The Meaningful Use program provides for up to $44,000 in total incentives from Medicare for Meaningful Use of a certified EHR starting in 2011 by eligible professionals. Under the Medicaid incentive program, eligible professionals can receive up to $63,750 starting in 2011, based on state-defined guidelines.

Eligible Hospitals and Critical Access Hospitals for Medicare and Medicaid Incentives

Hospitals and critical access hospitals can receive Medicare and Medicaid incentive payments based on the following.

Medicare eligible hospitals include:

➢ Subsection (d) hospitals in the 50 states or DC paid under the hospital inpatient prospective payment system,

➢ Critical access hospitals, and

➢ Medicare Advantage affiliated hospitals.

Medicaid eligible hospitals include:

➢ Acute care hospitals with at least 10% Medicaid patient population that includes critical access and cancer hospitals and

➢ Children's hospitals.

Table 7-2 provides a summary of hospital type and related incentive money eligibility.

Table 7-2. Eligibility by Hospital Type

Hospital Type	Medicare Incentive Eligible	Medicaid Incentive Eligible
Critical Access	Yes	Yes
Rehabilitation	No	No
Cancer	No	Yes
Psychiatric	No	No
Children's	No	Yes
Acute Care	Yes	Yes

Meaningful Use, Timeline Stages and Requirements

Initially, the Meaningful Use criteria were staged over a period of five years and contained both core (required) and menu set objectives specific to the eligible professionals and hospitals. On July 6, 2011, Farzad Mostashari, MD, ScM, National Coordinator for Health Information Technology (HIT) announced his support for delaying Stage 2 of the Electronic Health Records Meaningful Use program by one year to 2014 for providers who attested to Stage 1 in 2011, based on recommendations from the HIT Policy Committee. The rationale is that Stage 1 pioneers who attested in 2011 should not be penalized by the tight timelines for getting prepared for Stage 2, which starts in fiscal year 2013. A current timeline (as of the release of the final Stage 2 rules) is provided in Table 7-3. The table illustrates, for a Medicare provider, the steps through the meaningful use stages from the time they start in the program.

Table 7-3. Payment and Participation Timeline for Stages of Meaningful Use[217]

First Payment Year	2011	2012	2013	2014	2015	2016	2017	2018	2019	2020	2021
2011	1	1	1	2	2	3	3	TBD	TBD	TBD	TBD
2012		1	1	2	2	3	3	TBD	TBD	TBD	TBD
2013			1	1	2	2	3	3	TBD	TBD	TBD
2014				1	1	2	2	3	3	TBD	TBD
2015					1	1	2	2	3	3	TBD
2016						1	1	2	2	3	3
2017							1	1	2	2	3

Eligible providers that participate in the Medicaid EHR Incentive Program would follow the same overall structure but do not have the same requirement to demonstrate meaningful use in consecutive years.

The final Stage 2 rules were released on August 23, 2012 (Additional information regarding Stage 2 rules and criteria can be found at www.bridgingthedivide.info). Measures for Stage 1 were finalized and announced July 13, 2010.[218] For eligible professionals, 20 of 25 objectives and six clinical quality measures must be met in Stage 1. Eligible hospitals and critical access hospitals are required to meet 19 of 24 objectives. Figure 7-2 from Flareau and colleagues, *Clinical Integration: A Roadmap to Accountable Care*, provides an example of the reporting path for eligible professionals for Stage 1.[219] Forty-four clinical quality measures can be found on the CMS Web site[220] and focus on providing insight to patient care outcomes. For Stage 1, eligible professionals only have to meet six of 44 measures.

Figure 7-2. Stage 1 Meaningful Use Reporting for Eligible Professionals

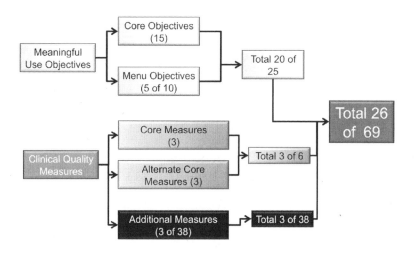

Appendix C provides a listing of the core objectives and the menu objectives and their associated measures from Stage 1. One of the core measures is maintaining an up-to-date problem list of current and active diagnoses. The measure requires that more than 80% of unique patients seen by an eligible professional or admitted to the eligible hospital or CAH's inpatient or emergency department (POS 21 or 23) have at least one entry recorded as structured data for an indication that no problems are known for the patient. The problem list is a key element of the patient's medical record, as it denotes the most critical health issues facing a patient.[221] Reducing variation in problem lists will be achieved through standardizing of language used (ICD-9 and, eventually, ICD-10), gaining support from senior clinical leadership for these initiatives as noted in the following case study.

Case Example: Managing Problem List Documentation in a Meaningful Way

A 400-bed, urban academic medical center in Brooklyn, New York, implemented the processes necessary to achieve many of the Stage 1 Meaningful Use requirements in 2010, via their computerized provider order entry (CPOE) implementation. CPOE addressed the requirements of not only medication order entry but also of allergy documentation, drug-formulary checks, drug/drug and drug/allergy checks, active medication list, and medication reconciliation at transitions in care. While in most provider organizations, medication reconciliation is a challenge, the biggest challenge came with the introduction of problem list documentation.

Because the patient's history was cited in the paper-based history and physician note, providers were challenged to remember to use a one-off process to document the required problems on the problem list, from which the certified EHR technology pulled for Meaningful Use reporting. Even if the patient's problems were presented elsewhere in the medical record, the challenge of the hybrid environment of paper and the EHR required providers to implement new processes to document the problems in the EHR.

The challenge of problem list documentation became paramount as the Meaningful Use compliance reports were run; compliance rates for some service lines were well below the 80% Meaningful Use target. It became apparent that daily intervention would be needed to communicate leadership's commitment to ensuring problem list documentation in the EHR. Senior hospital and medical staff leadership collaborated by reviewing detailed problem list documentation compliance reports daily and notifying the section chair of outstanding problem list documentation needs by patient. This effort continued over a 6-month period with performance across all service lines well above the 80% requirement.

Case Example: Managing Problem List Documentation in a Meaningful Way (cont.)

Of note is that problem list documentation differs depending on the environment of care. Hospital providers are focused on differential diagnosis, but they must consider the patient's history as well. Ambulatory providers are more likely to document problems more fully, as they interact with the patient, not only in times of illness but also when well working to manage chronic health issues or wellness factors. This challenge of appreciating and sharing problems across the continuum of care offered by an ACO must be addressed and fully understood by all involved in the care of the patient.

There are many other measures as listed in Appendix C along with the 44 clinical quality measures identified by CMS. As Table 7-3 illustrates the timeline for meeting the requirements for reporting on these measures by eligible professionals, eligible hospitals, and critical access hospitals extends out over several years. Many changes, system modifications and implementation of new applications may well be needed as the industry strives to address current and future challenges.

Stage 1 Implementation Challenges

The challenges associated with implementing each of the Meaningful Use requirements are complex. The impact of modifying the underlying clinical and technical workflows that impact caregiver processes and patient health outcomes must also account for the multidimensional aspect of some measures, and it requires dynamic post-implementation monitoring and process optimization.

As an example, the full process of medication reconciliation across the continuum of care is addressed in Figure 7-3 below. The patient has prescribed medications, which he or she may or may not actually take, as well as other possible medications. A discussion with the patient upon hospital admission, as well as knowledge of allergies and problems, allow the provider to order hospital medications via computerized physician order entry. This same process is revisited upon hospital discharge, with communication then to the ambulatory provider to monitor for effectiveness and ongoing adjustment via computerized physician order entry and e-prescribing.

Figure 7-3. Interdependency of Meaningful Use Requirements

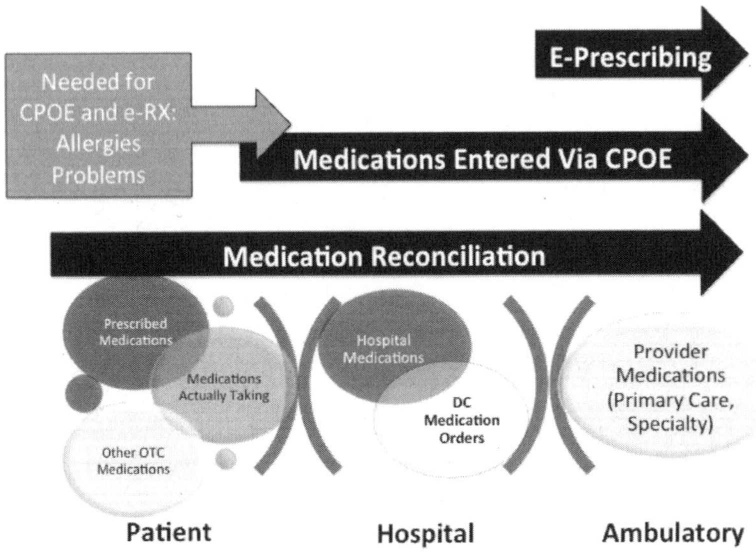

The process is complex, to say the least. The challenge of integrating and sharing information across an ACO in a manner that allows for accurate and timely communication to ensure quality patient outcomes requires particular attention to the data collection process, notwithstanding the workflow implications of such.

Computerized physician order entry implementation decisions have to address the full process of order management, not only the process of entering an order. The following areas must be addressed with ordering providers as part of a comprehensive computerized physician order entry/order set design process:

➢ Order and order set content;

➢ Heuristics of how the order entry content and process will be rendered on the screen, including alerts and reminders;

➢ Quality measure data elements;

➢ Order completion process, including incomplete orders;

➢ Order entry correction process;

➢ Order discontinuation;

➢ Recurring orders; and

➢ Desired alerts and reminders.

Coming to agreement on disease and population health management in a manner that ensures care coordination across the ACO, bringing together caregivers in a new business relationship that holds each accountable to each other and the patient to ensure quality outcomes and cost containment. Computerized physician order entry was chosen to highlight an example that demonstrates a basic challenge, but one of utmost importance in the overall care management process. The intent is to show that each of the Meaningful Use requirements affects another; the complexity of demonstrating Meaningful Use of health information technology; that Meaningful Use is a driver in the ACO structure, and, while not required, it holds great benefits and promise for supporting advancement in quality of care for the future. In light of many of these challenges within the final Stage 2 Meaningful Use rule, CMS identified a set of changes for Stage 1 that are provided in Appendix D.[222]

Meaningful Use Stage 2

On January 12, 2011, CMS released draft Stage 2 and Stage 3 Meaningful Use criteria for comment through February 25, 2011. However, it was a year later, on February 24, 2012, when CMS released a Notice of Proposed Rule Making for Stage 2 Meaningful Use with expectations of publishing a final rule in the fall of 2012.[223] Then on August 23, 2012 CMS released the final Stage 2 Meaningful Use rules.[224] The progression is clear - move from Stage 1 efforts to capture and utilize foundational levels of data, to Stage 2 criteria of expanding data collection and EHR utilization as well as enhancing the sharing of data across settings of care, to Stage 3 criteria focusing on using data to improve quality of care and clinical outcomes. Stage 2 implementation is not scheduled to begin until 2014 with projected implementation of Stage 3 in 2016.

Highlights of the final rules for Stage 2 include:[225]

➢ Increased percentage and/or scope compliance with Stage 1 core objectives,

➢ Virtually all Stage 1 core and menu objectives are finalized with Stage 2,

➢ In Stage 2, "test of the exchange of key clinical information" core objective from Stage 1 was replaced by a "transition of care" core objective in Stage 2.

➢ The requirement "provide patients with an electronic copy of their health information" objective is replaced by a new core objective for "electronic / online access."

➢ A new eligible provider Core Objective requiring use of secure electronic messaging to communicate with patients on relevant health information.

➢ A new eligible hospital/CAH Stage 2 Core Objective requiring automatic tracking of medications from order to administration using assistive technologies in conjunction with an electronic medication administration record (eMAR).

A summary of changes to the objective requirements from Stage 1 to Stage 2 include:

➢ Eligible hospitals and critical access hospitals have core objectives increased to 16 from 14 and must meet three of six menu objectives,

➢ Eligible professionals now have 17 core objectives, increased from 15 and must meet three of five menu objectives,

➢ Required percentages of compliance with core objectives are increased substantially and items previously requiring proof of concept (transmission or submission of data) now require ongoing transmission or submission. Proposed use of electronic medication administration record (eMAR) shifts to be a core objective.

The full set of final Stage 2 core and menu set objectives can be found in Appendix E.

Changes to Clinical Quality Measures in Stage 2

The Stage 2 rules established that reporting of clinical quality measures (CQM) would be required for core objectives and the Stage 2 rules align well with the clinical quality goals of the Medicare Shared Savings Program across six domains that measures fall within:

1. **Patient and Family Engagement.** Measures that reflect the

potential to improve patient-centered care and the quality of care delivered to patients. They are focused on the importance of collecting patient-reported data and the ability to impact care at the individual patient level and the population level through greater involvement of patients and families in decision making, self-care, activation, and effective management of their health condition.

2. **Patient Safety.** Measures that reflect the safe delivery of clinical services in both hospital and ambulatory settings including processes that may reduce harm to patients and the burden of illness. These measures will enable a longitudinal assessment of condition-specific, patient-focused episodes of care.

3. **Care Coordination**. Measures that demonstrate appropriate and timely sharing of information and coordination of clinical and preventive services among care team members and with patients and families to improve appropriate and timely communication.

4. **Population and Public Health**. Measures that reflect the use of clinical and preventive services and achieve improvements in the health of the population served, focused on the leading causes of mortality. Outcome-focused measures that support longitudinal measurement and demonstrate improvement or lack of improvement in the health of the US population.

5. **Efficient Use of Healthcare Resources**. Measures that reflect efforts to significantly improve outcomes and reduce errors. These measures benefit a large number of patients and emphasize the use of evidence to best manage high priority conditions and determine appropriate use of healthcare resources.

6. **Clinical Processes/Effectiveness.** Measures that reflect clinical care processes closely linked to outcomes based on evidence and practice guidelines.

The final CQM Stage 2 reporting requirements are as follows:[226]

➤ Eligible hospitals and critical access hospitals must report on 16 CQMs across at least three of the six national quality strategy domains.

➤ Eligible professional must report on:

    o A core set of nine CQMs from at least three of the six National Quality Strategy domains focused on adult populations and controlling blood pressure;

    o A core set of nine CQMs for pediatric populations.

The final set of CQMs for eligible hospitals, CAHs, and eligible providers can be found in the Stage 2 final rule issued by CMS in Section II.B. Reporting on Clinical Quality Measures Using Certified EHRs Technology by Eligible Professionals, Eligible Hospitals, and Critical Access Hospitals.[227]

As the final Stage 2 rules were released near the completion of this book, early reviews of the final Stage 2 rule, offered two early perspectives per an August 23, 2012 Modern Healthcare article:[228]

➤ "The final rule still puts providers at risk of not demonstrating meaningful use based on measures that are outside their control, such as requiring 5% of patients to view, download or transmit their health information during a 3-month period," per College of Healthcare Management Executives, President and CEO, Richard Correll.

> "They've decreased the thresholds for some meaningful-use requirements, in particular: providing online access for the patient to get a hold of their medical records" per Robert Tennant, senior policy adviser at Medical Group Management Association (MGMA).

The effect of the Stage 2 rules will be significant on the eligible physicians and eligible hospitals. With a priority of increasing physician adoption, the regulatory impact analysis in the final Stage 2 rule provided a projection of Medicare EPs projected to demonstrate Meaningful Use of CEHRT and the forecast is provided in Table 7-4.

Table 7-4. Medicare EPs 2014-2019 Projected Meaningful Users[229]

	Calendar Year					
	2014	**2015**	**2016**	**2017**	**2018**	**2019**
EPs who have claims with Medicare (thousands)	568.9	574.8	580.8	586.8	592.7	598.6
Nonhospital based EPs (thousands)	491.0	496.1	501.3	506.4	511.5	516.7
EPs who are both Medicare and Medicaid EPs	98.2	99.2	100.3	101.3	102.3	103.3
Percent of EPs who are Meaningful Users	37	46	52	57	62	67
Meaningful Users (thousands)	147.1	184.2	206.5	229.3	252.5	276.1

Achieving significant rates of adoption is forecasted with a degree of uncertainty given other factors that will impact the rate. Legislative actions such as future payment reductions to physicians under the sustainable growth rate (SGR) formula for Medicare payments will have a more significant impact on physician behavior in terms of adoption rates for EHRs.[230]

As the industry works through implementation of Stages 2 and 3, our nation will continue on its path toward establishing the digital infrastructure needed for the US healthcare system[231] and strengthening its characteristics as a learning health system in being better able to provide tighter information linkages to engender better apprised decision making and more real-time reporting of quality and outcomes as denoted by the Institute of Medicine in 2011.[232]

Meaningful Use HIPAA Security Risk Assessment

As health information technology utilization by providers and patients increases, the need for information security and privacy protections has continued to grow. The Meaningful Use program "broadens HIPAA's reach and strengthens its privacy and security standards, in addition to adding new provisions related to enforcement and entities not covered by HIPAA."[233] As such, included in the Meaningful Use Stage 1 rule is the core requirement to revisit information security protections via a formal risk analysis process. The challenge of ensuring information security and privacy protections within an ACO, given its multiple stakeholder organizations, can cause even greater challenges. As a rule, every healthcare provider organization and physician must comply with HIPAA; however, because HIPAA allows for interpretation, each may have different levels of assumed risk and management of said risk. Organizations participating in an ACO must have assurances and agreements for information sharing that ensures HIPAA compliance, including policies on how breaches will be handled. Because of the importance of ensuring information security and privacy protections, the following segment provides an overview of the scope of a formal assessment process.

HIPAA Security Rule Overview

The HITECH Act expanded the privacy and security provisions of HIPAA to apply to business associates of a covered entity in addition to the covered entity itself that included the requirement to conduct a risk analysis annually with oversight from DHHS's Office of Civil Rights.[234] This analysis is to determine security risks and implement measures "to sufficiently reduce those risks and vulnerabilities to a reasonable and appropriate level" as set forth in the Code of Federal Regulations in 2007.[235] The Meaningful Use requirements state that eligible hospitals (EH) and eligible professionals (EP) must "conduct or review a security risk analysis per 45 CFR 164.308(a)(1) of the certified electronic health record (EHR) technology, and implement security updates and correct identified security deficiencies as part of its risk management process." The Meaningful Use attestation requirement states that a risk analysis and gaps are addressed as part of the eligible hospital and eligible professional's risk management process; it does not state that any gaps must be resolved prior to Meaningful Use compliance attestation. While eligible hospitals and eligible professionals may have a certified EHR in place to meet the requirements of the HIPAA security rule for applications, the rule goes well beyond vendor compliance to address an eligible hospital's organizational policies, procedures and practices that ensure information security.

The added availability and use of EHRs in the patient care process and across the continuum of care of an ACO poses significant risks related to information security and privacy. Now, more than ever, eligible hospitals and eligible professionals must ensure prudent steps are taken to ensure the security and privacy of electronic patient health information. Beyond the requirement to conduct an information security risk assessment, section 13402(e)(4) of the HITECH Act,[236] the Secretary is required to post a list of breaches of unsecured protected health information affecting 500 or more individuals. Therefore covered entities, including business associates, must have a process in place to monitor for such breaches and respond accordingly.

The HITECH Act contained several new security provisions including:

➢ Requirement to notify patients and DHHS of electronic protected health information security breaches,

➢ New HIPAA regulations regarding business partners and enforcement of penalties,

➢ Restrictions on the sale and marketing of electronic protected health information,

➢ Ensuring that patients have access to their electronic health information, and

➢ Accounting of disclosures of electronic protected health information to patients.

The challenge of ensuring security across the ACO is not insignificant and poses tremendous privacy implications should a security breach occur. Table 7-5 outlines the requirements[237] per the Code of Federal Regulations for the HIPAA security rule that should be addressed as part of an overall information security risk analysis process.

Table 7-5. HIPAA Security Rule (Rev. 2007)

HIPAA Requirement	Description
ADMINISTRATIVE SAFEGUARDS	
Security Management Process (§164.308(a)(1))	Implement policies and procedures to prevent, detect, contain, and correct security violations.
Assigned Security Responsibility (§164.308(a)(2))	Identify the security official who is responsible for the development and implementation of the policies and procedures required by this subpart for the entity.
Workforce Security (§164.308(a)(3))	Implement policies and procedures to ensure that all members of its workforce have appropriate access to electronic protected health information, as provided under paragraph (a)(4) of this section, and to prevent those workforce members who do not have access under paragraph (a)(4) of this section from obtaining access to electronic protected health information.
Information Access Management (§164.308(a)(4))	Implement policies and procedures for authorizing access to electronic protected health information that are consistent with the applicable requirements of subpart E of this part.
Security Awareness and Training (§164.308(a)(5))	Implement a security awareness and training program for all members of its workforce (including management).
Contingency Plan (§164.308(a)(7))	Establish (and implement as needed) policies and procedures for responding to an emergency or other occurrence (for example, fire, vandalism, system failure, and natural disaster) that damages systems that contain electronic protected health information.
Security Incident Procedures (§164.308(a)(6))	Implement policies and procedures to address security incidents.

HIPAA Requirement	Description
Evaluation (§164.308(a)(8))	Perform a periodic technical and nontechnical evaluation, based initially on the standards implemented under this rule and, subsequently, in response to environmental or operational changes affecting the security of electronic protected health information, which establishes the extent to which an entity's security policies and procedures meet the requirements of this subpart.
Business Associate Contracts and Other Arrangements (§164.308(b)(1))	A covered entity, in accordance with §164.306, may permit a business associate to create, receive, maintain, or transmit electronic protected health information on the covered entity's behalf only if the covered entity obtains satisfactory assurances, in accordance with §164.314(a), that the business associate will appropriately safeguard the information.
PHYSICAL SAFEGUARDS	
Facility Access Controls (§164.310(a)(1))	Implement policies and procedures to limit physical access to its electronic information systems and the facility or facilities in which they are housed, while ensuring that properly authorized access is allowed.
Workstation Use (§164.310(b))	Implement policies and procedures that specify the proper functions to be performed, the manner in which those functions are to be performed, and the physical attributes of the surroundings of a specific workstation or class of workstation that can access electronic protected health information.
Workstation Security (§164.310(c))	Implement physical safeguards for all workstations that access electronic protected health information, to restrict access to authorized users.

HIPAA Requirement	Description
Device and Media Controls (§164.310(d)(1))	Implement policies and procedures that govern the receipt and removal of hardware and electronic media that contain electronic protected health information into and out of a facility, and the movement of these items within the facility.
TECHNICAL SAFEGUARDS	
Access Control (§164.312(a)(1))	Implement technical policies and procedures for electronic information systems that maintain electronic protected health information to allow access only to those persons or software programs that have been granted access rights as specified in §164.308(a)(4).
Audit Controls (§164.312(b))	Implement hardware, software, and/or procedural mechanisms that record and examine activity in information systems that contain or use electronic protected health information.
Integrity (§164.312(c)(1))	Implement policies and procedures to protect electronic protected health information from improper alteration or destruction.
Person or Entity Authentication (§164.312(d))	Implement procedures to verify that a person or entity seeking access to electronic protected health information is the one claimed.
Transmission Security (§164.312(e)(1))	Implement technical security measures to guard against unauthorized access to electronic protected health information that is being transmitted over an electronic communications network.

HIPAA Requirements	Description
ORGANIZATIONAL SAFEGUARDS	
Business Associate Contracts or Other Arrangements (§164.314(a)(1))	The contract or other arrangement between the covered entity and its business associate required by §164.308(b) must meet the requirements of paragraph (a)(2)(i) or (a)(2)(ii) of this section, as applicable. A covered entity is not in compliance with the standards in §164.502(e) and paragraph (a) of this section if the covered entity knew of a pattern of an activity or practice of the business associate that constituted a material breach or violation of the business associate's obligation under the contract or other arrangement, unless the covered entity took reasonable steps to cure the breach or end the violation, as applicable, and, if such steps were unsuccessful—(A) Terminated the contract or arrangement, if feasible; or (B) If termination is not feasible, reported the problem to the Secretary.
DOCUMENTATION SAFEGUARDS	
Policies and Procedures (§164.316(a))	Implement reasonable and appropriate policies and procedures to comply with the standards, implementation specifications, or other requirements of this subpart, taking into account those factors specified in §164.306(b)(2)(i), (ii), (iii), and (iv). This standard is not to be construed to permit or excuse an action that violates any other standard, implementation specification, or other requirements of this subpart. A covered entity may change its policies and procedures at any time, provided that the changes are documented and are implemented in accordance with this subpart.
Documentation (§164.316(b)(1))	(i) Maintain the policies and procedures implemented to comply with this subpart in written (which may be electronic) form; and (ii) if an action, activity or assessment is required by this subpart to be documented, maintain a written (which may be electronic) record of the action, activity, or assessment.

Threats and Vulnerabilities

A complete HIPAA information security assessment should address each of the following threats and vulnerabilities of the mission critical systems containing electronic protected health information.

Threats:

- ➢ Loss of network
- ➢ Loss of power
- ➢ Loss of air conditioning
- ➢ Vandalism
- ➢ Water in basement
- ➢ Fire
- ➢ Natural disaster

Vulnerabilities:

- ➢ Hardware/server failure
- ➢ Data corruption
- ➢ Application failure or incorrect operation
- ➢ Vendor disruption
- ➢ Disgruntled IT employee
- ➢ Disgruntled non-IT employee
- ➢ Inappropriate access by an employee or contractor
- ➢ Unencrypted backup files
- ➢ Change control

The challenge of ensuring security and privacy protections across an ACO becomes significantly greater as organizations increase their level of clinical practice, administrative, and infrastructure integration. Blending technologies, policies, and procedures along with integrated patient health records increases the potential for harm from vulnerabilities and threats.

Regional Extension Centers

In addition to the incentives allocated for those demonstrating Meaningful Use, the HITECH Act authorized $677 million in funding for a national Health Information Technology Extension Program consisting of Regional Extension Centers (RECs) and a national Health Information Technology Research Center (HITRC). As of January 31, 2012, 62 RECs have been funded across the country to help providers become meaningful EHR users. RECs are available to:

➢ Focus on providing support to individual physicians and small practices,

➢ Provide training and support services to assist providers in adopting EHRs,

➢ Offer information and guidance to help with EHR system selection and implementation, and

➢ Provide technical assistance as needed.

Efforts of these organizations led to mixed results through 2011. Some have encountered challenges with staffing, community/regional marketing to their physician communities, and system upgrade issues to help physician practice clients in achieving Stage 1 Meaningful Use.[238]

Meaningful Use Attestation

While each eligible professional and eligible hospital and critical access hospital involved in an ACO is required to complete its own Stage 1 Meaningful Use attestation, there is a need to ensure completeness in meeting all criteria and objectives before attestation. One issue to consider is the potential for CMS to conduct Meaningful Use audits.[239] Figure 7-4 provides a step-by-step guide to the activities each entity must complete to make a successful attestation.

Figure 7-4. Process for Attestation of Stage 1 Meaningful Use

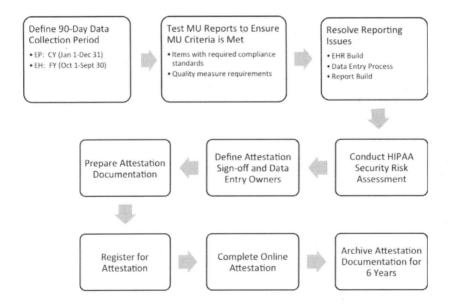

Accountable Care Organizations, Meaningful Use and Health Information Technology

In the final Medicare Shared Savings Program rule published October 20, 2011, CMS lightened its position on the requirement for an ACO to demonstrate that achieving Meaningful Use of EHRs is part of the overall Care Coordination domain (Table 7-6).

Table 7-6. Proposed vs. Final ACO Rule and Meaningful Use

Proposed Rule on ACO	Final Rule on ACO
• Percent of all physicians meeting Stage 1 Meaningful Use requirements • Percent of PCPs meeting Stage 1 Meaningful Use requirements • Percent of PCPs using clinical decision support • Percent of PCPs who are successful electronic prescribers under the eRx incentive program	• Percent of PCPs who successfully qualify for an EHR incentive program payment

The e-prescribing requirement was removed from the final ACO rule but remains as a Stage 1 Meaningful Use requirement for eligible professionals. While the utilization of health information technologies is not a specific requirement to participate in the Medicare Shared Savings Program (or other ACO-related initiatives), the implementation of EHRs and becoming meaningful users will only help eligible professionals and hospitals in achieving financial, operational, and clinical outcome goals for the population they serve.[240] Additionally, such tools have the potential to improve the quality of healthcare and work toward achieving the six specific quality aims for quality improvement from the Institute of Medicine Report, *Crossing the Quality Chasm,* in 2001:

1. Safety
2. Timeliness

3. Efficiency

4. Effectiveness

5. Equitability

6. Patient-Centeredness

Working toward achieving Meaningful Use of EHRs will help physicians and provider organizations across the United States with meeting these aims and the Three-Part Aim for Medicare ACOs: better care for individuals, better health for populations, and lower growth in expenditures. ACOs will be a vital part of our health system's evolving architecture of care delivery entities and, as stated by the President's Council of Advisors on Science and Technology in 2010,

> Information technology has the potential to transform healthcare as it has transformed many parts of our economy and society in recent decades. Health information technology can allow clinicians to have real-time access to complete patient data, and provide them with support to make the best possible decisions.[241]

Achieving the requirements for clinically integrated and quality-driven operations will be more realizable for public and commercial ACOs with Meaningful Use of EHRs as part of the culture of the stakeholders engaged.

Bridging the Divide

The Stage 1 Meaningful Use requirements set the foundation for the use of EHRs in collecting and reporting health information, while the proposed Stage 2 requirements are focused on expanding EHR utilization and moving the industry toward integration and interoperability across levels of care. This expansion includes the introduction of a robust patient health record approach. In August of

2012, the preliminary Stage 3 criteria were presented to the ONC-HIT Policy Committee with the intent of having final recommendations ready for DHHS by May 2013.[242] While these were early draft concepts, several new criteria were recommended for Stage 3 that included:[243]

➤ Reporting on the use of 15 clinical decision support interventions;

➤ Collecting and reporting on additional patient demographic data to include occupation, disability status, gender identity, and language;

➤ Expanding use of CPOE for referrals and transition-of-care orders;

➤ Allowing patients to submit various types of patient-generated health information electronically;

➤ Improving EHR functionality for maintaining problem lists, medication lists, and medication allergies; and

➤ Increasing capabilities within EHRs for public health reporting on immunizations, hospital acquired infections (HAI), and adverse events.

Many challenges exist across the industry to meet the Stage 2 criteria. Stage 3 will present new challenges to be addressed over the coming years.

As discussed in Chapter 1, three themes are driving the need for a national and coordinated effort in the use of EHRs aligned with payment and health care service delivery reform offered by the ACO model:

➤ Health system complexity,

➤ Influence of the aging population on the health system, and

➢ Need for innovation and the continuous drive in health information technology.

In relation to the Meaningful Use program, successful implementation will mitigate some of the complexity and communication challenges experienced by eligible professionals and hospitals in today's environment. For the Medicare ACO program, the Meaningful Use program will strengthen capabilities for ACOs to provide electronic health information to their beneficiary population as stakeholders work through achieving the objectives of Stage 1 and eventually Stages 2 and 3. There is clear alignment of the ACO requirements with the Stage 1 Meaningful Use quality measures for eligible professionals, further supporting the importance of health information technology in improving quality and reducing costs. Besides the measure regarding the "% of PCPs who successfully qualify for an EHR incentive program," the following clinical quality measures are cited within both the ACO and Meaningful Use rules:

➢ Medication reconciliation upon transition in care

➢ Hypertension: blood pressure measurement

➢ Controlling high blood pressure

➢ Smoking and tobacco use cessation

➢ Breast cancer screening

➢ Colorectal cancer screening

➢ Influenza immunization for patients 50 and older

➢ Pneumonia vaccination for patients 65 and older

➢ Diabetes

- o HbA1c poor control

- o Blood pressure management

- o Urine screening

- o LDL management and control

➢ Ischemic vascular disease

- o Use of aspirin or other antithrombotic

- o Complete lipid panel and LDL control

➢ Coronary artery disease: drug therapy for lowering LDL-cholesterol

➢ Heart failure: beta-blocker for left ventricular systolic dysfunction

➢ Adult weight screening and follow-up

This commitment by the federal government to implement evidence-based guidelines across the country is commendable, and the implications for information technology utilization to collect, share, report and improve upon such data cannot be overstated. The direction for federal health IT initiatives has America on a path to move toward CMS's value-based and quality-driven healthcare culture. While Meaningful Use of EHRs will provide the foundation for collecting, managing, and reporting of electronic protected health information for an ACO, as CMS described, simply meeting the requirements of Meaningful Use will not provide ACOs with the data sharing capabilities and analytics needed to effectively manage and coordinate care as well as measure cost savings and distributions for all stakeholders.

Case Example: Medication Reconciliation- What's Real and Whose Job is it?

Maintaining an active medication list, a required element for Stage 1 Meaningful Use, and the ability to reconcile medications upon transitions in care, a menu item, should be viewed by an ACO as a primary goal in ensuring quality of care. The challenge of medication reconciliation is extreme, no matter what type of organization or relationship is involved. Patients see multiple providers, who prescribe based on what the patients have said they are taking. But unless the patients bring in the bottles themselves, how do we really know everything we need to know? Does the provider call the pharmacy? Does the generalist call the specialist? Even if providers are using the same EHR in the same organization, we know what was prescribed, but not necessarily what patients are actually taking.

With the ACO structure focused on the Medicare population, we have patients who are usually on multiple medications to manage multiple chronic conditions. In an ACO relationship, reconciliation of medications in a manner that supports patient compliance is key to managing disease, wellness, and expenses. So whose job is it? What guidelines will be set up within the ACO to ensure effective communication of medication prescribing to allow for providers across the continuum of care to reinforce medication compliance as well as manage issues that can result from poly-medication interactions?

What processes and tools will be put in place to proactively share medication information across the ACO? How will providers work with patients to ensure medication compliance accountability? After all, an ACO structure includes that patient, correct?

It is important to cite the work of the ONC-HIT's report, *Federal Health Information Strategic Plan 2011-2015*. The ONC-HIT's mission is to "improve health and health care for all Americans through the use of information and technology." Figure 7-5 is the Federal Health IT Strategy Map, which clearly aligns with the goals of both the Meaningful Use and the Medicare ACO's final rule issued in October 2011.

Figure 7-5. Federal Health IT Strategy Map

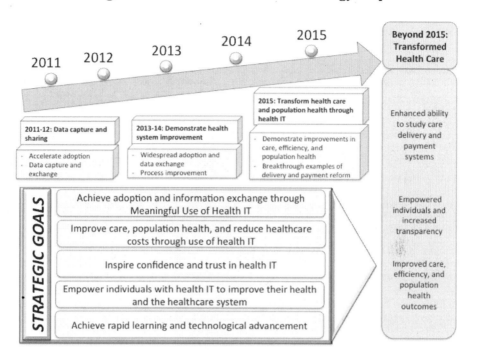

The integration of disparate data sources from those participating in a Medicare ACO, in addition to the challenge of integrating home-based health monitoring, telehealth, and remote care technologies, moves well beyond the prescriptive Meaningful Use regulations and forces organizations toward greater health information technology integration strategies. In Chapter 1, ACORM was introduced as a comprehensive model for ACOs to consider as a building block guide in establishing their health information technology infrastructure. Driving toward the achievement of Meaningful Use from Stage 1 through Stage 3 will be important for all healthcare provider organizations to help support these national strategic goals provided in Figure 7-5. Meaningful Use is not specifically identified in ACORM, but it is a foundational requirement that touches every information technology component and those that enable their capabilities within the model. A final quote summarizes the essence and importance of the Meaningful Use program to Medicare ACOs.

ACOs create incentives for providers to work together to treat Medicare patients across care settings, including physician offices, hospitals, and long-term and rehab facilities, coordinate their care and apply standards to improve their performance. Healthcare providers will need the capabilities of electronic health records, health information exchanges and other tools so they can share patients' data wherever they seek treatment, distribute decision support about treatment and communicate securely to coordinate patient care.[244]

Chapter 7: Takeaways

✓ The final ACO rule includes the use of an EHR as one of the 33 quality performance measures; therefore, those ACOs with providers who are meaningful users will have the opportunity to boost performance scores over those performing at the same level of clinical quality but not considered meaningful users.

✓ The need for information security and privacy protections follows the path of increasing use of health IT by providers and patients. To support this need, the Meaningful Use Stage 1 rule calls for a formal risk assessment and management process.

✓ The challenge of ensuring security and privacy protections across an ACO increases as stakeholders blend technologies, policies, and procedures and integrate patient health records.

✓ The challenges associated with implementing each of the Stage 1 Meaningful Use requirements are simply the beginning; the impact of each measure on others in the caregiver process drives the need for dynamic post-implementation monitoring and process optimization.

✓ The Meaningful Use progression is clear—move from Stage 1 efforts of capturing and utilizing foundational levels of data, to Stage 2 where data collection and EHR utilization is expanded, along with the sharing of data across settings of care, to Stage 3, which will focus on using data to improve quality of care and clinical outcomes. ACOs will find the ability to manage and improve care across the continuum more efficient by leveraging the industries evolving EHR capabilities.

[203] Center for Medicare and Medicaid Services. Overview of EHR Incentive Programs. Accessed online April 7, 2012 at http://www.cms.gov/Regulations-and-Guidance/Legislation/EHRIncentivePrograms/index.html?redirect=/EHRIncentivePrograms/.

[204] Office of the National Coordinator for Health Information Technology. HITECH Programs. Accessed online April 7, 2012 at http://healthit.hhs.gov/portal/server.pt/community/healthit_hhs_gov__hitech_programs/1487.

[205] Ford EW, Menachemi N, Peterson LT, Huerta TR. Resistance is futile: but it is slowing the pace of EHR adoption nonetheless. *J Am Med Inform Assoc.* 2009;16(3):274-281.

[206] Transcript: Obama's Speech on the Economy. *New York Times.* January 8, 2009. Accessed online April 7, 2012, at http://www.nytimes.com/2009/01/08/us/politics/08text-obama.html?pagewanted=all.

[207] Landrigan CP, Parry GJ, Bones CB, Hackbarth AD, Goldmann DA, Sharek PJ. Temporal Trends in Rates of Patient Harm Resulting from Medical Care. *N Engl J Med.* 2010 Nov 25;363(22):2124-2134.

[208] American Recovery and Reinvestment Act. Public Law 111-5. February 17, 2009. Title IV-Medicare and Medicaid Health Information Technology; Miscellaneous Medicare Provisions. Sec. 4101. Incentives for Elegible Professionals. (a) Incentive Payments. Accessed online April 8, 2012 at http://www.gpo.gov/fdsys/pkg/PLAW-111publ5/pdf/PLAW-111publ5.pdf.

[209] Centers for Medicare and Medicaid Services. CMS Meaningful Use of EHRs Registration and Payment Update for June 2012. Accessed online August 3, 2012 at https://www.cms.gov/Regulations-and-Guidance/Legislation/EHRIncentivePrograms/DataAndReports.html.

[210] CMS. CMS Meicare and Medicaid EHR Incentive Programs. Milestone Timeline. Accessed online April 9, 2012, at https://www.cms.gov/Regulations-and-Guidance/Legislation/EHRIncentivePrograms/Downloads/EHRIncentProgtimeline508V1.pdf.

[211] CMS Medicare and Medicaid EHR Incentive Programs. Milestone Timeline.

[212] Blumenthal D. Stimulating the Adoption of Health Information Technology. *N Engl J Med.* 2009;360:1477-1479.

[213] American Recovery and Reinvestment Act. Public Law 111-5. February 17, 2009. Title XXX-Health Information Technology and Quality. Sec. 3001. Office of the National Coordinator for Health Information Technology. (b) Purpose.

[214] American Recovery and Reinvestment Act. Public Law 111-5. February 17, 2009. Title XXX-Health Information Technology and Quality. Sec. 3001. Office of the National Coordinator for Health Information Technology. (c) Duties of the National Coordinator.

[215] Office of the National Coordinator for Health Information Technology. Electronic Health Records and Meaningful Use Webpage. Accessed online April 8, 2012, at http://healthit.hhs.gov/portal/server.pt?open=512&objID=2996&mode=2.

[216] Center for Medicare and Medicaid Services. EHR Incentive Programs Eligibility Requirements for Professionals and Hospitals. Accessed online April 10, 2012, at http://www.cms.gov/Regulations-and-Guidance/Legislation/EHRIncentivePrograms/Eligibility.html#BOOKMARK1.

[217] Center for Medicare and Medicaid Services. EHR Incentive Programs. Stage 2. Accessed online August 27, 2012 at http://www.cms.gov/Regulations-and-Guidance/Legislation/EHRIncentivePrograms/Stage_2.html.

[218] Blumenthal D, Tavenner M. The "Meaningful Use" Regulation for Electronic Health Records. *N Engl J Med.* 2010 Aug;363(6):501-504.

[219] Flareau B, et al. Chapter 7. The Quality Continuum—Continuous Improvement. In: *Clinical Integration: A Roadmap to Accountable Care, Second Edition.* Virginia Beach, VA: Convurgent Publishing; 2011;220-221.

[220] Centers for Medicare and Medicaid Services. Meaningful use clinical quality measures. Accessed online April 11, 2012, at http://www.cms.gov/QualityMeasures/03_ElectronicSpecifications.asp.

[221] Holmes C. The Problem List beyond Meaningful Use. Part I: The Problems with Problem Lists. *J AHIMA.* 2011 Feb;82(2):30-3; quiz 34.

[222] Centers for Medicare & Medicaid Services. 42 CFR Parts 412, 413, and 495. Medicare and Medicaid Programs; Electronic Health Record Incentive Program--Stage 2. Final Rule. August 23, 2012. Section 3 (b). Changes to Stage 1 Criteria for Meaningful Use. pp. 41-43.

[223] Center for Medicare and Medicaid Services. Press Release. Secretary Sebelius Announces Next Stage for Providers Adopting Electronic Health Records. CMS Press Release February 24, 2012. Accessed online August 23, 2012, at http://www.cms.gov/apps/media/press/release.asp?Counter=4291&intNumPerPage=10&checkDate=&checkKey=&srchType=1&numDays=3500&srchOpt=0&srchData=&keywordType=All&chkNewsType=1%2C+2%2C+3%2C+4%2C+5&intPage=&showAll=&pYear=&year=&desc=false&cboOrder=date.

[224] Center for Medicare and Medicaid Services. Secretary Sebelius Announces Next Stage for Providers Adopting Electronic Health Records. CMS Press Release August 23, 2012. Accessed online August 24, 2012, at http://www.cms.gov/apps/media/press/release.asp?Counter=4441&intNumPerPage=10&checkDate=&checkKey=&srchType=1&numDays=3500&srchOpt=0&srchData=&keywordType=All&chkNewsType=1%2C+2%2C+3%2C+4%2C+5&intPage=&showAll=&pYear=&year=&desc=&cboOrder=date.

[225] Centers for Medicare & Medicaid Services. CMS Medicare and Medicaid HER Incentive Programs: Stage 2 Final Rule. Press Release. August 23, 2012. Accessed online August 24, 2012, at http://www.cms.gov/apps/media/press/factsheet.asp?Counter=4440&intNumPerPage=10&checkDate=&checkKey=&srchType=1&numDays=3500&srchOpt=0&srchData=&keywordType=All&chkNewsType=6&intPage=&showAll=&pYear=&year=&desc=&cboOrder=date.

[226] Centers for Medicare & Medicaid Services. 42 CFR Parts 412, 413, and 495. Medicare and Medicaid Programs; Electronic Health Record Incentive Program--Stage 2. Final Rule. August 23, 2012. Section 2. Summary of Major Provisions. p. 15.

[227] Centers for Medicare & Medicaid Services. 42 CFR Parts 412, 413, and 495. Medicare and Medicaid Programs; Electronic Health Record Incentive Program--Stage 2. Final Rule. August 23, 2012. Section II.B. Reporting on Clinical Quality Measures Using Certified EHRs Technology by Eligible Professionals, Eligible Hospitals, and Critical Access Hospitals. Table 8: CQMs Finalized For Medicare and Medicaid Eps Beginning With CY 2014; Table 10: CQMs Finalized for Eligible Hospitals and CAHs Beginning with FY2014. pp. 354-400.

[228] Zigmond J. AHIMA, MGMA welcome Stage 2 rule; AHA airs concerns. Modern Healthcare. August 23, 2012. Accessed online August 25, 2012, at http://www.modernhealthcare.com/article/20120823/NEWS/308239955/ahima-mgma-welcome-stage-2-rule-aha-airs-concerns.

[229] Centers for Medicare & Medicaid Services. 42 CFR Parts 412, 413, and 495. Medicare and Medicaid Programs; Electronic Health Record Incentive Program--Stage 2. Final Rule. August 23, 2012. Section V.C.3.a. Regulatory Impact. Medicare Eligible Professionals. Table 22: Medicare Eps Demonstrating Meaningful Use of Certified HER Technology. pp. 580-581.

[230] Centers for Medicare & Medicaid Services. 42 CFR Parts 412, 413, and 495. Medicare and Medicaid Programs; Electronic Health Record Incentive Program--Stage 2. Final Rule. August 23, 2012. Section V.B. Regulatory Impact. Overall Impact. p. 565..

[231] Yu P. Why Meaningful Use Matters. *J Oncol Pract.* 2011 Jul;7(4):206-209.

[232] Roundtable on Value & Science-driven Health Care. Institute of Medicine. Summary: Introduction and Overview. Box S-1 Learning Health System Characteristics. In: *Digital Infrastructure for the Learning Health System. The foundation for Continuous Improvement in Health and Health Care.* (Prepublication Copy). Washington, DC: The National Academies Press; 2011:2.

[233] Goldstein MM, Jane HT. The First Anniversary of the Health Information Technology for Economic and Clinical Health (HITECH) Act: The Regulatory Outlook for Implementation. *Perspect Health Inf Manag.* 2010 Summer; 7(Summer):1c.

[234] P.L. 111-5. American Recovery and Reinvestment Act. February 17, 2009. Title XIII-Health Information Technology. Subtitle D-Privacy. Part 1—Improved Privacy Provisions and Security Provisions. Sect. 13401(c). Application of Security Provisions and Penalties to Business Associates of Covered Entities Annual Guidance on Security Provisions. Annual Guidance; Department of Health and Human Services. Guidance on Risk Analysis Requirements under the HIPAA Security Rule, July 14, 2010. Accessed

online April 15, 2012, at
http://www.hhs.gov/ocr/privacy/hipaa/administrative/securityrule/rafinalguidance
pdf.pdf.

[235] Code of Federal Regulations, 45 CFR §164.308(a)(1)(ii)(B) Administrative
safeguards and Risk Management. Revised October 1, 2007. Accessed online April 15,
2012, at
http://www.gpo.gov/fdsys/search/pagedetails.action?collectionCode=CFR&searchPa
th=Title+45%2FSubtitle+A%2FSubchapter+C%2FPart+164%2FSubpart+C&granuleId
=CFR-2007-title45-vol3-toc-id2&packageId=CFR-2007-title45-
vol3&oldPath=Title+45%2FSubtitle+A%2FSubchapter+C%2FPart+164&fromPageDet
ails=true&collapse=true&ycord=507.

[236] P.L. 111-5. American Recovery and Reinvestment Act. February 17, 2009. Title XIII-
Health Information Technology. Subtitle D-Privacy. Part 1—Improved Privacy
Provisions and Security Provisions. Sect. 13402(e)(2). Notification in the Case of
Breach. Media Notice.

[237] Code of Federal Regulations, 45 CFR §164. Security and Privacy. Sections 308-316.
Revised October 1, 2007.

[238] Hirsch MD. Regional extension centers struggling to help docs meet Meaningful
Use. *FierceEMR article*. November 17, 2011. Accessed online April 16, 2012 at
http://www.fierceemr.com/story/regional-extension-centers-struggling-help-docs-
meet-meaningful-use/2011-11-17; Dimick, Chris. RECs on a Mission: Assessing the
Regional Extension Center Program. *Journal of AHIMA*, 2011 November-
December;82(11):26-30.

[239] Tate J. Meaningful Use Attestation and Audits: A Word to the Wise. Medcity News.
February 10, 2012. Accessed online April 17, 2012, at
http://www.medcitynews.com/2012/02/meaningful-use-attestation-audits/; Scheps
L. MU Attestation: Save Your Documentation—Meaningful Use Monday. EMR and
HIPAA Website. March 26, 2012. Accessed online April 17, 2012, at
http://www.emrandhipaa.com/lynn/2012/03/26/mu-attestation-save-your-
documentation-meaningful-use-monday/.

[240] Nguyen J, Choi B. Accountable care: are you ready? *Healthc Financ Manage*. 2011
Aug;65(8):92-100.

[241] President's Council of Advisors on Science and Technology. *Realizing the Full
Potential of Health Information Technology to Improve Healthcare for Americans: The
Path Forward.* December 2010. Accessed April 16, 2012, at
http://www.whitehouse.gov/sites/default/files/microsites/ostp/pcast-health-it-
report.pdf; Chaudhry B, Wang J, Wu S, Maglione M, Mojica W, Roth E, Morton SC, and
Shekelle PG. Systematic review: impact of health information technology on quality,
efficiency, and costs of medical care. *Annals of Internal Medicine*. 2006 May
16;144(10):742-752.

242 Conn J. IT policy committee gets Stage 3 recommendations. *Modern Healthcare.* August 3, 2012. Accessed online August 4, 2012, at http://www.modernhealthcare.com/article/20120803/NEWS/308039981?AllowVie w=VW8xUmo5Q21TcWJOb1gzb0tNN3RLZ0h0MWg5SVgra3NZRzROR3l0WWRMVGJY UDBDRWxiNUtpQzMyWmVqNTM4WUpiU2c=&utm_source=link-20120803-NEWS-308039981&utm_medium=email&utm_campaign=hits#.

243 Hall SD. Stage 3 Meaningful Use to focus on better coordination, more clinical decision support. *FierceEMR.* August 2, 2012. Accessed online August 4, 2012, at http://www.fierceemr.com/story/stage-3-meaningful-use-focus-better-coordination-more-clinical-decision-sup/2012-08-02; Office of the National Coordinator for Health Information Technology Policy Committee meeting, August 1, 2012. Meeting transcript. Accessed online August 9, 2012, at http://www.healthit.gov/policy-researchers-implementers/hit-policy-committee-0.

244 Mosquera M. CMS: Want ACO Savings? *Government Health IT.* April 4, 2011. Accessed online April 17, 2012, at http://www.govhealthit.com/news/cms-want-aco-savings-start-meaningful-use.

Chapter 8. Revenue Cycle Management Implications for ACOs

Tim Webb

... through our own decisions rather than our conditions, if we carefully learn to do certain things, we can accomplish those goals.

Stephen R. Covey, PhD, MBA
American Author and Public Speaker

In the first decade of the 21st century, the US healthcare system has faced unprecedented financial challenges. Landmark federal legislative reforms including ARRA, the Affordable Care Act, CMS Meaningful Use initiative, Medicare Shared Savings Program (MSSP) , and mandates for preparation for ICD-10 conversion, along with the nationwide economic downturn in 2007/08, stringent credit markets, and fluctuations in health systems investment portfolios have all contributed to the continued need for focus on health system financials and revenue cycle management. With the industry shift underway to public and private accountable care organization models of operation there will be new partnerships and expanded groups of stakeholders with the requirement to have clinical integration programs in place driving tighter operational connectivity between ambulatory care operations and those of hospitals, physician hospital organizations, and integrated delivery networks. To maintain staffing, facilities, information technology infrastructure, and regulatory compliance for these new models of care, ensuring that effective revenue cycle management tools and applications are in place will continue to be a high priority for chief financial officers, physician executives, chief information officers, and chief executive officers presiding over healthcare organizations for decades to come.

With all the discussion about ACOs, it seems revenue cycle is being largely ignored. One recent article put it this way

> We're starting to feel like revenue cycle is the red-headed step child of healthcare IT priorities and accountable care organization (ACO) conversations.[245]

The "Accountable" in ACO means two things: a group of healthcare providers and payers is responsible for the quality of the care provided; and the ACO is at risk for the cost of the care provided. Much of the focus has been on the quality of care and the data and systems required to support the sharing of clinical data to support the clinical functions. However, most of the same discussions have not addressed the changes necessary in revenue cycle to support ACOs.

> An ACO could technically have all the measures in place that make it appear destined for success—integrated care, core measures to assess quality delivery, a competent information technology plan that allows for data sharing—but if the organization fails to revolutionize the way it pays physicians, it is in serious jeopardy.[246]

Given the changing landscape, what lies ahead and what health IT issues impact the effectiveness of revenue cycle management?

This chapter will address how the current reimbursement models will need to change and the new functions organizations will take on to support the planning and successful operations (i.e., profitability) of ACOs. There are two fundamental changes in revenue cycle that must be addressed by ACOs:

➢ Developing new economic incentives compatible with the intent of an ACO[247] and

➢ Performing new care management and coordination functions that relies on existing and new clinical and financial data.

To manage the changes coming for all stakeholders in healthcare effectively, understanding and managing the revenue cycle is essential. Figure 8-1 illustrates the traditional four major phases in revenue cycle management of a program's life cycle.

Figure 8-1. Traditional Revenue Cycle Management: The Life Cycle—Its Major Phases and Key Players

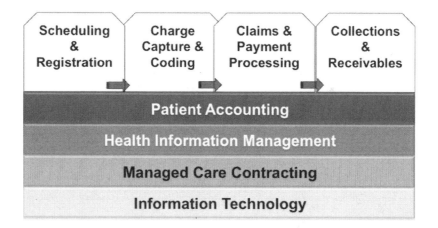

There are hundreds if not thousands of processes and procedures that must take place with the involvement of each of the key players (e.g., ACO support operation departments). But one thing is certain: the necessary changes in revenue cycle management to support ACOs will be profound for all healthcare organizations, from the perspective of cultural change, financial impact, and, most importantly, for the effects felt by their patient populations. With revenue cycle management systems, there is a need for integration with clinical health information technologies, as well as other administrative and financial applications. As noted in a 2011 article, John Glasser stated, "revenue cycle system forms the foundation of a provider's response to accountable care and payment reform. As the reimbursement environment becomes more complex, revenue cycle systems must evolve to support payments based on quality and performance."[248]

Given the importance to the lifeblood of each ACO and its stakeholders, it is critical to evaluate the performance of the revenue cycle management approach and systems. Providing measurements of key performance indicators (KPI) gives leadership insights for corrective action in administrative, financial, contracting, and health information management operations, along with a status on hard (i.e., dollars savings) and soft (i.e., quality and process efficiency gains) return on investment. In 2010, the HIMSS Financial System Revenue Cycle Task Force identified three areas and metric categories for tracking key performance indicators based on best practices in the industry (Table 8-1).[249]

Table 8-1. Metric Areas and KPI Categories for Revenue Cycle Management

Metric Area	Metric Category
Upstream	Revenue sharing model development
	Patient risk modeling
	Contracting
	Scheduling
	Patient access
	Pre-authorization and insurance verification
	Financial counseling
Midstream	Case management
	Disease management
	Care coordination
	Charge capture and clinical documentation
	Charge description master (CDM) maintenance
	Health information management (HIM)
Downstream	Billing and claim submission
	Cashiering, refunds, and adjustment posting
	Third-party and guarantor follow-up, processing, and payment posting
	Customer service
	Collections and outsourcing

Examples of KPI's can include:[250]

➢ **Upstream**. Predicted medical expense based on risk (Risk modeling); Percent tests scheduled in system (scheduling);

➢ **Midstream**. Late charges as a percentage of total charges (charge capture);

➢ **Midstream**. Inpatient charts coded per coder/day (health information management);

➤ **Midstream.** Discharged Not Final Billed (DNFB) accounts work in process as a percentage of revenue (health information management);

➤ **Midstream.** Coding denials in terms of percentage of total accounts or total charges for a given time period (health information management); and

➤ **Downstream.** "Self-pays" as a percentage of total collections (collections and outsourcing).

To support early stage ACOs and their stakeholders, maintaining a grasp on financial performance will be essential. This is only a sample of indicators to be tracked; organizations should invest the time and resources in comprehensive revenue cycle management strategies and systems to provide physicians, executives, and other stakeholders with meaningful insights on their return on investment. Information technologies help ensure the accuracy and completeness of patient health information that reinforces the validity and value in the metrics above. In today's healthcare organizations, high quality patient information can significantly impact the organization's revenue cycle

> When patient information is not captured or input correctly, the whole revenue cycle for that individual is at risk. Conservatively speaking, 1%–3% of a hospital's revenue is lost to third-party claim discrepancies, according to industry experts. This often is due to lackluster insurance eligibility verification efforts prior to the service. It could be the result of poor registration and coding activities. [251]

Financial Goals/Challenges of ACOs

The primary financial goal of ACOs is to reduce medical expense. However, the challenges are not trivial and can include the following:

➢ **Managing population health status.** The health status of the population covered by the ACO;

➢ **Open networks for beneficiaries.** The ability of the population to seek care from providers outside the control of the ACO;

➢ **Risk/reward modeling.** The ability to write a contract with sufficient information to understand the risk/reward model;

➢ **Data integration and care coordination.** The tools to integrate data from multiple sources, including claims and clinical data and support risk modeling and care coordination; and

➢ **ACO performance.** The processes and measurements for ACO performance, delivered in a timely manner.

Let us take a closer look at each of these challenge areas.

Health Status of the Population

For the Medicare ACOs, populations have been identified as Medicare beneficiaries. While this represents a traditionally higher cost group, the numbers of required members are small (15,000 for Pioneer ACOs and 5,000 for the basic Medicare Shared Savings Program participants). These small populations make it difficult to use traditional actuarial models with any effect. Therefore, in order to mitigate the risk, using historical claims information and health status to tune the model will be an important strategy.

Depending on other factors, such as economic demographics and health status, if the ACO does not have prior knowledge of care, the ACO will be in a greater financial risk position. CMS has promised to provide historical claims information on beneficiaries. While this is helpful for initial modeling, it will be incomplete. Claims information under ICD-9 and CPT codes lacks sufficient detail to provide accurate information on health status and is minimally required to do any risk modeling.

Pharmaceutical information is also required, and it must be combined with medical information in order to understand the severity of key diseases. Most organizations will be entering into ACO contracts with very little understanding of the health of the population for which they are assuming risk. A whole new level of clinical analytics/informatics will be required to understand the financial risk the ACO is assuming.

Open Network for Beneficiaries

For the Medicare ACOs, CMS has been clear that the ACO pilots are not closed models. Freedom of choice of providers creates complications for the ACO in trying to improve health and control cost. CMS has provided clauses to reduce the risk significantly to ACOs if patients go outside. However, this places an additional challenge on the ACO to create a provider-patient relationship such that the beneficiaries do not go outside the network. Patient centered medical homes support this relationship building; however, most providers do not have experience with the processes and customer-centric attitudes necessary to create this type of environment. Successful ACOs will create strong relationships with patients to keep them in the network and compliant with their care plans.

Risk/Reward Modeling

The type of modeling, tools and expertise required to understand the financial implications for entering into ACOs, are sometimes scarce in provider organizations. There are many tools in the market that have varying degrees of performance for risk-modeling using claims data.[252] In addition, health risk assessment tools and methodologies for collecting additional information from beneficiaries to determine health status, chronic disease, and additional risk factors can be used. Selecting, implementing, and obtaining high quality data (not always 100% accurate) to populate these tools is expensive. Even if the tools are optimized, the best accuracy possible may be 85%. After ACOs implement use of these tools and processes, the imperfect data and analysis will still have uncertainties and financial risk. Developing a contract based on the model is only the first step. Additionally, CMS provides two options for contracting: prospective or retrospective. Using the prospective model, Medicare ACOs will have predictive information on the potential population to model. Using the retrospective model, an ACO will not know the population risk until after the first performance period (year 1).

Data Integration and Care Coordination

One of the biggest challenges with revenue cycle management will not be in the finance department, but in the clinical care processes. The ability of the ACO to qualify for bonuses will depend on the improvement in the health of its beneficiaries. The patient care team members will need constant data on their patients. If one of the patients is admitted to the hospital through the emergency room, the data about the event will need to move from the hospital to the primary care physician or specialist in real-time or near real-time speed. Under the shared savings model, delivery of care cannot continue as business as usual. The clinical care team will need the tools and applications to monitor their patient's condition in near real-time. This will enable continuous clinical analysis using risk modeling tools, beneficiary encounters/claims, and monitoring health condition indicators for negative changes in health status (e.g., onset of diabetic symptoms). When issues are identified, the care team can take proactive steps to quickly mitigate negative changes in the patients' health status and reduce potential negative financial impact to the ACO. Improving the health of a beneficiary can take years; hence, the reason why CMS ACO pilots are for three years. If an ACO allows itself to get behind in quality indicator performance in year 1, making up the lost revenue could be impossible in the following 2 years.

ACO Performance

Keeping up with ACO performance will place new demands on the finance department. Revenue cycle will fundamentally change from a process focused on correctly billing for services to capturing accurate data about the health of the members.

Financial teams may need to examine each beneficiary as an investment over a period of time, not as episodic revenue. The objective will be to ensure each beneficiary incurs less medical expense than the predicted expense based on his or her health. Examples of the types of new activities that ACOs may have to perform may include tasks traditionally performed by payers. The implications of the following activities will require new technology, new processes, and new staff.

More importantly, these changes will alter the patient-care provider relationship.

Managing Patients With Gaps in Care. Understanding gaps in care requires information about preventative care and disease-specific tests (e.g., diabetic's annual vision test). Making sure the patient has the tests performed will be key to improving the health of the patient and avoiding predicted medical expense to support achieving shared savings and bonus payments to the ACO.

Identifying Patients Using Inappropriate Services. Ensuring an ACO's patients stay "in the network" will require evaluating claims information for each beneficiary monthly, routine contact with the patient, and intervening when the patient uses inappropriate services (e.g., goes to the ED when a primary care visit may have been more appropriate).

Identifying Physicians With Non-optimal Utilization Patterns. Traditionally, physician utilization has been the purview of hospitals and payers. In an ACO, physicians will need to monitor utilization rates themselves and adapt to a new payment model focused on managing cost and improving population health outcomes.

Managing High Risk Patients. Understanding who the high-risk patients are and developing appropriate interventions for them will represent a significant investment. Monitoring the expense versus the "return" will be a key financial activity. This will require new systems and processes.

Reviewing Drug Utilization. Pharmaceutical cost is one of the highest expenses in healthcare today. The ACO will need to incorporate pharmaceutical information into the overall patient care model. CMS is encouraging ACOs to partner with pharmacy benefit managers (PBMs) to find ways to work together. This is new for providers, and it may represent both opportunities and risks to the ACO.

ACOs are bringing about cultural transformation as previously separate entities are being clinically and administratively integrated through both process and technological change. During the course of a transformation, decisions are made about information technology applications to be used for the merged cultures within each ACO. Types of applications affected that will impact revenue cycle management activities include patient accounting, risk modeling, health information management, claims clearinghouses, coding, case management, managed care eligibility, claims submission, billing, and scheduling—to name a few. From the external environment, the revenue cycle is impacted by reductions in reimbursements from Medicare and Medicaid, rising numbers of self-pay patients, and the increasing population of uninsured and underinsured patients who require care that ends up being uncompensated.

One of the key challenges faced by many healthcare organizations in regards to revenue cycle management in this transition to the ACO model is evaluating and determining the acceptable level of risk sharing among the provider, patient, and payers. Four types of risk have been identified and each serves as an element of new payment model risk and reason for gravitating away from the traditional fee-for-service contracting. Those four types of risk are: bonus payment risk, market share risk, baseline revenue loss risk, and patient population (whole or partial) financial risk.[253]

For Medicare ACOs, their ability to manage clinical risk associated with individual patients while focusing on population health management may directly correlate to their incentive payments received in the future. One of the factors that can impact this risk is intensity of medical coding (i.e., the completeness of diagnostic codes assigned to beneficiaries). When ACOs increase coding intensity, there is the potential for increases in the risk score associated with the beneficiary. CMS proposed to retain the option of auditing ACOs for appropriate coding practices and risk adjustment methodologies.[254] In addition to these issues for the Medicare ACO, CMS introduced two risk-sharing options: a one-sided model and a two-sided model. The one-sided model is for new Medicare ACO entities in the early stages of maturing their infrastructure, health information technology systems, and physician relations. This model gives ACO participants a lower level of risk in the first and second year performance periods and the ACO is not responsible for losses, in exchange for a lower percentage of shared savings (up to 50%) based on quality performance scores plus a lower potential shared savings rate (up to 2.5%) for the inclusion of rural health clinics or federally qualified health centers in their network.[255]

Likewise, the two-sided model is for mature organizations with strong infrastructure, advanced health information technologies, DOJ/FTC-approved clinical integration programs, strong physician relations, and advanced quality improvement programs and processes. With a greater degree of risk comes greater potential for a larger percentage of shared savings (up to 60%) plus an increased potential shared savings rate (up to 5.0%) based on the inclusion of rural health clinics or federally qualified health centers in their network. [256]

However, the financial risk of loss is very real for the Pioneer ACOs. According to the CMS application

> CMS will enter into Agreements with Pioneer ACOs only if they provide enforceable assurances that they can reimburse Medicare for all potential losses. This assurance could take the form of an irrevocable letter of credit for the full amount of risk undertaken or any similarly enforceable mechanism that covers the full amount of risk.[257]

Risk Shifting in ACOs

The CMS goals for ACOs are to improve care for individuals, improve population health, and reduce expense for Medicare and Medicaid programs. Achieving the reduced expense, means the revenue model must fundamentally change from "fee-for-service" to a "fixed fee." In order to make the financial aspect of the ACO model work, risks have to be shared.

The risk for the one-sided savings model is on CMS, not the ACO, initially. Pioneer ACO participants are built primarily on the two-sided shared savings model, also considered a shared risk model. CMS offered participants three options, with managing risks ranging from 5% to 15%. This limited participation in the Pioneer ACO program is for those organizations with the financial resources to take on the level of risk associated with the two-sided model. In order to minimize the loss to CMS or the ACO due to a lack of experience, CMS required Pioneer ACO participants to have experience managing risk (e.g., at least 50% of revenue must come from risk-based contracts).[258]

This is in contrast to the fact that most Medicare Shared Savings Program (MSSP) participants are one sided (25 of the 27 initial ACOs operating under the MSSP[259] are one-sided). The one-sided risk model reduces the risk for the ACOs. If the costs exceed budget, the providers will be reimbursed.

However, the Pioneer ACOs assume greater risk, in return for greater reward. Although the benefit may be 75% of savings going back to the ACO from Medicare, there is downside risk on the ACO. Although there is a phase-in period for various aspects of reimbursement, in year 1, the ACO will assume some downside risk (e.g., at-risk reimbursement). One of the fundamental differences in ACO reimbursement is the aspect of population management; therefore, modeling risk will require a stable population of beneficiaries.

The impact of risk-sharing arrangements on revenue cycle management is important to note. When greater risk is taken on by the provider there is a need for better information technology infrastructure; improved documentation capture in coding operations; closing gaps in charging efforts for medications and procedures; and employing internal audit procedures to review billing activities and claims processes, among many other proactive initiatives.[260] Without ensuring that steps are taken to reduce risk of failure points throughout the financial, administrative, and health information management operations, the provider organization will be at a greater risk of loss due to poor controls and inadequate measures taken.

Bundled Payment Methodologies and Regulatory Impacts

One of the most discussed alternative payment models in the industry is bundled payments. This type of payment model, also called episode-based payments, can be described as

> ...reimburses multiple providers (hospitals, physicians, and post-acute care) in a single, comprehensive payment that covers all of the services

involved in the patient's care. An "episode" can take many forms, from a single rate for all services relating to a particular procedure, combining hospital care and post-acute care, to all treatment associated with a chronic condition for a defined period of time.[261]

In 2011, the Center for Medicare and Medicaid Innovation announced a Bundled Payments for Care Improvement Initiative.[262] Within this new program are four different bundled payment models characterized by separate and distinct episodes of care:

➤ Inpatient stay in the general acute care hospital;

➤ Inpatient stay and post-acute care for at 30 or 90 days after discharge;

➤ Begins at discharge from inpatient stay and ends no sooner than 30 days after discharge; and

➤ All services furnished by the hospital, physicians and other practitioners.

As part of the process for bundled payments, the payer provides a set amount for a particular episode of care, starting from the point of hospital admission for a specified procedure through discharge and possibly post-acute care requirements based on the terms set for the payment bundle, which includes an adjustment factor for severity of the case. This type of payment bundle may be determined by the physician and provider organization, agreeing to a package of services for treating specific conditions that returns a single payment that is allotted on the basis of the agreement.[263] Managing and sharing bundled reimbursements will also require new methodologies for sharing baseline and bonus payments.

Regulatory Impact

Two federal programs noted throughout this book that will have a significant impact on revenue cycle management activities are ICD-10 and CMS's Meaningful Use of EHRs program. First is ICD-10. The industry-wide transition to ICD-10 for the US healthcare market is set for October 1, 2014.[264] ACOs and physician practices, in preparing for the implementation of ICD-10, will need to ensure it is covered in managed care payer negotiations for annual contracts to offset or mitigate risks they may face regarding claims denials and authorization delays. Additionally, health information management departments should consider increasing specificity requirements in coding documentation to prepare for future billing and quality reporting requirements.[265] ICD-10 will have the potential to alter realization and capture of revenue for the healthcare organization and its physicians, thereby, potentially impeding efforts in providing optimal patient care. In addition, ICD-10 will complicate the analysis of data, requiring analytics systems to be upgraded and staff to be trained. However, the additional specificity of ICD-10 will provide new clinical information that will be of benefit to the ACO.

Second is the impact of CMS's Meaningful Use of EHRs program. As described in detail in Chapter 7, this program is having long-term effects on ACOs, physician practices, and hospital organizations across the country in terms of multiyear capital expenditure plans for acquisition and implementation of EHRs. More importantly, from a long-term revenue cycle perspective there are significant financial incentives to the hospital organizations and professionals who are eligible for them. After 2015, incentives start to transition to incrementally larger decrements to Medicare and Medicaid reimbursement rates that shall have a definite negative impact on revenues for future years. For those working in revenue cycle management activities, the key issue to plan for is understanding your organization's risk mitigation plans for ensuring that requirements are met in future years to avoid the decremented reimbursements to come from the impending increases in Medicaid beneficiaries and the growth in the Medicare beneficiaries as a result of the aging Baby Boomer population. With the effects of reduced reimbursement from Medicare and Medicaid, combined with revenue at risk, the opportunities to lose reimbursement will be significant.

Technology Implications

The revenue cycle management services market sector for healthcare is becoming more tightly integrated with the transformation occurring across the clinical systems sector. As physician practices, hospitals, integrated delivery networks, and ACOs go through the processes for acquiring, implementing, adopting, and or upgrading EHRs to keep pace with regulatory requirements and quality objectives, the need to replace or upgrade revenue cycle management systems is also increasing. Even if an organization is not replacing the revenue cycle system, the ability of the ACO to handle the accounting for shared reimbursement will create new requirements for configuration. A few of the health IT vendors in this market sector are Siemens, Lawson, RelayHealth, McKesson, Emdeon, Zirmed, MedAssets, and GE Healthcare.

Risk areas that technology solutions can aid physician practices, ACOs, and other provider organizations will include:[266]

➤ Need for staying current with payer requirements for claims submission,

➤ Inadequate monitoring of the organization's full claims process,

➤ Having suboptimal resources to manage resubmission of rejected claims,

➤ Poor verification of patient eligibility for insurance claims and the need to improve cycle times,

➤ The need to reduce denials, and

➤ Need for addressing patient population level trends in claims processing.

To address these risks, executives, physicians, and stakeholders involved in acquisition decisions for new and upgraded systems should recognize the need to have questions answered about how any new technology solution will reduce or hopefully eliminate these risks and others. From the buyer and stakeholder perspective, there is a number of issues to be considered in selecting a vendor and solution for revenue cycle management requirements. Any selected revenue cycle management solution should integrate and interface with other clinical and administrative systems. Having a data warehouse in place as part of the infrastructure will provide a central repository for all in-house systems that require interfacing. In addition to interfacing, selection and implementation planning criteria should consider the projected total cost of ownership, training requirements for staff, licensing requirements (e.g., time period of initial license and how often it must be renewed), and the revenue cycle management vendor's track record with customer service post-implementation.[267] After a system is in place, data mining and analytics tools will be crucial to help increase the real-time operational and administrative decision making for those responsible for activities throughout the revenue cycle management life cycle.

Bridging the Divide

Going forward, as ACOs evolve, their needs for greater and more timely insights to the financial health of their organization and its stakeholders will continue to be a high priority. The more functions that can be automated, the lower the risk of human errors that may occur with data entry or manipulation of data sets, financial records, or a patient's protected health information (PHI). Large industry-leading health IT vendors will likely continue to acquire small to mid-size revenue cycle management companies to provide more comprehensive coverage of ACOs that need information technology services within their own suite of technology solutions. For the healthcare executives evaluating and deciding on acquisitions of these systems that will be relied upon by their organizations for years to come, remember to consider the organizational change impact on the people.

The integration of new systems and processes in the finance and revenue cycle management functions will fundamentally transform how revenue cycle management is conducted. The most profound changes may include:

➢ Understanding the financial risk of a patient population,

➢ Determining appropriate investments in care coordination and preventative care in addition to the delivery of care services, and

➢ Measuring the results of those investments to improve patient health outcomes.

Consideration will also need to be given to the analysts, staff, and administrators who will shoulder the burden of implementing a new system that is adopted by physicians and clinical staff. Providing leadership and support for the workforce in these situations will show the urgency and attention needed to ensure effective and efficient implementation of revenue cycle management systems across all healthcare settings.

Improving revenue cycle management will be key to delivering the predictive financial insights needed for managing and leading ACOs in the future. Ensuring that revenue cycle management systems are integrated with EHRs and other clinical and administrative systems should be a high priority for ACOs and those stakeholders in health IT governance roles who can help their organizations manage these changes in the years ahead.

Chapter 8: Takeaways

✓ Reimbursement models and functions will need to be changed in healthcare organizations to ensure profitable operations for ACOs. Two fundamental changes in revenue cycle management for ACOs are:

   o New economic incentives based on ACO intent and

   o New care management and coordination functions that rely on existing and new clinical and financial data.

✓ There are four phases to traditional revenue cycle management: (a) scheduling and registration, (b) charge capture and coding, (c) claims and payment processing, and (d) collections and receivables. Patient accounting, health information management, managed care contracting, and information technology support these phases.

✓ Revenue cycle management systems require integration with clinical health information technologies and other administrative and financial applications.

✓ Healthcare organizations should invest the resources to provide physicians, executives, and other stakeholders with meaningful insights on their return on investment from comprehensive revenue cycle management strategies and systems.

✓ CMS has established that ACO pilots are to allow freedom of choice of providers to its beneficiaries. Successful ACOs will create strong relationships with patients to keep them in the network and compliant with care plans.

✓ ACOs and physician practices, in preparing for the implementation of ICD-10, will need to ensure it is covered in managed care negotiations for annual contracts to mitigate risks in claims denials and authorization delays.

Chapter 8: Takeaways (cont.)

✓ The impact of risk-sharing arrangements on revenue cycle management is important. When greater risk is taken on by the provider there is a need for better information technology infrastructure, improved documentation capture in coding operations, closing gaps in charging for medications and procedures, and internal audits to review billing activities and claims processes among many other proactive initiatives.

✓ As physician practices, hospitals, integrated delivery networks, and ACOs implement or upgrade EHRs, the need to replace or upgrade revenue cycle management systems increases.

✓ Revenue cycle management technology solutions can aid physician practices, ACOs and other provider organizations by mitigating risks that include:

- o Claims submission payer requirements,

- o Monitoring of the organization's full claims process,

- o Verification of patient eligibility for insurance claims,

- o Reducing denials.

✓ Address patient population level trends in claims processing.

[245] Mathur S, Lorusso K. Revenue Cycle: The Red-Headed Step Child of ACO Conversations. *Executive Insight.* March 2012. Accessed online May 15, 2012, at http://healthcare-executive-insight.advanceweb.com/Features/Articles/Revenue-Cycle-The-Red-Headed-Step-Child-of-ACO-Conversations.aspx.

[246] Spoerl B. 8 Biggest Mistakes an ACO Can Make. *Beckers Hospital Review.* April 27, 2012. Accessed online May 15, 2012, at http://www.beckershospitalreview.com/hospital-physician-relationships/8-biggest-mistakes-an-aco-can-make.html.

[247] Spoerl B. 2012.

[248] Shaw G. 6 technologies to support ACOs. *FierceHealthIT.* April 12, 2012. Accessed online July 26, 2012, at http://www.fiercehealthit.com/story/6-technologies-support-acos/2012-04-12.

[249] Healthcare Information and Management Systems Society (HIMSS). *Revenue Cycle Management: A Life Cycle Approach for Performance Measurement and System Justification.* May 2010. HIMSS Financial Systems Revenue Cycle Task Force. Accessed online April 26, 2012, at www.himss.org/ASP/ContentRedirector.asp?ContentID=78492.

[250] HIMSS. 2010.

[251] The Future-Proof Revenue Cycle. *Health Leaders Media.* June 2011. Accessed online April 19, 2012, at http://www.healthleadersmedia.com/content/HOM-266944/The-FutureProof-Revenue-Cycle.html.

[252] A Comparative Analysis of Claims-Based Tools for Health Risk Assessment. The Society of Actuaries. 2007. Accessed online July 30, 2012, at www.soa.org/Files/Research/Projects/risk-assessmentc.pdf.

[253] Anderson C. The 4 approaches to ACO payment models. *Government Health IT.* July 27, 2011. Accessed online April 25, 2012, at http://www.govhealthit.com/news/4-approaches-aco-payment-models.

[254] Flareau B, et. al. Financial Perspectives. In: *Clinical Integration: A Roadmap to Accountable Care*, 2nd Ed. Virginia Beach, VA: Convurgent Publishing; 2011:270-271; Fed. Reg. Vol. 76, No. 67. April 7, 2011. II(F)(4). Establishing an Expenditure Benchmark. pp. 19604-19606.

[255] Flareau B, et. al. 2011:273.

[256] Flareau B, et. al. 2011:273.

[257] Center for Medicare and Medicaid Services. Pioneer ACO Model Application. Accessed online May 14, 2012, at http://innovations.cms.gov/Files/x/Pioneer-ACO-Model-Request-For-Applications-document.pdf.

[258] Centers for Medicare and Medicaid Services. Pioneer ACO Model Application.

[259] CMS New Affordable Care Act Program to Improve Care, Control Costs, Off to a Fast Start. CMS Press Release April 10, 2012. Accessed online May 14, 2012, at https://www.cms.gov/Medicare/Medicare-Fee-for-Service-Payment/sharedsavingsprogram/News.html.

[260] Degaspari J. Mastering Revenue Cycle Management. *Healthcare Informatics*. April 22, 2011. Accessed online April 24, 2012, at http://www.healthcare-informatics.com/print/article/mastering-revenue-cycle-management.

[261] Proskauer Rose LLP. *United States: Latest Accountable Care Act Initiative: Bundled Payments For Care Improvement*. September 23, 2011, article. Accessed online April 26, 2012, at http://www.mondaq.com/unitedstates/x/146466/Healthcare/Latest+Accountable+Care+Act+Initiative+Bundled+Payments+for+Care+Improvement.

[262] Center for Medicare and Medicaid Innovation. Bundled Payments for Care Improvement Initiative. Accessed online April 26, 2012, at http://innovations.cms.gov/initiatives/bundled-payments/index.html.

[263] Evans J. Current state of bundled payments. *American Health and Drug Benefits*, August 2010. Accessed online July 23, 2011, at http://www.ahdbonline.com/article/current-state-bundled-payments?page=0,1.

[264] American Medical Association. Press Release. AMA Response to CMS Proposal to Postpone the ICD-10 Implementation Date. April 9, 2012. Accessed online April 26, 2012, at http://www.ama-assn.org/ama/pub/news/news/2012-04-09-cms-postpone-icd-10-implementation.page.

[265] Bosanko-Cera R. The I10 Impact: Preparing for ICD-10 in Physician Practices. *Journal of AHIMA*. November–December 2011:82(11);38-40.

[266] Riley J. Top 5 provider mistakes in revenue cycle. *Healthcare IT News*. December 16, 2010. Accessed online April 26, 2012, at http://www.healthcareitnews.com/blog/top-5-provider-mistakes-revenue-cycle.

[267] Keller M. RCM: Out with the Old, In With the New. *For The Record*. February 27, 2012;24(4):8. Accessed online April 28, 2012, at http://www.fortherecordmag.com/archives/022712p8.shtml.

Chapter 9. The Role of Patient Centered Tools

Laishy Williams-Carlson

Whether used for checking case-management records, consulting with a colleague, or any number of other important daily activities, mobile solutions empower people to generate efficiencies and reduce costs in the healthcare setting, but most importantly contribute to higher-quality patient care.

Steve Shihadeh
Vice President, Microsoft Health Solutions Group

When the US Department of Health and Human Services released new rules to help healthcare providers better coordinate care for Medicare patients through ACOs, involving patients was an important issue. "The Affordable Care Act is putting patients and their doctors in control of their health care," said HHS Secretary Kathleen Sebelius.[268]

Since the goal of an ACO is to deliver seamless, high-quality care for patients – a model that will eventually be adapted more widely—it is difficult to conceive of an ACO without significant patient involvement. The name "Accountable Care Organization" implies accountability and therefore, participation on the part of the patient. According to the Department of Health and Human Services, "the ACO would be a patient-centered organization where the patient and providers are true partners in care decisions."[269]

The idea that patient involvement is a key aspect of ACOs is broadly accepted. Two of the core values set forth by the American Medical Group Association embrace this concept:

➢ The timely sharing of information between patients and physicians to allow patients to become active participants in their own care and to receive services based on their individual needs and preferences; and

➢ Openness to adoption and adaptation of evolving health care delivery models, including modern infrastructure, patient registries and electronic prescribing.

According to the Medicare Shared Savings Program (MSSP), proposed quality measures used to establish quality performance standards will include health promotion and education and shared decision making, both of which will be supported by involving patients in these systems.

Under the federal rules, in order to share in savings, ACOs must meet quality standards in five key areas, four of which will benefit by providing patients with tools to help manage their care:

➢ Patient/caregiver care experiences

➢ Care coordination

➢ Preventive health

➢ At-risk population/frail elderly health

Looking ahead, it is likely that patient health records (PHRs) will be included in Stage 2 Meaningful Use. PHRs, like computerized provider order entry (CPOE) and barcoded medications, are considered to be part of the right answer for our healthcare system. PHRs fit in perfectly with the spectrum of care offered by ACOs; just as providers are connected in an ACO, these systems offer an avenue for patients to connect as well. They are destined to become the tools that will be utilized to help make patients accountable for their care.

Patients Want Control

Not only do PHRs and patient portals already exist, but increasingly, patients want to use them and expect their healthcare providers to share in their enthusiasm.

A survey conducted in 2006 by the Markle Foundation found that two-thirds of the public was interested in accessing their own personal health information electronically because it gave them more control. According to the survey, Americans believe that the online services enabled by such access will increase the quality of their care. They also view online records as a way to increase healthcare efficiency by reducing unnecessary and repeated tests and procedures.[270] In 2008, about 80% of the public believed using an online PHR would provide major benefits to managing healthcare services.[271] More recently, a Markle survey found that roughly two out of three members of the public and doctors agree that patients should have the option to view and download their personal health information online.

Younger and more technically savvy patients are especially likely to embrace the use of PHRs and patient portals. Given their propensity to utilize technology, these tools might be the only way young people conceive of maintaining such records.[272] Not surprisingly, a 2010 survey of healthcare consumers by Deloitte found that more Generation X and Generation Y consumers are interested in accessing their PHRs than Baby Boomers and seniors.[273]

Physicians are also getting on board with the concept of their patients using PHRs. A national survey conducted in 2008-2009 found that 42% would be willing to use a patient's electronic PHR. At integrated delivery networks such as Kaiser Permanente and the US

Department of Veterans Affairs, PHRs gained favor among physicians after initial skepticism.[274]

The public's perception that consumer health IT applications can improve healthcare holds up to scrutiny. A 2009 literature review by the Agency for Healthcare Research and Quality (AHRQ) found that these applications had a positive effect on outcomes for breast cancer, diet/exercise/physical activity, alcohol abuse, smoking cessation, diabetes, mental health issues, and other clinical areas.[275]

A 2010 Deloitte survey found that one in five consumers rate their interest in PHRs as high, would switch physicians to obtain access and would be very likely to use a mobile communication device to maintain them.[276] So far, adoption rates for PHRs have been low, but they are gradually increasing.

As of 2009, 3 million out of 8.6 million members used Kaiser's My Health Manager personal health record system.[277] More generally, a 2010 survey found that 10% of the public reported use of PHRs, up from 3% in 2008.[278] Wellness programs, which could be facilitated easily by PHRs and patient portals, are used by one in five consumers, with increasing numbers of seniors and those with one or more chronic conditions participating.[279] Kaiser has reported that Medicare beneficiaries who use their system—all 65 and older—are overwhelmingly satisfied with using the Internet to manage their healthcare online.[280]

It is clear that use of this type of technology will continue to grow as more and more patients and healthcare providers become increasingly comfortable with managing their health online. With the built-in concept of harnessing patients to take responsibility for their healthcare, ACOs are poised to take advantage of this trend.

Motivating Patients to Take Control

Accountability is at the heart of the ACO model, but it extends beyond the healthcare provider. Personal responsibility on the part of the patient is integral to the success of these systems, which are designed to better equip patients to take ownership of their healthcare. "We must create a platform for innovation that allows patients to get what information they need so that they may use it in a meaningful way," said Farzad Mostashari, MD, ScM, National Coordinator for Health Information Technology at DHHS. The capabilities of PHRs, patient portals and mobile applications discussed in this chapter empower patients, allowing them to assume responsibility and become partners in managing their care. These tools also play an important role in the drive to interconnectedness that determines how well ACOs will work.

Right now, most Americans' protected health information is scattered across many sources: doctors, hospitals, insurance companies, and personal files. Not many people have a complete, comprehensive set of their health records at their disposal or easily accessible to their healthcare providers. This lack of updated medical records means that patients are disconnected from their medical conditions, and their ability to perform health maintenance is impaired. Health problems from otherwise manageable conditions escalate from lack of information. A lack of a comprehensive PHR leads to the duplication of paperwork and a high possibility of losing or forgetting crucial information. This could—and often does—keep patients from getting proper treatment.[281]

In an accountable care model, providers are connected to one another. PHRs and patient portals fit in perfectly with this spectrum of care because they offer a way for patients to connect as well. When implemented and utilized properly, they have the potential to transform the healthcare experience. ACOs aim to improve chronic disease management, increase the focus on preventive medicine, improve healthcare quality and outcomes, and decrease costs. For these goals to be realized, all healthcare constituents—including patients—need to be motivated.

Health information technology tools such as PHRs and patient portals integrate data and workflows, with the ultimate goal of consumer access to support a patient-centered care model.[282] They bring patients into the equation, motivating them to take responsibility and play a leading role in their health and healthcare.

Personal Health Records vs. Patient Portals

Different groups have created their own definitions of PHRs that include varying elements, but the underlying concept remains the same:

➤ The Key Health Information Technology Terms Project defines a PHR as

> [A]n electronic, record of health related information on an individual that conforms to nationally recognized interoperability standards and that can be drawn from multiple sources while being managed, shared, and controlled by the individual.[283]

➤ In its *Connecting for Health* report, the Markle Foundation defined a PHR as

An electronic application through which individuals can access, manage and share their health information, and that of others for whom they are authorized, in a private, secure and confidential environment.[284]

In reality, electronic PHR systems are provider-linked—available through the patient's employer, doctor, or insurer—or stand-alone. But consumers who choose to maintain their PHRs on their own are faced with a considerable task, especially for older patients who have a longer health history and would need to round up data—a time-consuming job. Consumers who go it alone may see gaping holes in their data—missing dates of procedures and absent medication names, for example.[285]

Patient portals, on the other hand, are Web-based platforms created and maintained by healthcare organizations that allow patients to access portions of their EHRs and communicate with their healthcare providers. They are customized according to the organization's requirements and are often marketed as a service to attract patients and increase patient loyalty, but their benefits, outlined later in this chapter, are numerous.

In the case of ACOs, it is clear that the provider-linked model makes more sense. The concept of an ACO requires providers within the system to work together, a task that is facilitated by PHRs and patient portals managed by the ACO. This avoids the pitfalls of "information islands," where information exists in different formats and from different sources but is not linked together.

Some organizations, such as Kaiser and Cleveland Clinic, already offer their own PHRs. There are also numerous other platforms available that offer approaches to PHRs (Table 9-1). While some of these are quite innovative, they are not always successful. Google Health announced in 2011 that it was shutting down because it failed to attract the large number of users hoped for when the service began in 2008. When considering implementing a PHR and/or patient portal, ACOs will need to take into account interoperability with other systems such as electronic medical records and health information exchanges. In many cases, it may be preferable to build their own platforms to ensure that these tools meet the needs of both providers and patients. Table 9-1 identifies a number of electronic PHRs in the market today:

Table 9-1. PHR Platforms

Platforms
Access My Records
ER Card
Keas
MedKey
My HealtheVet (Veterans Administration)
My Health Info / Health Vault (Microsoft)
My Revolution
NoMoreClipboard
Peoplechart
Shared Care Plan (Congral)
The Bartlett Personal EHR
Trip Mate
VitalKey
WebMD Health Record

An Array of Functionality

Patients are already accustomed to turning on their computers to access health information. In 2010, more than half of consumers said they looked online for information about treatment options. This was true for seniors, Baby Boomers, and members of Generation X and Y. [286] Making the leap to using an online PHR or patient portal is the next logical step.

As healthcare management tools, PHRs and patient portals offer a variety of options that patients and providers can take advantage of and use to improve the quality of care. It is important for ACOs to examine the individual capabilities of these systems to determine what functionalities they will want to incorporate into the systems they implement.

There are four types of interactions between PHRs and patients, each of which has the potential to affect how patients will use these platforms:[287]

- ➤ PHR-to-patient interactions, in which the system interacts with individuals using automated alerts, reminders, information and education;

- ➤ Patient-to-PHR connections, which enable patients to update their records with new data;

- ➤ Patient-to-patient connections that include applications such as e-mail, social networking, and online discussion boards and support groups; and

- ➤ PHR-to-PHR connections that allow for the transfer of health information to maintain accurate and up-to-date records.

In the context of ACOs, it makes sense to combine PHRs and patient portals in a single platform that coordinates the myriad functions offered by these technologies. The capabilities of these platforms that facilitate patients' participation—and therefore responsibility—in their healthcare include:

Disease Management

➤ Decision support capabilities and tools (e.g., care guides) that allow patients to view and share in the development of care plans to help manage chronic conditions;

➤ Behavioral data entry tools can track information such as food, activity, and weight diaries. Data entered could indicate trends, trigger alerts and reminders about next steps, and alert providers so that they could intervene if appropriate;

➤ Information about clinical trials and clinical trial research tools;

➤ Pharmacy interfaces for prescription renewals;

➤ Input and integration of data from stand-alone or implanted medical devices such as pacemakers, pedometers, or glucometers;

➤ A platform for care coordination by linking patients with providers electronically via e-mail or messaging. Secure electronic communication allows for a confidential exchange of information between patient and provide[288];

➤ Chronic care reminders and alerts based on patients' health conditions and status;

➤ Tools to manage and coordinate transitions when patients leave hospitals and other health care settings; and

➤ Health information and health information search tools,

➤ Ability to connect multiple providers and family members with patients to communicate across all disciplines and among all members involved in the patient's care.[289]

Prevention

➤ Access to wellness programs and guides,

➤ Online health risk assessment tools,

➤ Health libraries, and

➤ Health news feeds.

Health Management

➤ Complete and up-to-date medical history;

➤ Smartphone and mobile applications, which will become increasingly important as devices become more sophisticated and vendors provide mobile solutions. Mobile phones could also introduce an opportunity to support behavior change through direct and customized text reminders[290];

➤ Access to health information about family members (e.g., elderly parents or children) for whom there is a designated caregiver, as well as contact information for caregivers;

➤ Information about home and work environments that affects health;

➤ Insurance information;

➤ Portability of medical information when switching health care providers, travelling, or during emergencies;

➢ Interactive communication tools that allow for messaging, appointment scheduling, and reminders;

➢ Medication (including vitamins and supplements) reconciliation between care providers;

➢ Tools to make information such as test results comprehensible to patients;

➢ Opt in/opt out capability so that both patients and physicians can control the sharing of sensitive information (e.g., mental health issues or certain test results); and

➢ Harnessing the power of peer support through the construction or ability to connect with social networks to help support behavior change.[291]

The Importance of Integration

The information contained in a PHR is most valuable if it is integrated into the clinician's electronic medical record; otherwise, it exists as isolated data with limited usefulness. A lack of integration translates into a missed opportunity to engage the patient in his or her care and creates more work for the provider. Data exchange that is automated or "pushed," to the end user is preferable to data that is "pulled" from another system.[292] This type of integration creates a seamless interface in which information is shared in a timely manner. The ideal PHR will receive health data from multiple sources and integrate the data points that are necessary to manage health.[293] This demonstrates clearly the important role of health information exchanges as our healthcare system evolves from a transaction-based reimbursement system to a value-based purchasing system. Systems will need to be integrated more fully so that care can be coordinated effectively with resulting improvements to safety and quality.

Benefits

Consumer health informatics (CHI) in the form of PHRs and patient portals can benefit providers and individual patients as well as improve public health. One of the most important benefits to these systems is greater patient access an array of credible health information, data, and knowledge. This information can be highly customized, allowing patients with chronic diseases to track their conditions in conjunction with their providers, promoting earlier interventions when a problem develops. The ongoing connection between patients and providers changes encounters from episodic to continuous, which could shorten the time it takes to address problems that may crop up.[294] It could also reduce the risk of medical errors and prevent unnecessary repetition of diagnostic tests and procedures.

Patients who are more engaged in their health are more active participants in their care, resulting in improved medication adherence, for example, or improved outcomes.[295] In this regard, PHR adoption has the potential to influence patients' behavior. This may include behaviors such as smoking cessation, regular exercise, and dietary changes that play an important role in overall health.

PHRs and patient portals also enable caregivers and family members to collaborate with healthcare providers on a loved one's care. For example, an adult child involved in an elderly parent's care could regularly and more easily communicate with his or her healthcare provider if an issue arises. This is especially important as grown children are increasingly geographically distant from their parents. It allows them to be involved in their care in a more meaningful way than would otherwise be possible.

PHRs can also benefit clinicians. Data entered into a PHR could be pushed to the provider's EHR, enabling better decision making and facilitating increased efficiency. The greater access to clinicians provided by PHRs and patient portals may also play a factor in increasing patient loyalty.

According to a report from AHRQ, "there may be a role for CHI applications to reach consumers at a low cost and obviate the need for some activities currently performed by humans."[296] Consider the following examples of providers who have demonstrated cost savings by providing their patients with PHRs:

➤ HealthPartners reported saving 63 cents every time it did not have to mail a lab result;

➤ Northshore University Health System reported saving $17 every time a billing query was handled online rather than by phone and $7 for every appointment scheduled online; and

➤ Geisinger Health System reported a 25% reduction in the number of patient visits for surgical follow-up and a reduction in 12,000 phone calls per month due to the fact that patients transacting business and getting questions answered online.[297]

The AHRQ report concluded that, "CHI applications may hold significant future promise for improving outcomes across a wide variety of diseases and health issues."[298] But these applications do more than benefit individuals; they also have the potential to improve public health by providing information and resources, promoting healthier living, strengthening the continuum of care and being a source of health monitoring data to supplement traditional public health activities. Research has shown that 75% of the US population would share personal health information with public officials to speed outbreak investigations and other public health activities.[299]

How PHRs and Portals Can Integrate to Improve Care

More than half of Medicare beneficiaries have five or more chronic conditions such as diabetes, arthritis, hypertension, and kidney disease.[300] The concept of coordinated care, which is built into the ACO model, is a boon to these patients. Involving them through online PHRs and patient portals takes coordination a step further by handing the patients tools to engage actively in their healthcare.

Consider the hypothetical case of a 45-year-old woman with hypertension who has asthma. Like many patients with comorbid conditions, she sees several physicians. All of these physicians take her blood pressure during office visits. She also owns a blood pressure cuff and periodically checks her blood pressure at home. If she were to populate a PHR with these readings, she and her physicians could easily chart trends over time and determine if periodic spikes were a cause for concern or an anomaly in an otherwise controlled condition. Populating the PHR with her medications would allow each physician easy access to her entire medication history, potentially avoiding adverse events due to contraindications. If the PHR were combined with a patient portal, she could also renew prescriptions and communicate with her pulmonologist regarding questions or concerns about her asthma care plan and track to see if, or how, her asthma is related to her blood pressure. The patient's access to all of her health information, coupled with the ability to easily communicate with her providers, could potentially empower her to take a more active role in her health, seeking out information (conveniently available on the portal) to make lifestyle changes that could positively influence her health and then tracking those changes to see their effect. As she heads into menopause, the usefulness of these functionalities increases further. In the future, the blood pressure readings she takes at home will be transmitted via Bluetooth technology directly to her PHR, a convenience that will only encourage her to monitor this condition more closely.

PHRs and Portals Are Already Successful

In reality, a number of healthcare organizations already offer PHRs and patient portals and are seeing increasing adoption rates and positive changes. Kaiser Permanente reports 35% adoption for its HealthConnect, with features that include built-in treatment guidelines, secure e-mail to doctors, and online checking of lab test results. Seattle-based Group Health Cooperative (GHC) reports more than 60% patient adoption of its patient portal, along with 29% fewer emergency visits and 6% fewer hospitalizations.[301]

My HealtheVet, the Veteran Administration's free online PHR, has features that include wellness reminders, appointment tracking, and secure messaging. As of March 2010 there were almost 1 million registered users and the site had received almost 39 million visits.

In early 2011, Norton Healthcare in Louisville, Kentucky and Humana Inc. formed an ACO that used Microsoft HealthVault® for its PHR applications. In the pilot program, patients are able to record and share health status measures, such as blood pressure and glucose levels, and have access to portions of their electronic health records.

The Cambridge Health Alliance (CHA) , a Harvard-affiliated integrated public healthcare system, launched the MyChart® patient Web portal in late 2010, enabling patients to access their medical records; review immunizations, lab results, and medications; seek medical advice; request appointments; and communicate securely online with their care team. "Enabling patients to access their health information and communicate online through MyChart is a key step in CHA's transformation," said Hilary Worthen, MD, CHA's Chief Medical Information Officer. A case example on MyChart use and application by Sentara Healthcare is provided.

Case Example: Sentara MyChart®

In 2008, Sentara Healthcare, a regional integrated delivery system comprised of 9 hospitals, 10 long-term care/assisted living centers, an extended stay hospital, the 520-provider Sentara Medical Group and a 432,600-member health plan introduced MyChart through its eCare Health Network. MyChart is a Web-based patient portal that allows patients access to their health care providers and portions of their medical records.

Patients who utilize MyChart can:

- View lab or test results;
- Renew prescriptions;
- Schedule appointments and get appointment reminders;
- Communicate with physicians and staff members;
- Manage the healthcare of a child, spouse, or parent after release forms and verification have been completed;
- Print out a wallet-sized health ID card that contains their health information;
- Utilize an online health reference library that is also linked to their medical conditions, prescriptions, and immunizations; and
- Utilize an iPhone application to access the portal.

"Patients are becoming savvier, they want to participate in their own healthcare, they're more educated, and they are starting to demand these tools," said Elise Spoto, Information Technology Director at Sentara. By 2011, MyChart had an adoption rate of about 16%, with almost 60,000 patients using it. "The more patients use it, the more they love it," said Spoto.

Some practices have adoption rates as high as 40% and the key seems to be the recommendation of the physician. "Patients like that endorsement from the doctor," said Spoto. "In fact, some providers who don't use MyChart are getting asked why they don't offer it."

Case Example: Sentara MyChart (cont.)

For Sentara, one the biggest challenges involved in implementing MyChart was the fear on the part of physicians that they would be overwhelmed with communication from patients. To address this issue, Sentara implemented a workflow that allowed the majority of messages to be handled by staff, just as phone messages were typically handled. In reality, providers are noticing more efficiency because they are not constantly interrupted by phone calls all day. Instead, they carve out time to go to their MyChart mailbox and manage messages logically. After this barrier was overcome, physician response to the system was positive.

Not surprisingly, Sentara has had to find solutions to address delicate issues that crop up with tools such as MyChart. For example, providers can attach comments explaining test results and sensitive results, such as cancer markers, that are not released through MyChart. Regarding the availability of data, Sentara created a Physician Advisory Group to determine which parts of their medical record patients can access. Interestingly, rather than wanting to opt out of including information, patients have expressed a desire to include more types of data, such as information that predates the existence of MyChart.

Right now, patients cannot self-report information on MyChart but Sentara is working toward including this function, as well as other features that will appeal to patients. Although different functionalities may appeal to different demographics, and there will always be a need to include two ways of doing things (for example, phone and e-mail), Sentara expects that, over the next few years, the overall adoption rate of MyChart will approach 40%. "MyChart allows for a truly patient-centric healthcare delivery model," said Spoto.

A second case example comes from the Howard University Hospital's Diabetes Treatment Center.

Case Example: HUH Urban Diabetes Treatment Center

The PHR initiative at Howard University Hospital's Diabetes Treatment Center shatters several myths regarding PHRs and the urban poor. There are currently 1,000 patients enrolled at the center, divided evenly into elderly patients receiving Medicare, those with commercial insurance through their employer, and those on Medicaid. In 2008, the center launched a PHR initiative creating a patient portal using NoMoreClipboard that was linked to the clinical diabetes EHR (CliniPro from NuMedics). The PHR contains features such as access to vital signs; medications; and lab results, including A1C results, which can be tracked to spot trends.

By late 2010, 26% of the center's patients used the PHR, with enrollment on the rise. Considering that PHR adoption rates nationally were about 10% in 2010, this is an astounding figure. Even more surprising is the fact that the highest adoption rates and use of the PHR were among Medicaid patients, who comprised 87% of all users. For this group of patients, which receives fragmented care from different providers, the PHR effectively serves as their "medical home." Furthermore, the PHR is proving to have clinical value. In a small group of patients using the mHealth App that sends smartphone alerts to upload glucose readings and other reminders, there have been more self-reported glucose readings, and A1C values are trending downward faster than for those using just the online PHR.[302]

Challenges

Incorporating a PHR into a healthcare organization is a major transformation that brings many challenges. First and foremost are the issues of privacy and security. Many Americans fear that data in electronic records will be used for purposes other than their healthcare, such as marketing.[303] There is an even larger concern about health information being used in a manner that could affect insurance premiums or job security. However, the American Recovery and

Reinvestment Act (ARRA) includes changes to health information privacy and security requirements under HIPAA that may allay some of these fears. The HITECH Act expands HIPAA to include business associates, such as entities contracted to provide PHRs. These entities are directly responsible for compliance with the safeguards, policies and procedure requirements of the Security Rule and are subject to penalties if they do not comply. Entities using electronic health records are required to provide a full accounting of disclosures of a patient's personal health information upon request. As more and more protected health information is maintained and shared in an electronic manner, healthcare organizations will have to become very proficient in the use of best practice information security and privacy practices, something that has not necessarily been at the forefront of healthcare spending plans.

Beyond security issues, other barriers stand in the way of patients using this technology. Not everyone has Internet access or has the computer literacy and skills required to use a PHR. That such platforms should be designed with user friendliness at the forefront is a given. But PHRs also face the challenge of patients having to input data initially from various sources. Furthermore, the value of data that is input by patients is questionable, because patients are not always truthful about health issues, especially if those issues reflect on their behavior (e.g., weight, smoking, or alcohol consumption). A PHR can only be as good as the information that is put into it.

Likewise, staff members may also need to be convinced of the value of PHRs and patient portals. They may fear that such platforms will mean an increased workload, such as for example an unmanageable amount of e-mail messages. Another challenge is the source of the information contained in a PHR. Will a healthcare organization accept the patient's assessment that he or she has an allergy, or will it require some other form of documentation? How is the data in the PHR updated, and how is it shared across the ACO? These questions and others need to be considered in planning for implementation of a PHR.

ACOs will also need to drive through the obstacle of interoperability in order to adopt PHR technology. All of the different members will need to be able to push and pull information from a patient's PHR. For example, the Continuity of Care Document (CCD) is an important component that should be incorporated into the PHR automatically. One of the greatest challenges may be ensuring that patients keep their health information up-to-date in their PHRs and are accountable for using them to manage their health.

Utilization of PHRs by ACO beneficiaries faces other barriers as well. Automated data entry, inability to allow for back entry of old data, and lack of adequate user customization could significantly affect the ease with which these systems are adopted.[304] Healthcare organizations will need to ensure that they will be able to quickly address issues if the system is not working properly.

Developing, implementing and maintaining PHRs and patient portals in ACOs is a costly undertaking that is likely to be born by the ACO. One of the reasons PHR adoption rates have been low is that consumers are not willing to pay for them. However, if these tools are being provided by the ACO, patients may be more likely to use them. For the ACO, it will be necessary to carefully evaluate vendor offerings and customize them to meet their needs. While considerable, the cost may be offset by reductions in administrative fees, improved patient satisfaction, and improved health management. In the end, the cost of providing this technology is an expense ACOs will ultimately have to assume if they want to remain competitive and meet the quality standards that are required of them.

Mobile Health Applications (mHealth)

Mobile health applications (mHealth) are another example of patient-centered tools that will be employed in an accountable care model. One in five mobile phone owners today owns a smartphone,[305] a trend that is on the rise as consumers increasingly use these devices as handheld computers. Not surprisingly, the number of consumer smartphone applications (apps) that were downloaded went from 300 million in 2009 to five billion in 2010.[306] With mobile devices outnumbering personal computers,[307] we are approaching the point where they will be the most common way to access data.

For healthcare, the explosion of the smartphone market is an unprecedented opportunity. More than 200 million mHealth apps are in use today, and that number is expected to increase threefold by 2012.[308] Worldwide, 70% of people are interested in having access to at least one mHealth app.[309] According to the Global Mobile Health Market Report 2010-2015, smartphone applications will enable the healthcare industry to reach out to 500 million users in 2015.[310]

The remainder of this chapter discusses what is driving the mHealth industry, strategies that healthcare organizations are employing to reach consumers, and developing best practices for apps that can be used across various devices and that appeal to consumers.

Top Drivers for mHealth Apps

Most health consumers regularly seek health information online, so it makes sense that they are turning to their smartphones for their health questions and needs. Health care organizations have an advantage here, because they are already a trusted source of information. While patients may not be doing in-depth research on their mobile devices, they are looking for action-oriented information, according to Scott Eising, Director of Product Management for Mayo Clinic Internet Services.[311] As discussed previously, many healthcare organizations already have personal health records and/or patient portals that can easily be adapted to smartphone technology.

ACOs will increasingly want to connect more directly with patients as a means of providing efficient, high-quality care. With features such as mobile scheduling, the ability to check wait times in offices and emergency rooms, and mobile prescription refills, mHealth apps make it easy for patients to interact with healthcare providers.

Beyond the ability to connect, mHealth apps make it easy for patients to do business with healthcare providers. In today's world, people will pay money to buy back their own time. Just as innovations such as E-ZPass let customers save time and get where they are going faster, mHealth apps have the potential to provide faster, more efficient healthcare.

Mobile health apps offer the opportunity to:

➤ Build brand equity through frequent contact,

➤ Increase consumer loyalty by providing a broader range of services,

➢ Improve customer service through the range of options available to patients,

➢ Drive differentiation by providing a competitive advantage,

➢ Improve customer service through an array of options to serve patients, and

➢ Increase the availability and access to healthcare so patients can take ownership of their data and have increased responsibility for their own health.[312]

Smartphones have advantages over other information and communication technologies, including portability, continuous uninterrupted data stream, and the capability to support multimedia software applications.[313] With the potential to provide cost-efficient care delivery to patients and improve health outcomes, the value proposition for mHealth is strong.[314]

Healthcare providers are getting into the mHealth apps market. Consumers demand it. Providers who have mobile apps give patients back their own time and have a better chance of becoming providers of choice.

mHealth Strategies for Improving Care

A number of strategies are being employed by healthcare organizations to involve patients in their care through mHealth apps. They are aimed at providing patients with the tools to manage their health with the goal of improving it.

Chronic Disease Management

For patients with chronic health conditions such as asthma, diabetes, or heart disease, sound health management involves making good health "micro decisions" every day.[315] Smartphone apps facilitate this process when and where decisions are made. This can prevent situations from escalating to the point where more costly and time-consuming interventions are required. Apps that track asthma flare-ups or blood glucose, for example, let patients know their health status without an office or hospital visit. Or, if a patient with chronic obstructive pulmonary disease (COPD) experiences a sudden weight gain, for example, an app that tracks that information and communicates it to the physician can raise a red flag that allows measures to be taken before the patient's health deteriorates to the point that he or she has to be hospitalized.

Some apps connect patients with caregivers on a continuous basis. Examples of sensor technologies that can be combined with smartphones to track health measurements and monitor patients with chronic conditions include:

➤ Peak flow meters and pulse oximeters for respiratory conditions,

➤ Digital blood pressure monitors for hypertensive patients, and

➤ Glucometers to measure blood glucose for those with diabetes.

PHR Applications

As previously mentioned, the majority of the public believes that using an online PHR would provide major benefits to managing healthcare services. Two out of three members of the public and doctors agree that patients should have the option to view and download their personal health information online.[316] Use of personal health records has been slow to take off but is on the rise. Coupled with the proliferation of smartphones, this means that patients increasingly expect this option to be available and are more likely to utilize it. The ability to schedule appointments, communicate with providers, view test results, and request prescription refills meshes perfectly with the trend toward using a smartphone to manage many aspects of one's life. Furthermore, many hospitals already have online PHRs and patient portals that can be converted easily to smartphone platforms.

Behavioral Change

Consumers are already using apps to track and manage their behavior and there is no reason why healthcare providers should not benefit from this trend. Apps that help patients adhere to treatment regimens, offer diet assistance, or track exercise have the potential to help keep patients healthy and to prevent disease.

Health Information

Providing health information is another strategy that echoes the online presence maintained by many hospitals. Apps that provide health news and information coupled with other functionality have the potential to attract consumers and increase their loyalty. For example, Mayo Clinic's Symptom Checker lets users search MayoClinic.com for more information about thousands of health topics and provides access to information about care at Mayo Clinic.

Remote Monitoring

One of the key factors that is expected to contribute to the growth of mHealth apps is the increase in remote patient monitoring devices. The market for wearable devices will exceed 100 million units annually by 2016, driven by devices for both consumer and clinical settings.[317] In 2009, nearly 50,000 blood pressure monitors were used in telehealth apps, and this is expected to hit 500,000 by 2013. In addition, global shipments of home digital blood glucose meters, blood pressure monitors, weight scales, pulse oximeters and peak flow meters used in mHealth apps will grow to more than 1.6 million, according to a 2010 InMedical Report.[318] Providers that offer remote monitoring linked to a smartphone app will offer a valuable service to their patients that will also give them a competitive edge.

Hospitals Using Apps to Connect With Patients

➢ Southcoast Hospitals Group has an iPhone app that helps patients keep track of their medications, find a physician and stay connected with news and events;

➢ Akron Children's Hospital's Care4Kids app offers general health and hospital information, as well as allowing parents to store their family's medical history;

➢ DMC Children's Hospital of Michigan developed an app that answers common pediatric health-related questions and provides a child safety checklist; and

➢ Mayo Clinic's Meditation, based on the research of Amit Sood, MD, helps patients use the mind-body connection to stay healthy, while its Symptom Checker helps patients manage acute problems and provides guidance on practicing self-care at home.

Best Practices for mHealth Apps

Providers should keep the consumer in mind when designing mHealth apps to ensure ease of use. Tech-savvy professionals build many of these apps, so providers should make sure that they are conceived from a patient-centric perspective. If properly designed, mHealth apps will be targeted to those who want to engage in managing their health. For example, apps for chronically ill patients need to be designed so they will be easily used in the already complicated lives of these individuals and their caregivers.[319] "A badly designed application is like a badly designed Web site," said Sai Chanderraju, General Manager for Products at iSpace, a leading developer of mHealth applications. Optimizing the user experience is paramount to launching an app that people will come back to again and again.

Designing an mHealth app can be a complex undertaking, but there are a few characteristics that providers should always keep in mind.

Make It Broad

mHealth apps can range from low complexity to high and can be used in SMS/Text, browser-based, mobile websites, or on devices. SMS/Text has simple functionality and ubiquitous access, while Mobile Web presents standardization issues. On-device applications are more complicated to develop but offer a sharper interface and better graphics. Providers should consider developing solutions in all three areas.

Make It Simple

In terms of optimizing the user experience, the fewer clicks the better. Users should be able to get where they want to go quickly and easily.

Consider the features patients most want to use and include those. After patients are using the app, they can always go to the Web site for more in-depth information and features. The key is to attract them with an easy-to-use interface.

Make It Useful

Consider the features that patients will be most interested in while they are on the go. For example, the ability to schedule or change appointments and locate provider facilities is a useful feature for patients while they are out and about. Additional options, such as a GPS feature that provides directions from the user's current location, can be a bonus. According to Sentara's Bert Reese, the best way to determine what features will be appealing is to crowd source—bring patients and employees together and ask them what features to include or change to add value. If an idea fits in with the value proposition, then it is worth pursuing.

Make It Unique

Smartphone apps are an opportunity to differentiate from other providers. Providers should consider functionality that no one else is offering to make it more appealing for patients to do business with them.

Make It Easy

Developing mHealth apps can be challenging because they need to be usable on different platforms, such as Android, IOS, or Windows. Solutions should be able to be delivered simultaneously via SMS/Text, Mobile Web, and on-device. Furthermore, new smartphones are coming to the market quickly, and it is difficult to keep pace. The fact that an app works on one device does not mean it will work on all of them. Providers who cater to one platform will be leaving potential consumers behind. Vendors must devise methods of overcoming this obstacle without compromising value or ease of use.

A case example on mobile application development comes from Cancer Care of Ontario.

Case Example: Mobile Application Development for Cancer Care

Cancer Care Ontario (CCO) is the agency of the Provincial Government of Ontario responsible for managing cancer and other chronic diseases for the Province of Ontario. Ontario is about the size of the US state of Texas, with a population of 13 million, more than150 hospitals, and more than 14,000 active physicians. Managing a chronic disease like cancer, across such a population and geography, and across the continuum of care, from prevention to screening, diagnosis, treatment, recovery, and/or end of life is a daunting challenge. To be at all successful requires accurate, timely, and tailored information, distributed to patients and providers in a useful and actionable manner.

CCO has relied heavily on traditional means of communicating best practices, guidelines, and clinical evidence, through a large and representative network of clinicians that meets regularly and communicates amongst members even more frequently. In recent years, the CCO Web site has served as an additional means of communications, hosting almost all guidelines, evidence and provider- and patient-relevant information available from CCO. However, a meeting, an e-mail, or even access to a Web site is not the most efficient means of equipping patients or providers with information they need at the moment, wherever they happen to be. So, beginning in 2010, CCO began to think about the use of mobile applications to improve communications with patients and providers.

As in any new endeavor, it took a while for CCO to determine an appropriate first use of mobile technology and to develop the internal capability to create, publish, and distribute a mobile application. The agency undertook both tasks simultaneously, believing that when the clinicians decided on an appropriate use for a first mobile application, they would not want to wait to see it. After shopping around many ideas and soliciting even more from customers, CCO decided to take a set of guidelines for assessing the clinical status of palliative care patients (previously developed by CCO and widely agreed to in the clinical community) and make it into a mobile application. These guidelines use a patient's self-assessed symptoms (using a score based on the Edmonton Symptom Assessment System) and provide clinicians with pharmacological and nonpharmacological symptom management information required to support clinical decision making, leading to the best possible symptom control for patients.

Case Example: Mobile Application Development for Cancer Care (cont.)

By starting with content, the agency already had, without involving patient information, and making it available much more conveniently than from the Web site, CCO thought these guidelines would be a quick win for its first foray into application development. While deciding on the first "app," CCO also set about building the capability to produce it. The organization first found a manager with mobile application experience and assisted him in building a team, cross training some existing development staff members, and supplementing the team with contracted resources when necessary.

When CCO's mobile development team was in place, developers and clinicians joined forces to create workflows of each guideline and to test the user experience to ensure that this application would be intuitive for healthcare providers and easy to use while interacting with the patient at the time of care.

The first app was created for the iPhone, initially, and then ported to Windows Phone 7. The developers had intended to also make it available on Blackberry, but could not find the expertise nor the methodology to do so. The short timeline to develop the "app", and its rapid adoption amazed everyone. After only 2 months of development and signing up with the various apps stores, they had the "Symptom Management Guidelines Application" was published; within 1 month, the app had hundreds of downloads and, within 4 months, more than a thousand, from countries all over the globe. CCO now has a number of additional apps: a drug formulary application available for both patients and providers to act as an information resource on systemic cancer treatment and symptom management, and, an internally focused news application for CCO staff to keep informed of organizational-wide technology developments.

Case Example: Mobile Application Development for Cancer Care (cont.)

CCO also recognized that download rat" was not an in-depth enough metric to determine if the applications were truly being utilized by the target audiences, so the development team embedded analytics into the application to measure true usage data, for example, length of time spent in the application. These analytics will help to inform future app development at CCO.

These numbers show that healthcare providers are demanding the same information as consumers across all industries: multiple channels of delivery, instantaneous access to information, and without the constraints of a wired piece of equipment. "We are now convinced, and have the evidence to prove it, that mobile applications are an effective, secure, and responsive method of delivering information to patients and providers in healthcare," said Rick Skinner, CIO of Cancer Care Ontario.

An increasing number of patients are using mHealth apps on their smartphones to manage their health. As a trusted source of information, healthcare providers can take advantage of this opportunity to connect with patients. Apps that help patients manage chronic diseases, update their health records, institute behavioral change, find health information, and connect to remote monitoring devices have the potential to improve health outcomes, reduce costs, and help differentiate providers from the competition. Providers should aim to develop easy-to-use apps that can be extended across a variety of devices and platforms and offer functionality that patients can use on a regular basis. In many cases, mHealth apps can become an extension of the Web presence already established by providers.

Bridging the Divide

PHRs, patient portals, and mHealth apps can play an important role in the success of ACOs and are necessary components of their IT infrastructure. Healthcare organizations should expect a slow and growing adoption period before these tools are widely utilized by their patients. Bundling PHRs, portals, and mHealth applications together could drive adoption as ACOs strive to offer their patients an increasing array of services and options. Customization and interoperability are key aspects that will determine success and ensure that these platforms work well with other IT platforms required by ACOs.

Chapter 9: Takeaways

✓ Patient accountability is a critical success factor for the ACO model.

✓ Providers must give patients the tools necessary for them to manage their own care and assume a higher degree of accountability.

✓ A personal health record is an electronic record of health-related information on an individual that conforms to nationally recognized interoperability standards and can be drawn from multiple sources while being managed, shared, and controlled by the individual.

✓ Patient portals are Web-based platforms created and maintained by healthcare organizations that allow patients to access portions of their EHRs and communicate with their health care providers.

✓ It is likely that personal health records will be required in upcoming stages of Meaningful Use.

✓ For ACOs, a provider-linked model makes the most sense to avoid the "data island" scenario.

✓ It makes the most sense to combine PHRs, patient portals and mHealth applications in a single platform that coordinates the myriad functions offered by these technologies.

✓ The information contained in a PHR is most valuable when integrated into the clinician's EMR.

✓ With more than 200 million total applications in use today, the number of mHealth apps is also increasing rapidly.

✓ Best practices for mHealth apps include: make it broad, make it simple, make it useful, make it unique and make it easy.

268 US Department of Health and Human Services. Press Release. Affordable Care Act to improve quality of care for people with Medicare. March 31, 2011. Accessed online April 5, 2011, at http://www.hhs.gov/news/press/2011pres/03/20110331a.html.

269 US Department of Health and Human Services. Accountable Care Organizations: Improving care coordination for people with Medicare. March 31, 2011. Accessed online April 1, 2011, at http://www.healthcare.gov/news/factsheets/accountablecare03312011a.html.

270 Markle Foundation. Survey finds Americans want electronic personal health information to improve own health care. November 1, 2006. Accessed online April 5, 2011, at http://www.markle.org/sites/default/files/research_doc_120706.pdf.

271 Markle Foundation. Americans overwhelmingly believe electronic personal health records. June 1, 2008. Accessed online April 6, 2011, at http://www.markle.org/publications/401-americans-overwhelmingly-believe-electronic-personal-health-records-could-improve-t.

272 Konschak C, Jarrell LP. Personal Health Records. In: *Consumer-Centric Healthcare Opportunities and Challenges for Providers*. Chicago, IL: Health Administration Press; 2011:66.

273 Deloitte Center for Health Solutions. 2010 US healthcare consumerism survey. Accessed online April 6, 2011, at http://www.deloitte.com/view/en_US/us/Insights/centers/center-for-health-solutions/consumerism/2010-survey-health-consumers/index.htm?id=USGoogle%20Consumerism%20_HC_510&gclid=CO6Premo 3qECFYNd5Qod9DjKIw.

274 Wynia MK, Torres MK, Lemieux J. Many physicians are willing to use patients' electronic personal health records, but doctors differ by location, gender and practice. *Health Aff (Millwood)*. 2011 Feb;30(2):266-273.

275 Gibbons MC, Wilson RF, Samal L, Lehman CU, Dickersin K, Lehmann HP, Aboumatar H, Finkelstein J, Shelton E, Sharma R, Bass EB. Impact of consumer health informatics applications. *Evid Rep Technol Assess (Full Rep)*. 2009 Oct;(188):1-546. Review.

276 Deloitte Center for Health Solutions. 2010.

277 Kaiser Permanente Press Release. Kaiser Permanente honored for electronic health record implementation: HIMSS Analytics awards another 11 Kaiser Permanente hospitals. EMR and EHR News; February 22, 2011. Accessed May 5, 2011, at http://xnet.kp.org/newscenter/pressreleases/nat/2011/022211stage7.html.

278 Markle Foundation. Survey. The Public and Doctors Largely Agree Patients Should Be Able To View, Download and Share Their Health Info. January 31, 2011. Accessed April 6, 2011, at http://www.markle.org/publications/1460-public-and-doctors-largely-agree-patients-should-be-able-view-download-and-share-t.

279 Deloitte Center for Health Solutions. 2010.

280 Campbell S. Kaiser Permanente survey shows seniors embrace Internet to manage their health. *EMR Daily News*. July 14, 2009. Accessed online May 10, 2011, at

http://emrdailynews.com/2009/07/14/kaiser-permanente-survey-shows-seniors-embrace-internet-to-manage-their-health/.

281 Konschak C, Jarrell LP. 2011.

282 Miller HD, Yasnoff WA, Burde HA. *Personal Health Records The Essential Missing Element in 21st Century Healthcare*. Chicago, IL: Healthcare Information and Management Systems Society; 2009.

283 Defining key health information technology terms. The National Alliance for Health Information Technology Report to the Office of the National Coordinator for Health Information Technology; April 2008:19.

284 Markle Foundation. Connecting for health: the personal health working group final report. July 1, 2003. Accessed online May 10, 2011, at http://www.providersedge.com/ehdocs/ehr_articles/The_Personal_Health_Working_Group_Final_Report.pdf.

285 Konschak C, Jarrell LP. 2011.

286 Deloitte Center for Health Solutions. 2010.

287 Kahn JS, Aulakh V, Bosworth A. What It Takes: Characteristics of the Ideal Personal Health Record. *Health Aff (Millwood)*. 2009 Mar-Apr;28(2):369-376.

288 Nace DK, Jenrette JE, White A. Creating value: Better health IT. In: *Better to Best: Value-Driving Elements of the Patient Centered Medical Home and Accountable Care Organizations*. Vienna, VA: Health2Resources; March 2011:28-34. Accessed online August 1, 2012, at http://www.pcpcc.net/guide/better_to_best.

289 Nace DK, Jenrette JE, White A. 2011.

290 Kahn JS, Aulakh V, Bosworth A. 2009.

291 Kahn JS, Aulakh V, Bosworth A. 2009.

292 Miller HD, Yasnoff WA, Burde HA. 2009.

293 Kahn JS, Aulakh V, Bosworth A. 2009.

294 Tang PC, Ash JS, Bates DW, Overhage JM, Sands DZ. Personal health records: dDefinitions, benefits, and strategies for overcoming barriers to adoption. *J Am Med Inform Assoc*. 2006 Mar-Apr;13(2):121-126.

295 Tang PC, et al. 2006.

296 Gibbons MC, et al. 2009.

297 Gardner E. Will patient portals open the door to better care? *Health Data Management Magazine*. March 1, 2010. Accessed online May 10, 2011, at http://www.healthdatamanagement.com/issues/18_3/will-patient-portals-open-the-door-to-better-care-39853-1.html.

298 Gibbons MC, et al. 2009.

299 Bonander J, Gates S. Public health in an era of personal health records: opportunities for innovation and new partnerships. *J Med Internet Res*. 2010 Aug 10;12(3):e33.

300 US Department of Health and Human Services. Fact Sheet. Accountable Care Organizations: Improving care coordination for people with Medicare. March 31, 2011.

301 Reid RJ, Coleman K, Johnson EA, Fishman PA, Hsu C, Soman MP, Trescott CE, Erikson M, Larson EB. The group health medical home at year 2: cost savings, higher patient satisfaction, and less burnout for providers. *Health Aff (Millwood)*. 2010 May;29(5):835-843.

302 Moore J. Smashing myths and assumptions: PHR for urban diabetes care. Chilmark Research; November 10, 2010. Accessed online June 15, 2011, at http://chilmarkresearch.com/2010/11/12/smashing-myths-assumptions-phr-for-urban-diabetes-care/.

303 Miller HD, Yasnoff WA, Burde HA. 2009.

304 Agency for healthcare Research and Quality. Impact of consumer health informatics applications. Evidence Report/Technology Assessment Number 188; 2009.

305 Mobile Marketing Association. Press Release. One in five US consumers now using mobile commerce. *PRNewswire*, May 19, 2011. Accessed online September 1, 2011, at http://www.prnewswire.com/news-releases/one-in-five-us-adult-consumers-now-using-mobile-commerce-94244549.html.

306 Boulos MNK, Wheeler S, Tavares C, Jones R. How smartphones are changing the face of mobile and participatory healthcare: an overview, with an example from eCAALYX. *Biomed Eng Online*. 2011;10:24. Accessed online September 1, 2011, at http://www.biomedical-engineering-online.com/content/10/1/24.

307 Ingram M. Mary Meeker: Mobile Internet will soon overtake fixed Internet. *GigaOM*. April 12, 2010. Accessed online September 1, 2011, at http://gigaom.com/2010/04/12/mary-meeker-mobile-internet-will-soon-overtake-fixed-internet/.

308 Merrill M. mHealth apps forecast to increase threefold by 2012. *Healthcare ITNews*, December 30, 2010. Accessed online September 1, 2011, at http://www.healthcareitnews.com/news/mhealth-apps-forecast-increase-threefold-2012.

309 Merrill M. 2011.

310 Mikalajunaite E. 500m people will be using healthcare mobile applications in 2015. *Research2guidance*. November 10, 2010. Accessed online September 1, 2011 at http://www.research2guidance.com/500m-people-will-be-using-healthcare-mobile-applications-in-2015/.

311 Sarasohn-Kahn J. How smartphones are changing health care for consumers and providers. *California HealthCare Foundation*. April 2010.

312 Merrill M. 2011.

313 Boulos MNK, Wheeler S, Tavares C, Jones R. 2011.

314 Merrill M. 2011.

315 Sarasohn-Kahn J. 2010.

[316] Gullo C. Ten predictions for the mobile health market. *MobileHealthNews*. August 26, 2011. Accessed online September 2, 2011, at http://mobihealthnews.com/12751/ten-predictions-for-the-mobile-health-market/.

[317] Markle Foundation. Americans overwhelmingly believe electronic personal health records could improve their health. June 1, 2008.

[318] Gullo C. 2011.

[319] Gullo C. 2011.

Chapter 10. Comparative Effectiveness Research

Ken Yale, DDS, JD

We need to take medicine from empirical to evidence-based, and not just broad guidelines, but patient-specific medicine.

Janet Woodcock, MD,
Director, Food and Drug Administration (FDA),
Center for Drug Evaluation and Research (CDER)

This comment by the FDA/CDER Director symbolizes the challenge faced by the medical establishment in translating research into medical practice. This author recalls sitting at dinner with his father, a medical science researcher at the National Institutes of Health in Bethesda, Maryland, and being fascinated by stories of cutting-edge research being performed by world-renown scientists. When asked how soon the research findings would make it to the shelves of the local Peoples Drug Store, it was always perplexing to hear "that takes 17 years or more." That was 40 years ago. Curiously, today when asked how long it takes for bench science findings to become medical reality, the answer is still 17 years. Has nothing changed in the past 4 decades? Actually, much has changed, and change is accelerating with health information technologies that promise a revolution in medical practice that will evolve comparative effectiveness research from the exclusive realm of bench science research into popular science and culture.

Comparative effectiveness research (CER) evaluates different medical therapies to determine what works best in healthcare.[320] Until now CER has been relegated to large corporations (mainly health insurance and pharmaceutical companies) who could afford the enormous cost or bench science researchers who had the patience to wait for lengthy and expensive randomized, controlled clinical trials. With the advent of health reforms fomented by the Affordable Care Act, the field of comparative effectiveness research is morphing. Led by demand from nontraditional users (value-based suppliers such as accountable care organizations), and fueled by increasingly sophisticated technology tools, CER is being pushed into innovative territory where quick results are more important than perfect experimental design.

Health information technology plays a significant role in this new environment. In fact, government policy makers and legislators recognize the link between greater availability of data through health information technology and potential improvements in CER.[321] Various technology tools are needed to conduct CER, including technology for sharing data sets that will be transformed into value-adding knowledge in the research infrastructure.[322] To meet the needs of CER proposed by the federal government, significant resources will be needed, including the use of EHRs and other clinical databases to compile source data and information for CER studies and evidence compilation.[323]

So how is CER evolving in this new environment? We will explore that issue in this chapter. Provider-based organizations accountable or at-risk for a population of patients are increasingly asking which treatments are more effective and efficient. CER answers these questions, but traditional CER using expensive randomized controlled trials cannot provide answers in a timely fashion. To meet the growing demand there are other methods to identify effective treatments such as use of evidence-based medicine, enhanced by current medical research, to develop best practice protocols. Gaps in care may be identified and corrected when clinical practice is compared to these best practice protocols. This application of evidence-based medicine is one of the practical results of medical research and is widely used to identify what works best and to improve the quality and affordability of care.

Who performs CER, how the research is conducted, and the use of the results are questions being answered as the field of CER grows in visibility and importance. In addition, established methodologies comparing present physician practices to evidence-based medicine and identifying gaps in care will expand as providers become more accountable for care and seek out best practices.

Introduction

CER generally refers to any work that compares different medical devices, drugs, and treatment methods to determine which are more effective in treating a disease or condition. Essentially, CER attempts to determine "what works best" in healthcare by comparing different therapies meant to treat the same disease or condition.[324] There is an established medical research infrastructure, and a growing part of that infrastructure looks at the relative effectiveness of different treatments. The field of CER is receiving additional attention with the burgeoning availability of new medical technologies, increasing cost of healthcare, shift to value-base purchasing, growing risk and accountability at the hospital and physician level, with resulting demand for information on what works best. Practical application of comparative effectiveness research includes use of evidence-based medicine, best-practice protocols, and patient-centered outcomes. In this environment, patient preferences and preferred outcomes are increasingly important considerations.

The term "comparative effectiveness research" encompasses a wide range of activities and is almost as diverse as the universe of medical therapies being studied.[325] Payers, consumers, patients, providers, and other caregivers are increasingly interested in technologies that provide the greatest value. Value may be defined as the technologies, medicines, or treatment techniques that are most effective at treating diseases and disorders and that provide the greatest benefits while causing the least clinical harm, at the lowest economic cost. With reforms in the finance and delivery of healthcare, and with perspectives brought by such new players as the Patient-Centered Outcomes Research Institute, the field of comparative effectiveness is evolving and becoming increasingly important.

Comparative effectiveness may examine relative clinical benefits or harms (therapeutic effectiveness), may include discovery of relative cost-effectiveness, and increasingly is focused on patient preference. There is ongoing debate among industry observers and policy makers as to whether cost-effectiveness should be included when comparing different treatments, especially for government-funded research—in part, because of concerns about restricting the availability of costly treatments that benefit only a subpopulation or have marginal benefits over existing treatments. Restrictions on services with marginal clinical benefits and higher costs may satisfy government budget examiners, but clinicians and patients who see some benefit might object. There seems to be a general consensus among health services researchers about the importance of pursuing clinical comparative effectiveness, while leaving cost considerations to those in government and the private sector responsible for making decisions on how best to finance care.[326] As new models of care delivery shift risk to hospitals and physicians (such as clinically integrated networks and accountable care organizations), their interest in CER is increasing, as knowledge about the benefits and drawbacks of specific treatment options are needed to deliver quality care at an affordable cost. CER is a critical component of these models, which require performance evaluation based on quality and cost and directly impact reimbursement and compensation.

Clinical efficacy is sometimes confused with comparative effectiveness, but they are different activities with different purposes. Efficacy, according to the FDA, is a measure of whether a device or drug works better than doing nothing. Efficacy is usually determined through tightly structured and controlled clinical trials that compare a new drug or device to a placebo, although, in some situations, comparison may be made to existing treatments (such as pre-market notification for certain medical devices). Comparison to a placebo is a low threshold to meet and is not intended to compare different medical therapies that treat the same disease or condition. The FDA also weighs clinical benefits and risks of a new drug or device to determine its safety. After safety and efficacy must be proven before a drug or device is allowed by the FDA to be marketed and made available to the public.[327] Once safety and efficacy are established to the satisfaction of the FDA, the drug or device may be marketed to the public, even if the long-term effects of the treatment are unknown. This is a potentially fertile area for CER studies that can follow treatments after they are marketed, especially by using such health information technologies as EHR, and identify side effects, effectiveness, or off-label uses not evident in the narrowly focused clinical trials used for FDA approval.

ARRA and the Affordable Care Act created new CER programs with substantial increases in funding. Different approaches to CER, the wide range of activities related to comparative effectiveness, and confusion between efficacy and cost-effectiveness led Congress in the ARRA to request greater definition of CER. The IOM Committee on Comparative Effectiveness Research Prioritization, convened at the request of Congress, defined comparative effectiveness research as

> ...the generation and synthesis of evidence that compares the benefits and harms of alternative methods to prevent, diagnose, treat, and monitor a clinical condition or to improve the delivery of care. The purpose of CER is to assist consumers, clinicians, purchasers, and policy makers to make informed decisions that will improve health care at both the individual and population levels.[328]

It is not insignificant that this definition of CER adopted by the IOM does not specifically mention cost-effectiveness, because of the sensitivities of focusing on cost at the expense of quality.[329] Moreover, legislation increasing federal government funding has specifically mandated that findings of federally funded research cannot be used for coverage decisions.[330] It remains to be seen how long federally funded CER can be kept separate from economic effectiveness considerations in federal government healthcare programs (e.g., Medicare and Medicaid). In addition, the IOM definition favors applied research, rather than basic research. This emphasis reflects Congressional interest in care delivery and wide dissemination of research findings that could directly inform consumer and provider clinical decision making.[331]

Because of the lack of emphasis on cost-effectiveness, government-funded CER initiatives may not be immediately useful to new provider care models that focus on the financial impact of clinical actions, such as clinically integrated networks (CINs) and ACOs. All CER research findings, however, can help increase the body of knowledge of evidence-based medicine, improve best practice protocols and quality, and be used to strengthen clinical decision support for physician and patient benefit. It is unlikely that an individual hospital or physician will have the resources necessary to conduct research that compares different medical therapies. Nevertheless, new and more accountable provider organizations will make decisions on appropriate care and look to reduce inappropriate care. As the ACO and CIN models evolve and these organizations gradually assume greater degrees of risk (essentially operating more like health insurance payers), they may become more involved in medical coverage decisions, benefit design, and appeals of decisions about care provided. These decisions require an understanding of both therapeutic effectiveness and cost-effectiveness. Fortunately, there is a large body of work in this field and other organizations have developed evidence-based medical protocols and clinical decision support tools useful to ACOs and CINs as they face these decisions.[332]

History of Comparative Effectiveness Research

A wide range of organizations and individuals, for many different reasons, has performed research into the comparative effectiveness of medical drugs, devices, and treatment methodologies.[333] Life science companies (manufacturers of drugs and medical devices), health plans, healthcare providers, and other private sector organizations perform a variety of CER-related programs. Independent, private organizations have also been established to organize, support, or conduct such research.[334] Governments may compare different treatments for a variety of purposes, including basic scientific research to increase knowledge, identify the highest-value product or service (best outcome and quality for the cost) for government reimbursement or fulfill legislative fiat. Increasingly, federal government policy makers are looking to patients as the ultimate judges of value and to patients' preferences as an important consideration in comparative effectiveness research.

Research into comparative effectiveness in the United States has been limited for a number of reasons. First, research is expensive to conduct, especially randomized, controlled trials that are believed to be more accurate and valid. An organization would have to see a return or benefit for the investment made, such as a manufacturer of a drug or device who may benefit directly from a study's positive findings. If an organization does benefit—or worse, if the results show harm—the results may be proprietary and kept confidential, limiting the value to society of such research. Second, after results of CER are in the public domain, they may benefit other organizations that did not pay for the research and eliminate any return on the investment anticipated by the organization originally funding the research. Furthermore, advances in healthcare may cause the technology or medicine being researched to become obsolete before effectiveness can be compared or established, especially for more costly but potentially more valid research methodologies that take years to complete. For these and other reasons, CER is thought to be a public good, requiring government funding.[335]

The federal government has conducted CER but only sporadically. The National Center for Health Care Technology was created in 1978 to research and compare healthcare technologies. It evaluated a number of technologies and made coverage recommendations to the Medicare program, but it was controversial and no longer received funding after 1981. At the same time, the Congressional Office of Technology Assessment evaluated the costs and benefits of a variety of technologies but lost funding in 1995.[336]

As of 2011, a number of federal government agencies support or perform some form of CER, including the Agency for Healthcare Research and Quality (AHRQ), National Institutes of Health (NIH), CMS, FDA, Centers for Disease Control and Prevention (CDC), Department of Defense (DOD), and Department of Veterans Affairs (VA). Each agency has its own legislative requirements for conducting research, which are usually tied to its core mission.[337] For example, the VA compares various treatment options for recipients of Veterans Health Affairs services. This program helps ensure that veterans receive proper treatments that are cost-effective and within budget limits. The NIH has a broad mandate to fund basic research and has occasionally sponsored research to compare treatments. CMS has funded research comparing different treatments but usually to determine clinical effectiveness or whether to pay the same amount for two different treatments. It is outside the legislative authority of CMS to look at cost-effectiveness. A vast number of activities and resources are available from the federal government related to comparative effectiveness.[338]

ARRA increased total CER funding for federal government agencies by an additional $1.1 billion. The funding was divided among AHRQ ($300 million), NIH ($400 million), and the Office of the Secretary of DHHS ($500 million). The amount given to the Office of the Secretary of DHHS is discretionary funding that can be used for a variety of comparative effectiveness programs. The ARRA funds were targeted to CER within the government (intramural) or outside government (extramural). In addition, $268 million of the funds were required to be used to encourage development and use of "clinical registries, clinical data networks, and other forms of electronic health data that can be used to generate or obtain outcomes data." This financial support to develop and use health information technology to generate and capture data in CER programs demonstrates the importance of new technologies to the future of CER and the importance of coordinating with other government health information technology programs.[339] ARRA also funded the IOM to consult with stakeholders and report on priorities for comparative effectiveness research.[340]

AHRQ has the broadest mandate for comparative effectiveness studies; however, until 2009, only $15 million of the entire $300 million AHRQ budget was targeted to programs related to comparative effectiveness. Before 2009, AHRQ had run a national clearinghouse for medical guidelines, helped fund a number of "evidence-based practice centers," sponsored an "Effective Health Care" program, and funded private sector research. ARRA's funding increase to AHRQ doubled the entire AHRQ annual budget, thereby, strengthening substantially its emphasis on CER. Programs created or expanded by the new funding include "horizon scanning" for new and emerging issues: synthesis of evidence to compare effectiveness of medical treatments; identification of gaps in research; translation and dissemination of CER findings; coordination and prioritization of comparative effectiveness projects; training and career development; and a program to formally engage stakeholders.[341] As these new initiatives gain momentum at the same time ACO and CIN programs are maturing in the coming years, opportunities to leverage insights may materialize to help providers improve patient care.

Government agencies are subject to Congressional and public scrutiny, so great caution is exercised by these organizations to mitigate controversial actions or initiatives. AHRQ lost funding in the mid-1990s when research into back surgery resulted in controversial guidelines that were opposed by orthopedic surgeons.[342] Concern about the effect of CER and the potential to use such information to make reimbursement decisions has led to restrictions on the use of CER results. For example, the Affordable Care Act established a tax-exempt, private nonprofit organization called the Patient-Centered Outcomes Research Institute (PCORI) . PCORI is separate from the government to reduce the potential for political intervention and manipulation. In addition, PCORI research findings may "not be construed as mandates for practice guidelines, coverage recommendations, payment, or policy recommendations," nor may they be used for coverage or reimbursement decisions by "any public or private payor."[343]

The Patient Protection and Affordable Care Act of 2010

PCORI was created by the Affordable Care Act to identify priorities for comparative effectiveness research and to fund research comparing "health outcomes and clinical effectiveness, risks, and benefits of two or more medical treatments, services, or items."[344] PCORI takes a patient-centered approach and is designed to improve the interaction between patient and provider by increasing the availability of valid evidence-based medical information to enable meaningful discussion between patient and clinician. The "patient preference" approach is central as some policy makers believe most medical decisions fall somewhere between 25% of care that is based on evidence and 10% of procedures that should never be done. It is this middle 65%, according to industry observers, where information can be applied to better inform patient preference. According to a governing board member, PCORI expects to bring about a new era in which both patients and their caregivers have access to the best information and the tools to turn that information into knowledge, allowing both patient and clinician to make the best decisions.

The PCORI Web site describes the organization as

...an independent organization created to help patients, clinicians, purchasers and policy makers make better informed health decisions. PCORI will commission research that is responsive to the values and interests of patients and will provide patients and their caregivers with reliable, evidence-based information for the health care choices they face.[345]

The description is decidedly focused on patients and their decision making, which may limit the ability of PCORI to fund or participate in basic research that increases scientific knowledge, unless there is a connection with consumer health decisions. Of course, the argument can be made that all basic research increasing scientific knowledge should be related to consumer health decisions. In addition, PCORI may not "mandate coverage, reimbursement, or other policies for any public or private payor,"[346] limiting the organization's ability to keep from being involved in considerations of cost-effectiveness—a concern for organizations paying the costs of care, such as government health programs, employers, health insurance companies, and partially capitated CINs and ACOs. Nevertheless, the output of PCORI will add to medical knowledge and, if valid, the results will be used by healthcare stakeholders.

PCORI is required to establish and carry out a research agenda that focuses on "priority areas" of research. It is governed by a board of governors appointed by the US Government Accountability Office, from public nominations, and must appoint advisory panels and a methodology committee. PCORI does not itself perform research; rather, it supports research through a variety of activities, including funding; collaborating with other government agencies; establishing a peer-review process for primary research; adopting research priorities, standards, processes, and protocols; and disseminating and publishing research findings. PCORI is required to submit annual reports to Congress, the Administration, and the public, and there are requirements that increase the transparency of the work performed by PCORI—which helps to increase the validity of the process and projects funded.[347]

Funding for PCORI comes from a new Patient-Centered Outcomes Research Trust Fund that receives monies from several sources, including Medicare trust funds, private sector health plans, self-insured plans, pharmaceutical companies, and general funds of the federal government. Funding starts small, $10 million in 2011, rising to an anticipated $500 million by 2014. Funding slowly increases from 2010 to 2019, but the actual amount of funding available to PCORI depends on a complex set of formulas tied to the number of persons covered by public and private healthcare.[348] Some believe PCORI annual funding could be as much as $650 million, depending on the amount brought in by the health coverage surtax, and total $3 billion over 10 years.[349] Affirmation by the Supreme Court of the constitutionality of the Affordable Care Act in June 2012 establishes the viability of PCORI as a source of funding for new forms of CER and confirms its leadership role in the field.

National Institute for Health and Clinical Excellence

A number of organizations in other countries sponsor or perform CER. This factor is important, as it not only shows that comparative effectiveness is a global issue, but also because it provides lessons learned from comparative effectiveness activities in other countries. In the United Kingdom (UK), the National Institute for Health and Clinical Excellence (NICE) is widely recognized as a pioneer in comparative effectiveness research. NICE was created in 1999 by the government of the United Kingdom to evaluate the clinical and cost effectiveness of various drugs, devices, and procedures. Part of the UK National Health Service (NHS), NICE organizes systematic reviews of existing comparative effectiveness research (meta-analyses) and develops cost effectiveness models to arrive at cost-benefit conclusions. It does not fund primary research, nor does it directly decide which treatments to cover or how much to pay. If a drug, device, or methodology is approved by NICE as effective, it must be covered for reimbursement by the NHS health program. But the NHS decides how much to pay and, if a medical therapy is not approved by NICE, the NHS does not automatically reject it. With a staff of 200 and a budget of approximately $60 million, NICE does not have extensive resources, and it takes a while to develop studies and produce results. NICE has published about 250 recommendations on procedures, more than 100 studies on specific technologies, and 60 treatment guidelines. It is up to local government authorities to make coverage decisions on treatment technologies and methodologies not studied by NICE. Australia, Canada, France, and Germany have government agencies similar to NICE. All of these countries have some form of centralized government-funded and controlled healthcare finance and delivery system, perhaps making NICE and similar organizations not directly applicable to the US healthcare system.

Commercial Comparative Effectiveness Research

A number of private sector comparative effectiveness programs currently operate in the United States. Life science companies, such as drug and device manufacturers, commission CER to determine the effectiveness of their products to gain a competitive advantage, identify improved uses for their products, and potential new uses. As reimbursement becomes more restrictive and the market becomes more competitive, life science companies may find it increasingly important to engage in comparative effectiveness studies to understand cost and benefits of their products. Health plans, self-insured employers, and government payers are interested in CER to determine the quality of drugs, devices, and procedures and to better understand their overall value to patients. Hospitals and health systems review treatment methodologies in their pharmacy and therapeutic committees and quality committees to assist with quality and risk management, determine pharmacy formularies, and make capital allocation for new devices. As integrated delivery networks, physician-hospital organizations, and physician groups assume increased risk and greater responsibility and accountability for quality and cost in new provider organizations such as CINs and accountable care arrangements, CER and evidence-based medicine will increase in importance.[350] In addition, as this shift occurs, the federal government may reexamine regulations governing the use of comparative effectiveness studies to better align with such reformed delivery entities as ACOs, CINs, and other new models of care delivery.

Medical drug and device manufacturers are required by the FDA to conduct clinical trials when developing their products to demonstrate safety and efficacy and, in some cases, to show how one device compares to another. These studies focus on safety and efficacy, but not on relative clinical or cost effectiveness. Manufacturers are beginning to study clinical and cost effectiveness through CER and application of pharmacoeconomics, mainly, to inform the design and content of package inserts but also to determine how their products compare with competitors as they prepare to go to market and help identify differentiators in the marketplace. This activity becomes more critical as drugs and devices lose their patent protections and the protected drug and device portfolios of companies shrink. In addition, the FDA is beginning to use the results of CER in the regulation of products. Comparative effectiveness is also becoming more critical for manufacturers, as payers increasingly perform comparative studies to find drugs and devices that provide greater value. Providers, consumers, health plans, self-funded employers, governments, CINs, and ACOs are interested in proof that a more costly drug or device results in a commensurate increase in clinical benefit for patients and return on investment in the treatment.[351]

Health insurance plans have an interest in CER as they strive to improve quality and affordability. Not only are health insurance plans at risk for the cost of care, they are also legally accountable for the quality of care, required to justify coverage decisions, and must work with patients or physicians who challenge these decisions and adjudicate their appeals. Health plans also use the results of CER to increase their knowledge of evidence-based medicine, develop best practice clinical protocols, and provide clinical decision support tools and technologies to physicians, nursing care managers, and patients. These technologies are used for predictive modeling and risk stratification, care management, disease management, total population registries, quality measurement, specific care recommendations, and personal health records.[352] Many of these technologies and tools may be leveraged by CINs and ACOs as the industry evolves and these organizations are increasingly interested in evidence-based medicine.

While physicians and hospitals may assume more accountability and risk for the outcomes of care in the future, health plans are currently the predominant bearers of risk and have the greatest experience and largest array of tools for risk mitigation and care management. As a result, health insurance plans are at the forefront of researching the quality and effectiveness of various medical drugs, devices, and procedures, and they have sophisticated infrastructure for reviewing the findings of medical research and making decisions.[353] The result has been identification of optimal treatment methodologies[354] and processes that assist patients and physicians in understanding appropriateness of different treatment options. Many health plans publish the results of their research as medical coverage policies.[355] As the market evolves around risk-sharing between providers and health insurance plans, observers anticipated that many of these risk mitigation and care management strategies and tools may be shared with providers.[356] As CINs and ACOs become more experienced in managing risk and improving care outcomes, they may become key players in the US healthcare system's larger framework of comparative effectiveness capabilities.

Many of the provider organizations noted in Figure 1-5 in Chapter 1 use comparative effectiveness techniques to assist with quality and risk management, determine pharmacy formularies, and make capital allocations. New business models for healthcare delivery and finance, such as medical homes, CINs, and ACOs require providers to take greater clinical responsibility and financial risk for care delivered to their patients. As these organizations refine their clinical and business practices, their perspective on clinical effectiveness may become broader, looking not only at the quality of care, but at affordability as well. Managing these new models of care delivery will require providers to have greater awareness of the relative benefit and harm of different treatment methodologies. This information will increase the importance of and demand for CER and related evidence-based medicine and clinical decision support services.[357]

Life science companies, provider organizations, health plans, and other commercial entities also support broader efforts in CER, such as the government-funded PCORI, which focuses on increasing the ability of patients and physicians to make better informed treatment decisions and improve overall quality and affordability. Government policy makers maintain that the current health finance and delivery system allows treatments with marginal clinical benefit relative to their cost. They see the current situation as contributing to unsustainable cost growth, requiring greater information and transparency on clinical effectiveness and cost of care to address this national problem. It is therefore natural that a wide range of stakeholders supports organizations like PCORI and other private sector efforts to obtain up-to-date, objective, and credible information on the effectiveness and value of healthcare services.

Comparative Effectiveness and Coverage Decisions

Organizations with the responsibility and burden of risk for clinical and financial outcomes of care have an interest in comparing both clinical and cost effectiveness. These comparisons are used to determine benefit design and decide which therapies are covered in the benefit package. Coverage decisions are made by all organizations accountable for care of a defined population, including government agencies that fund health programs (e.g., Medicare, Medicaid, Veterans Health Administration, state indigent care and children's health programs), unions, self-insured employers, health insurance plans, and ACOs. All these organizations have developed a range of activities to determine which treatments provide the best clinical outcomes for the resources expended.

A variety of comparative effectiveness services has been created to assist with decisions on clinical and cost effectiveness. The Blue Cross and Blue Shield Association has operated the Technology Evaluation Center whose clients include many of the Blue Plans and the CMS.[358] Other organizations that support or perform clinical effectiveness research include the Center for Medical Technology Policy, Cochrane Collaboration; Drug Effectiveness Review Project; ECRI Institute; Hayes, Inc.; Institute for Clinical and Economic Review; and Tufts Medical Center Cost-Effectiveness Analysis Registry.[359]

CMS is the largest payer of healthcare services and products in the United States, with a total budget for fiscal year 2011 of $782 billion. Given the size of its budget, and continued growth of programs administered, funded, and regulated by CMS (e.g. Medicare, Medicaid, state children's health plans, and the new health insurance exchanges), CMS has a substantial interest in CER.[360] An example of a coverage decision-making process, which includes comparative effectiveness input from external technology assessment resources is shown in Figure 10-1.[361] The Medicare National Coverage decision-making process illustrates the level of complexity in evaluating medical therapies for coverage decisions.

Figure 10-1. Medicare National Coverage Process[362]

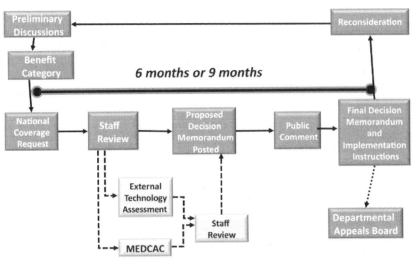

Source: Center for Medicare and Medicaid Services

For items and services required for the diagnosis and treatment of an illness or injury, Medicare covers decisions rendered through this process. The underlying methodology and program is run as an evidence-based process that even allows opportunities for public participation.[363] As CINs and ACOs continue to grow in their tolerance of clinical and financial risk and acceptance of responsibility, they will be more attuned to the decisions made by payer organizations such as CMS in their national and local coverage processes, and they may even begin to adopt these coverage determinations.

Comparative Effectiveness Research Methods

Various methods are used to research the effectiveness of medical therapies and arrive at conclusions about the best treatment for a condition. Each method has strengths and weaknesses and requires different levels of rigor and validity. Here we look at two different categories of research methods—randomized controlled trials and observational studies—and their usefulness in comparative effectiveness research.

The randomized controlled trial (RCT) is considered the gold standard of research methods. In an RCT, an experiment is designed in which research subjects are chosen and randomly assigned to a treatment group or a control group. The effects of the experiment on the treatment group are then isolated and observed and compared with the control group. The research subjects are chosen to minimize differences in their health status, and all other aspects of the study are controlled or accounted for as well as possible so that the only difference between the two groups is the treatment provided. By controlling as many variables as possible in the study, researchers attempt to isolate the cause-effect relationship between the treatment given and outcome recorded.[364]

Observational studies include a variety of research designs in which no experiment is set up in advance with random assignment or controls. Observational studies may be used in situations for which a controlled experiment may not be possible. Controlled trials are not possible, for example, where ethical standards prohibit the use of human subjects (e.g., effects of radon gas or cigarette smoking) or when setting up an RCT is difficult (e.g., rare occurrence of side effects or lack of resources to get a large enough experimental population). Observational studies make conclusions about the effects of the treatment in question based on educated guesses (inferences) from the data.[365] Observational studies include cohort studies, case-controlled studies, case series, and case reports.[366] Figure 10-2 illustrates progression through a hierarchy of evidence.

Figure 10-2. Hierarchy of Evidence for Intervention or Treatment Effectiveness [367]

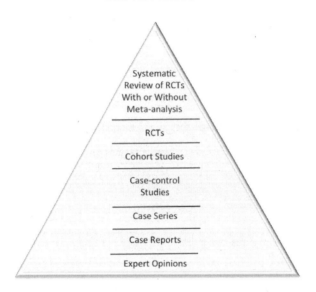

The RCT is considered the most rigorous and valid research design as it attempts to reduce errors and eliminate bias and extraneous effects (also known as confounding variables) by controlling the study as much as possible. A systematic review of a set of randomized controlled trials using meta-analysis may provide additional validity as because it assembles results of many RCTs and can cover larger populations, and filters out weaknesses of individual trials.

There are weaknesses to RCTs, however, especially in situations in which decisions that impact a large group of persons must be made quickly, such as coverage decisions that must be implemented in the short-term for a large population in a health plan, CIN/ACO, or clinical formulary decisions by one of these organizations. To begin, RCTs are more expensive to conduct and take much longer to set up, implement, and provide results—in many cases it takes years and millions of dollars. Second, because the population is controlled, the results apply to a defined population and may not be generally applicable. Finally, because the procedures used in an RCT are controlled and the experiment is carried out under optimal conditions, it may be difficult to replicate or implement in a real-life clinical setting.[368]

Observational studies have been criticized for being more prone to error, as they are perceived to be less rigorous or valid than an RCT. Perhaps not as rigorous as RCTs, observational studies can be designed to reduce errors and improve their validity. The lack of ability to control the situation rigorously and the potential for extraneous variables to affect the results leads to a need for adjustments to observational studies. After these adjustments are made, the effects of treatment can more reliably be determined.[369] Such techniques as propensity scoring and instrumental variables are used to correct for errors by adjusting observational studies to more closely replicate RCT experiments. Studies have shown that properly adjusted observational studies are almost as good as RCTs.[370]

Observational studies have important advantages for application of CER. Because they are less expensive and may use data already collected, they can be completed more rapidly. In addition, observational studies are usually done in real-world clinical settings on actual patients using real interventions rather than strict experimental controls.[371] Thus, the results can be obtained and applied more easily, which is important with situations in which decisions must be made quickly. Future improvements in observational study design will increase the availability of information on better medical therapies and help organizations with decision making on what works best, including which treatments should be used in clinical settings. The selection of one research methodology over another involves a number of issues. Table 10-1 provides a summary of some myths regarding each of these methodologies.

Table 10-1. Myths and Evidence on RCTs and Observational Studies[372]

Issue	Myth	Evidence
Gold standard	Randomized, controlled trials are always the gold standard in research design	Randomized trials on the same topic often contradict each other
Unknown confounders	Unknown confounders undermine all observational studies	If a factor is unknown, treatment will not be influenced and confounding is unlikely
Designed to replicate RCT	Novel strategies in designing and analyzing observational studies can replicate randomization	Purported benefits of new strategies to design and analyze are often conceptual rather than actual
Design vs. details	Study design matters more than specific details and attributes	Details of patients, interventions, and outcomes are highly relevant

Pragmatic randomized clinical trials (PCTs) have been proposed to combine the validity of RCT with the practical applicability of observational studies. In a PCT, the study design is set up specifically to address clinical quality and cost issues of interest to decision makers.[373] The Center for Medical Technology Policy has pioneered PCTs as a way to provide valid information to decision makers, such as patients, physicians, providers, policy makers, payers and healthcare administrators.[374] PCTs are designed to be more applicable and useful in real-world situations because they recruit a diverse set of participants from a wide variety of real-world clinical practices and focus on comparing specific medical therapies while collecting a wide range of outcomes.[375]

It is important for CINs and ACOs to understand the implications of these different research methodologies. As the use of CER expands, study results can benefit the patients and providers by bringing new intelligence into the shared decision-making process. This new information can improve patients' quality of care and ultimately their quality of life.

Health Information Technology and CER

The increasing availability of health information technology is creating tremendous new opportunities to advance knowledge and evidence while strengthening the healthcare industry's ability to study and compare the effectiveness of medical interventions. ARRA recognized the importance of the health information technology data infrastructure in advancing the national CER agenda and allocated $268 million to data infrastructure development.[376] In addition to such existing clinical study methods as RCT and observational studies, health information technology has created opportunities for new analyses by combining such traditional data sources as administrative claims with clinical information from electronic medical records, registries, and other clinical databases. These new combinations of data and information will enhance CER studies and medical evidence compilation.[377]

Claims data brings a number of advantages to comparative effectiveness studies. There is a large body of literature describing ways to analyze the data and established methods (such as propensity scoring) to adjust for potential errors. All health plans and self-insured employers have used claims data for years to analyze and improve the quality and affordability of healthcare. As discussed previously, health plans include claims data in their analyses of different treatment options when they develop medical coverage policies. Claims data is also used for a variety of quality, performance improvement, clinical decision support, and care management purposes. Some organizations have taken additional steps to develop sophisticated predictive models and advanced clinical decision support algorithms that yield accurate models of patients and their needed care. These systems can be used to improve quality by scanning both claims and clinical data to detect and correct errors in the care delivery process and deviations from best medical practices.[378] If you combine a clinical trial with subsequent claims data, you can also create a longitudinal record for a patient and continue to follow his or her progress even after the trial is completed. Use of such a longitudinal record could take trials out of the clinic and into daily life, identifying both beneficial and harmful effects in real-life situations.

There are disadvantages to only using claims data as the data may be specific to an episode of care and lack information necessary to understand the patient's full health status. Without additional information about the patient, it is difficult to identify similar patients or populations and compare the effectiveness of different medical therapies.[379]

Clinical information from health information technology, such as electronic health records, personal health records, and medical registries, can fill in the elements missing in administrative claims data, providing a more complete picture of a patient or population, and result in a more robust data set for CER. These technologies can provide such important data, including medical histories, measures of health status, laboratory test results, and treatment outcomes.[380] The additional data can give sufficient detail to allow proper research methodologies to compare medical therapies. Incorporating clinical data with claims data has been described as the "holy grail" of CER, but issues of federal government research priorities, privacy concerns, lack of information technology standardization, and difficulty in aggregating data are roadblocks to such integration.[381,382]

The private sector has advanced its comparative effectiveness research agenda and methodologies at a faster pace than the federal government. It is already aggregating and integrating administrative claims data with clinical-level data from health information technology. These efforts, in time, will allow ACOs and CINs to combine quality measures from clinical data with financial performance goals in their claims systems so they can monitor their performance against targets and annual goals in real-time.[383]

Comparative Effectiveness and Clinical Decision Support

Clinical decision support (CDS) refers to any methodical process used to assist clinicians or patients with medical decisions. Computer-based

CDS is further defined as the use of computers to bring relevant knowledge to bear on decisions about patients' healthcare and well-being.[384] Knowledge relevant to clinical care includes medical and pharmaceutical claims, clinical data, evidence-based guidelines, the most recent medical literature, personal values, and any other information that could help clinicians and patients make decisions and improve the quality of care. CER is part of the medical literature that goes into CDS.

Basic computer-based CDS technology combines data from a variety of sources, such as medical claims, pharmacy claims, and clinical data from EMRs and translates that data into information and knowledge applied by physicians, other clinicians, and multidisciplinary caregiver teams to improve the quality of care. The translation of data and resulting conclusions is often accomplished by comparing patient treatments to evidence-based guidelines and identifying gaps in care considering recommendations on appropriate care according to the evidence-based guidelines used. Comparing treatment recommendations to guidelines is a form of practical comparative effectiveness but has shortcomings.

Many EHRs have this basic CDS, which is a requirement for Meaningful Use under the CMS Meaningful Use of EHRs incentive program.[385] The CMS Meaningful Use regulation, however, requires only the implementation of "one clinical decision support rule . . . along with the ability to track compliance to that rule" for Stage 1.[386] One rule may be appropriate to prove the concept of delivering CDS, but is inadequate for ongoing decision support across a broad spectrum of diseases and conditions if you are looking for improved quality of care and outcomes. In addition, studies have shown that current EHRs do not deliver the features needed to improve patient care. Additional technologies are needed for EHRs to be effective, including registries, personal health records, and advanced clinical decision support.[387] A recent study on the use of basic clinical decision support in EHRs from 2005 to 2007 showed "no consistent association between EHRs and CDS and better quality."

Clearly, something is missing; additional clinical information from medical literature and CER is needed to improve and strengthen CDS. Advanced CDS technology is starting to become available, and it addresses the shortcomings of current EHR-based basic CDS by including a variety of additional data, tools, and techniques to improve decision support and care results. Advanced CDS is of great interest to ACOs and CINs, as it is more accurate in identifying appropriate care and allowing providers to mitigate and manage their risk and responsibility for clinical and economic outcomes.

Additional data not currently available to basic CDS in clinically focused EHRs but used in advanced CDS include pharmacy data, claims data, health risk assessments, patient-reported data, disability data, and other medical and demographic information. These additional elements help to provide a more complete picture of the patient, including medical history and future health risk.

Another feature of advanced CDS is the use of more recent medical findings, such as the latest peer-reviewed medical journal findings and results of CER. Basic CDS takes clinical information and compares it to evidence-based guidelines. By definition, evidence-based guidelines are consensus standards developed at a given point in time, using the medical literature then available. Industry experts recognize that medical research is constantly advancing and that "no physician can keep up with the literature and changing medical advances simply with intuition and top-of-mind memory."[388] Advanced CDS technologies, on the other hand, bring the capability to search the latest medical literature; present the latest medical findings identified by a team of experts; and update the evidence in real-time—presenting evidence-based medicine practices at the point of care.[389] One drawback of some advanced CDS is the level of effort and cost of human-intensive expert system techniques.[390]

A systematic review of studies of clinical decision support technologies identified specific features of CDS correlated with significant improvements in patient care. These features include: information that fits into clinician workflow; specific care recommendations; information at the point of care; periodic performance feedback; sharing recommendations with patients; and requesting documentation of reasons for not following recommendations.[391] The most advanced CDS tools and techniques build in all these features by using real-time care recommendations at the point of care, allowing bidirectional information sharing with the treating clinician, and utilizing such patient-facing tools as personal health records to allow patient self-management.[392]

Comparative Effectiveness and New Provider Organizations

Given current restrictions, government-funded CER results may not be directly useful to new care models, such as CINs and ACOs. Any CER findings, however, increase general medical knowledge and evidence-based medicine used by these organizations for decision support.

Whether directly or indirectly, improvements in medical knowledge improve best practice protocols. Thus, even government-funded CER, which is restricted from use in making coverage decisions, increases the body of medical knowledge, indirectly helping physicians and patients make more informed decisions about treatment options that improve patient care and quality of life.

CINs and ACOs do have commercially available advanced CDS tools to assist decision making on appropriate care. As these new provider organizations accept greater responsibility for clinical and financial outcomes, they will find themselves making medical coverage decisions, including benefit design, and responding to appeals of care decisions. Fortunately, there is a large body of work in this field and many tools on the market that allow providers to access this information.[393]

The success of such new provider organizations as ACOs and CINs will depend heavily on continued advancements in health information technology. Many organizations are establishing enterprise health information exchanges and are deepening their clinical integration in order to have the infrastructure necessary to operate in the new environment. Consider this possibility: properly established CINs and ACOs operating with appropriate health information technology and advanced CDS, and actively exchanging and aggregating data, may contribute to a "rapid-learning health system." Such a system would combine evidence from clinical and comparative effectiveness research with individual patients' information from electronic medical records to determine what works best for a patient.[394]

Another form of CER is comparing different healthcare finance and delivery models. For example, different ACO models (both public and private) could be evaluated and compared as their operations are established and as their results and outcomes tested. In fact, the Medicare Shared Savings Program ACO Proposed Rule noted that one of the ways competition could foster improvement would include

> **Provide better benchmarks for quality improvements**. For example, although a single ACO might claim that environmental or demographic factors limit what it can achieve in the treatment of certain illnesses, a comparison among multiple ACOs in the same service area could better ensure that the best standards possible under prevailing conditions are being met.[395]

This kind of initiative would focus on the effectiveness of variations in administrative systems, practice redesign, payment reforms, and related compensation models that would tie into opportunities for improving benchmarks to ensure comparability of results and savings achieved against targets. Ideally, different health finance and delivery models could be compared and help advance the study of health care quality, accessibility, and affordability.

Bridging the Divide

The field of CER covers a broader spectrum that includes federally funded programs and private sector initiatives. While federally funded CER holds promise, it brings challenges to the industry in terms of limits on the use of federal funds and maximizing the utilization of results and findings. Private sector CER studies and programs, such as those funded through the pharmaceutical and health plan industries, provide results more quickly, but are usually proprietary and may not be widely publicized. In addition, there may be an element of bias in pharmaceutical CER, especially when the studies are performed for marketing purposes. CER associated with health insurance plans can be more specifically targeted to both clinical and economic outcomes, but may not be readily available to providers unless there is a preexisting relationship.

Figure 1-2 in the first chapter addressed three factors influencing system change in healthcare, and each factor contributes to the need for CER studies. First, with the aging population, CER studies, both commercial and publicly funded, will support efforts of clinicians to improve care and quality of life for the Baby Boomers, Generation X and Generation Y segments of our population. Second, is the complexity of our US healthcare system. CER brings the opportunity to unwind complexities by increasing our understanding of relationships and relational patterns across clinical interventions when compared for optimal benefit to a patient population. Growing in our knowledge of these relationships results in overcoming barriers—that helps improve the health of our population. Last is innovation. Through CER we can better understand the need for new devices, technologies, biopharmaceuticals, and other interventions. The comparison of interventions holds the potential to discover new pathways to meeting unmet needs and lead us to a healthier America.

Finally, health information technology brings additional challenges. New technologies are arriving at a rapid pace, often faster than the industry can keep up with them. There are inherent risks in the development and implementation of new technologies, called "technology-related adverse events," identified by the Joint Commission's 2008 Sentinel Event Report Number 42.[396] EMRs, EHRs, and registries used in CER must address such risks, because the ability of society to develop new technologies may exceed the capacity of clinicians to use them safely and effectively.

Some of the most important challenges for CINs and ACOs involve effective and permissible use of CER study results to support improvements in the quality of patient care. It remains to be seen whether restrictions on the use of government-funded CER will persist. In addition, providers must consider whether it is worthwhile and economically viable to support CER. As both CER and new provider models continue to shape the future of healthcare services, new challenges will emerge, and stakeholders will find ways to meet them for the benefit of providers, patients, and the organizations that fund healthcare.

Chapter 10: Takeaways

✓ Funding for PCORI comes from a variety of sources, including a new Patient-Centered Outcomes Research Trust Fund expected to be $500 million in 2014 and as much as $3 billion over 10 years.

✓ Health reforms led by the Affordable Care Act are changing the field of comparative effectiveness research. Led by demand from nontraditional users (value-based suppliers such as accountable care organizations) and fueled by increasingly sophisticated technology tools, CER is being pushed into innovative territory where quick results are more important than perfect experimental design.

✓ *Commercial CER*—Life science companies, such as drug and device manufacturers, commission CER to determine the effectiveness of their products to gain a competitive advantage, identify improved uses for their products, and potential new uses.

✓ *Global CER*—A number of organizations in other countries sponsor or perform CER. This provides lessons learned from comparative effectiveness activities in other countries. In the UK the National Institute for Health and Clinical Excellence (NICE) is recognized as a pioneer in comparative effectiveness research.

✓ Methods used to research the effectiveness of medical therapies and arrive at conclusions about the best treatment for a condition include randomized controlled trials and observational studies.

✓ Health information technology has created opportunities for new analyses by combining traditional data sources such as administrative claims, with clinical information from electronic medical records, registries, and other clinical databases.

Chapter 10: Takeaways (cont.)

✓ Clinical information from health information technology can fill in elements missing in administrative claims data, provide a more complete picture of a patient or population, and result in a more robust data set for CER.

✓ Advanced CDS supports ACOs and CINs with more accuracy in identifying appropriate care and allowing providers to mitigate and manage their risk and responsibility for clinical and economic outcomes.

[320] Concato J, Lawler EV, Lew RA, Gaziano JM, Aslan M, Huang GD.. Observational Methods in Comparative Effectiveness Research, *Am J Med*. 2010 Dec;123(12 Suppl 1):e16-23. CER may also compare different delivery models, such as primary care physician compared to hospitalist care, or clinically integrated networks versus patient centered medical homes, but the main focus of this chapter is on comparison of therapies.

[321] Department of Health and Human Services Recovery Funding Page. Comparative Effectiveness Research. Accessed online July 15, 2011, at http://www.hhs.gov/recovery/programs/cer/index.html.

[322] Navathe A, Conway P. Optimizing Health Information Technology's Role in Enabling Comparative Effectiveness Research. *Am J Manag Care*. 2010;16(12):SP44-SP47. Accessed online August 12, 2011, at http://www.ncbi.nlm.nih.gov/pubmed/21314220.

[323] Etheredge L. Creating a High-Performance System for Comparative Effectiveness Research. *Health Aff (Millwood)*. 2010;29(10):1761–1767.

[324] Concato J, et al. 2010.

[325] Sean Tunis, Director, Center for Medical Technology Policy, personal discussion, May 2011.

[326] Wilensky GR. The Policies and Politics of Creating a Comparative Clinical Effectiveness Research Center. *Health Aff (Millwood)*. 2009 Jul-Aug;28(4):w719-29.

[327] Tunis SR, Stryer DB, Clancy CM. Practical Clinical Trials: Increasing the Value of Clinical Research for Decision Making in Clinical and Health Policy. *JAMA*. 2003 Sep 24;290(12):1624–1632.

[328] Committee on Comparative Effectiveness Research Prioritization. *Initial National Priorities for Comparative Effectiveness Research.* Institute of Medicine. Washington, DC: The National Academies Press; 2009:2–10.

[329] Wilensky GR. 2009.

[330] H.R. 3590, Patient Protection and Affordable Care Act, §6301(i) and (j), Patient-centered Outcomes Research . Rules and Rules of Construction; 2010:620.

[331] H.R. 3590, Patient Protection and Affordable Care Act, §937(a)(1), Dissemination and Building Capacity for Research; 2010:621.

[332] A description of one such service, and the results obtained, can be found in Javitt JC, et al. Using a Claims Data-based, Sentinel System to Improve Compliance with Clinical Guidelines: Results of a Randomized Prospective Study. *Am J Manag Care*. 2005;11:93-102; see also Javitt JC, Rebitzer JB, Reisman L. Information technology and medical missteps: evidence from a randomized trial. *J Health Econ*. 2008;27(3):585–602.

[333] See Congressional Budget Office, Research on the Comparative Effectiveness of Medical Treatments, Publication 2975, December 2007:7–9.

[334] For example, the Center for Medical Technology Policy, Cochrane Collaboration, Drug Effectiveness Review Project, ECRI Institute, Hayes, Inc., Institute for Clinical and

Economic Review, Technology Evaluation Center at BCBS Association, ActiveHealth Management, and Tufts Medical Center Cost-Effectiveness Analysis Registry.

[335] Congressional Budget Office, Research on the Comparative Effectiveness of Medical Treatments, Publication 2975, December 2007, p. 8.

[336] Congressional Budget Office, Research on the Comparative Effectiveness of Medical Treatments, Publication 2975, December 2007, p. 9.

[337] Committee on Comparative Effectiveness Research Prioritization. Existing CER Activities in the United States. In: *Initial National Priorities for Comparative Effectiveness Research*. Institute of Medicine. Washington, DC: The National Academies Press; 2009:46-51.

[338] Health Services/Technology Assessment Texts, National Library of Medicine, 1994. Accessed online August 11, 2011, at http://www.ncbi.nlm.nih.gov/books/NBK16710/.

[339] Department of Health and Human Services. Comparative Effectiveness Research Funding. Accessed online July 5, 2011, at http://www.hhs.gov/recovery/programs/cer/index.html.

[340] Committee on Comparative Effectiveness Research Prioritization. Preface. In: *Initial National Priorities for Comparative Effectiveness Research*. Institute of Medicine. Washington, DC: The National Academies Press; 2009:xv.

[341] Department of Health and Human Services. American Recovery and Reinvestment Act. Agency for Healthcare Research and Quality: Comparative Effectiveness Research Program Summary. Accessed online July 5, 2011, at http://www.hhs.gov/recovery/reports/plans/pdf20100610/AHRQ%20CER%20June%202010.pdf. See also http://www.ahrq.gov/fund/cerfactsheets/.

[342] Gray BH, Gusmano MK, Collins SR. AHCPR and the Changing Politics of Health Services Research. *Health Aff (Millwood)*. 2003 Jan-Jun;Suppl Web Exclusives:W3–283–307.

[343] H.R. 3590, Patient Protection and Affordable Care Act, §6301(d)(8), Release of Research Findings. §6301(i). Rules; 2010.

[344] H.R. 3590, Patient Protection and Affordable Care Act, §6301(a)(2)(A), Comparative Clinical Effectiveness Research; Research; 2010.

[345] Patient-Centered Outcomes Research Institute. Organizational description. Accessed online July 15, 2011, at http://www.pcori.org/about/.

[346] H.R. 3590, Patient Protection and Affordable Care Act, §937(a)(1), Dissemination and Building Capacity for Research; 2010.

[347] H.R. 3590, Patient Protection and Affordable Care Act, §6301(i) and (j), Patient-centered Outcomes Research. Rules and Rules of Construction; 2010.

[348] Clancy C, Collins FS. Patient-Centered Outcomes Research Institute: The Intersection of Science and Health Care. *Sci Transl Med*. 2010 Jun 23;2(37):37cm18.

[349] Leonard, D. Time for PCORI's Implementation. *National Pharmaceutical Council e-Newsletter*. April 2010. Accessed online July 20, 2012, at

http://www.npcnow.org/Public/Public/Newsroom/E-newsletter/2010_e-newsletters/April_2010_EVI/Time_for_PCORI_s_Implementation.aspx.

[350] Miller J. Aetna Manages Cancer Care. *Managed Healthcare Executive.* July 2011;21(7):18-21. Accessed online August 17, 2011, at http://managedhealthcareexecutive.modernmedicine.com/mhe/Thought+Leadership/Aetna-manages-cancer-care/ArticleStandard/Article/detail/728450.

[351] Committee on Comparative Effectiveness Research Prioritization. What Is Comparative Effectiveness Research? In: *Initial National Priorities for Comparative Effectiveness Research.* Institute of Medicine. Washington, DC: The National Academies Press; 2009:52.

[352] Juster IA. Technology-Driven Interactive Care Management Identifies and Resolves More Clinical Issues than a Claims-Based Alerting System. *Dis Manag* 2005;8(3):188–197.

[353] Kongstvedt, PR, ed. Essentials of Managed Health Care, 5th ed. Sudbury, MA: Jones and Bartlett Publishers; 2007:47–50.

[354] Javitt JC, et al. Using a Claims Data-based, Sentinel System to Improve Compliance with Clinical Guidelines: Results of a Randomized Prospective Study. *Am J Manag Care.* 2005;11:93–102.

[355] For example, see Aetna Clinical Policy Bulletins, which are detailed, technical documents explaining how decisions are made: http://www.aetna.com/healthcare-professionals/policies-guidelines/clinical_policy_bulletins.html.

[356] See *Aetna and Carilion Clinic Announce Plans to Collaborate on Accountable Care Organization.* Accessed online August 17, 2011, at http://www.aetna.com/news/newsReleases/2011/0310_Aetna_and_Carilion.html.

[357] Miller J. Aetna Manages Cancer Care. *Managed Healthcare Executive.* July 2011;21(7):18-21. Accessed online August 17, 2011, at http://managedhealthcareexecutive.modernmedicine.com/mhe/Thought+Leadership/Aetna-manages-cancer-care/ArticleStandard/Article/detail/728450.

[358] Wilensky GR. 2009.

[359] Institute of Medicine. Committee on Comparative Effectiveness Research Prioritization. *Initial National Priorities for Comparative Effectiveness Research.* Washington, DC: The National Academies Press; 2009:2-17 to 2-18; and Congressional Budget Office, Research on the Comparative Effectiveness of Medical Treatments, Publication 2975, December 2007:8.

[360] Wilensky GR. 2009.

[361] Jacques, LB, The stakeholder perspective. Presented at the third DEcIDE Symposium on Comparative Effectiveness Research Methods; June 6, 2011; Rockville, MD.

[362] Jacques, LB. Evidence for decision making: a Medicare perspective. Presented at third DEcIDE Methods Symposium: Methods for Developing and Analyzing Clinically Rich Data for Patient-Centered Outcomes Research; June 6, 2011; Rockville, MD.

363 Center for Medicare and Medicaid Services. Overview of Medicare Coverage Determination Process. Accessed online July 6, 2011, at https://www.cms.gov/DeterminationProcess/.

364 Agency for Healthcare Research and Quality. Glossary of Terms, definition of randomized controlled trials. Accessed online September 13, 2011, at http://www.effectivehealthcare.ahrq.gov/index.cfm/glossary-of-terms/?pageaction=showterm&termid=101.

365 ClinicalTrials.gov. Protocol Registration System. Protocol Data Element Definitions (DRAFT), definition of observational studies. Accessed online September 13, 2011, at http://prsinfo.clinicaltrials.gov/definitions.html.

366 Akobeng AK. Understanding Randomised Controlled Trials. *Arch Dis Child.* 2005 August;90(8):840–844.

367 Akobeng, AK. 2005.

368 Concato J. 2010.

369 ClinicalTrials.gov.

370 Horwitz RI, Viscoli CM, Clemens JD, Sadock RT. Developing improved observational methods for evaluating therapeutic effectiveness. *Am J Med.* 1990;89:630–638.

371 Concato J. 2010.

372 Concato J. 2010.

373 Tunis SR, et al. 2003.

374 Center for Medicare Technology Policy. Issue Brief: Pragmatic/Practical Randomized Controlled Trials.

375 Center for Medicare Technology Policy. Pragmatic Clinical Trials, Center for Medical Technology Policy.

376 Department of Health and Human Services. Recovery Programs. Comparative Effectiveness Research Funding. Accessed online July 15, 2011, at http://www.hhs.gov/recovery/programs/cer/index.html.

377 Etheredge L. 2010.

378 Javitt JC, et al. 2005.

379 Congressional Budget Office, Research on the Comparative Effectiveness of Medical Treatments, Publication 2975; December 2007:21–22.

380 Congressional Budget Office. 2007:22–23.

381 Navathe AS, Conway PH. 2010.

382 Congressional Budget Office. 2007:22.

383 Medicity. Technology Fundamentals for Realizing ACO Success. September 2010. Accessed online July 15, 2011, at http://www.himss.org/content/files/Medicity_ACO_Whitepaper.pdf.

[384] Greenes RA. Ed. *Clinical Decision Support, the Road Ahead*. Maryland Heights, MO: Academic Press; 2007:6.

[385] Fed. Reg. Vol. 75, No. 144, II(A)(2)(c). Stage 1 Criteria for Meaningful Use. p. 44350. CMS defines CDS in the context of meaningful use, as "HIT functionality that builds upon the foundation of an EHR to provide persons involved in care processes with general and person-specific information, intelligently filtered and organized, at appropriate times, to enhance health and health care."

[386] Fed. Reg. Vol. 75, No. 144, II(A)(2)(c). Stage 1 Criteria for Meaningful Use. p. 44328. Requirement for one clinical decision support rule as part of the core set of meaningful use objectives.

[387] Bates DW, Bitton A. The Future of Health Information Technology in the Patient-Centered Medical Home. *Health Aff (Millwood)*. 2010 Apr;29(4):614–621.

[388] Miller J. 2011.

[389] Jenrette J, Yale K. ACO technologies: performance and reporting tools. Presented at ACO West Conference; November 19, 2010; San Diego, CA.

[390] Greenes RA. 2007.

[391] Kawamoto K, Houlihan CA, Balas EA, Lobach DF. Improving clinical practice using clinical decision support systems: a systematic review of trials to identify features critical to success. *BMJ*. 2005 Apr 2;330(7494):765.

[392] Jenrette J, Yale K. 2010.

[393] A description of one such service and results obtained can be found at Javitt JC, et al. Using a Claims Data-based, Sentinel System to Improve Compliance with Clinical Guidelines: Results of a Randomized Prospective Study. *Am J Manag Care* 2005;11:93-102.; Javitt JC, Rebitzer JB, Reisman L. Information technology and medical missteps: evidence from a randomized trial. *J Health Econ.* 2008;27(3):585-602.

[394] Etheredge L. 2010.

[395] Fed. Reg. Vol. 76, No. 67. April 7, 2011. I.(4)(b). Competition and Quality of Care. p. 19630.

[396] The Joint Commission. Safely Implementing Health information and Converging Technologies. *Joint Commission on Accreditation of Healthcare Organizations, USA.* Sentinel Event Alert. 2008 Dec 11;(42):1-4. Accessed online July 15, 2011, at http://www.jointcommission.org/sentinel_event_alert_issue_42_safely_implementing_health_information_and_converging_technologies/.

Chapter 11. The New Horizon—A Network Transition to Individual and Population Health

John Reinhart, CPA, MBA *(Candidate 2012)*
and Robert Esterhay, MD

Western societies are moving towards a society of networks, i.e., a society, in which the formal, vertically integrated organization that has dominated the 20th century is replaced or at least complemented by consciously created and goal directed networks. [397]

Jörg Raab and Patrick Kenis
September 2009

A Network Transition Underway

The structure of every bridge consists of numerous foundational elements designed to support its type and level of usage. Bridges are conduits that enable connectedness. Health IT implemented over the past decades has accelerated the transformation of connected delivery systems by bridging the gaps in care coordination. Electronic communications and records empower delivery networks limited only by the speed of technology diffusion,[398] thus, eliminating traditional silos and barriers. One of the keys to the successful emergence of ACO models is the integration of health IT across the full continuum of care to enable real-time decision support for patients, physicians, providers, and payer organizations alike.

As described in Chapter 1, ACOs are collaborations between physicians, hospitals, and other providers of clinical services, accountable, both clinically and financially, for delivery of healthcare services to a designated patient population in a defined geographic market.[399] The ACO is physician led with a focus on population-based care management providing services to patients covered under both public and private payer programs. ACOs are part of the changing landscape of our healthcare system, and health IT is an enabler of change within and between these organizations. The revolution is now underway to transform processes, systems, organizations and the way we deliver health and healthcare universally: a *network in transition.*

The first five chapters of this book highlighted cornerstone technologies, including EHRs, HIEs, business intelligence, data analytics, PHRs, mobile health applications (mHealth apps) , and clinical decision support. In addition, the importance of comparative effectiveness research, CMS Meaningful Use of EHRs program, quality, and revenue cycle management were addressed in Chapters 6 through 10. Initiatives in these areas make full use of the range of technologies discussed throughout the text to support and improve patient care operations in both the public and private sector. Health IT individually implemented in silos is a tool that enables the sharing of information only within that silo. Our service delivery system is an ecosystem evolving from silos of care toward networked information platforms that effectively and efficiently connect networks. Chapters 4 and 5 addressed the importance of interoperability and standards as critical factors toward achieving efficient, effective, and integrated health information exchange to enable value-based decision making.

Chapter 1 established three emerging themes addressed throughout this text: global aging demographics, technology innovation, and the complexity of our healthcare system, impacted by consumerism and collaboration networks, which will be discussed in this chapter.

Are ACOs a bridge to the network transition for improving individual and population health? We believe they are. Enabled through innovations and advancement in technologies, structural changes to the healthcare system and improvement of processes will lead to better outcomes for the populations served globally.

Importance of Factors Influencing Transition

Many factors continue to impact the transition to better healthcare systems. The need for improved patient safety, investment in medical education training to address the physician and caregiver shortages, chronic disease management, and the overall financial costs of improving health are just a few. The three overarching factors addressed throughout this book are central challenges to address in improving the quality of care in America. Some concluding insights on each factor are offered.

Innovation.

West and Farr define organizational innovation as the intentional introduction and application (within a group or organization) of ideas, processes, products, or procedures, new to the relevant unit of adoption, designed to significantly benefit the individual, the group, organization, or wider society.[400] To meet the needs of patients, especially those with chronic conditions, innovations in technologies, processes, and the way we serve patients help drive the transition to better quality care. Figure 11-1, from a 2010 article by Omachonu and Einspruch titled *Innovation in Healthcare Delivery Systems: A Conceptual Framework*, illustrates at a high level the pathway and stakeholders for which innovations are generated and driven to the market.[401]

Figure 11-1. The Process of Healthcare Innovation[402]

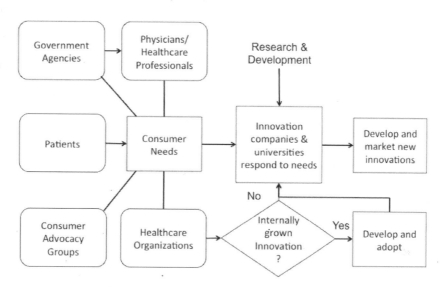

Stakeholders drive desires for innovations that are addressed through public and private sector research activities. The importance of consumerism cannot be overstated in regards to this drive for innovations in healthcare. As noted by Konschak and Jarrell in 2010, "Consumers . . . and their desires are prompting dramatic changes in how providers deliver healthcare."[403] To achieve a higher quality of care, consumer demands must be a factor in the design and development of innovative products and services, both disruptive and sustaining. In recent years, consumer-centric innovations have included virtual visits, patient portals (including PHRs), and behavioral economic tools [404] all of which help address needs of the consumer to improve the quality of their health and healthcare.

There have been attempts to classify innovation into categories. In a 2005 publication of the Organization for Economic Cooperation and Development (OECD) and EuroStat noted that "Innovation is the implementation of a new or significantly improved product (good or service), or process, a new marketing method, or a new organizational method in business practices, workplace organization or external relations."[405]

The OECD also made the distinction among four types of innovation, noted in Table 11-1.

Table 11-1. Four Types of Innovation

Product Innovation	Process Innovation
Marketing Innovation	Organizational Innovation

In healthcare today, innovative products and services support new process innovation, as we see with health IT enabling process changes and new interconnectivity among organizations. According to Varkey and colleagues, process innovation occurs in the production or delivery methods employed to get goods or services to the patient.[406] An example is described in the 2008 Health Affairs article *Continuous Innovation in Health Care: Implications of the Geisinger Experience*. Geisinger's Personal Health Navigator was described as one innovation of a health IT application developed for consumers that provided care coordination, a tool to increase access to specialty care, care coordination, and provided predictive analytics, and home-based monitoring.[407] Structural innovation usually affects the internal and external infrastructure and creates new business models. The impact of the patient-centered medical home (PCMH) is one such example of a structural innovation that, over the last few decades, has grown into a new model of operation for primary care and specialty care practices.[408]

According to Omachonu and Einspruch in their 2010 article,

> Healthcare innovation can be defined as the introduction of a new concept, idea, service, process, or product aimed at improving treatment, diagnosis, education, outreach, prevention and research, and with the long term goals of improving quality, safety, outcomes, efficiency and costs.[409]

This definition provides a bridge between the general notion of innovation across all industries and one that is refined to fit the domain of healthcare.

Within healthcare innovation there exists different dimensional elements that can affect the development and use of new products or service innovations. Two dimensions to consider are environmental and operational, as described by Omachonu and Einspruch in 2010. The environmental dimension involves elements that are challenging to measure but have a great impact on how a healthcare organization embraces innovations (e.g., leadership, culture, complexity, collaboration). The operational dimension has elements more readily measurable for their impact on an organization's capacity to generate and/or apply innovations (e.g., efficiency, effectiveness, stakeholder satisfaction, productivity, workforce levels, cost control). Figure 11-2 provides an illustration of these dimensions.

Figure 11-2. Dimensions of Healthcare Innovation[410]

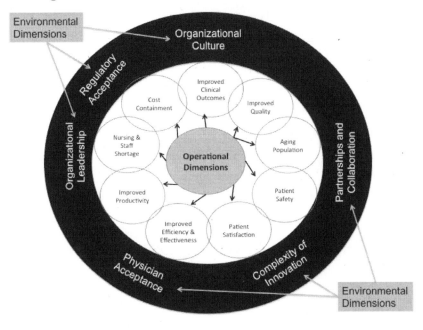

These various elements of healthcare innovation are impacting the shift to value-based and patient-centric healthcare. Recognizing the importance of each element and viewing these dimensions as a lens to derive greater insights on how we advance current care delivery models and technologies is crucial to achieving new levels of innovative thinking that benefits consumers and all stakeholders alike.

Aging Population—Trends, IT, and Financial Implications.

The post-acute sector provides healthcare services for our aging population, and many of these patients see between 7 and 16 different physicians annually, depending on their chronic health conditions. This fact stands in contrast to the intent of post-acute care services, where the goals are to decrease the length of costly hospital stays and to safely shift care to the lowest cost setting. As the "tech savvy" Baby Boomers reach retirement age daily (a generation of 78 million Americans),[411] healthcare service expectations are evolving rapidly.

Two fundamental shifts in philosophy are attributable to the Boomers and new demand for a coordinated continuum of care:

➢ Shift from a reactive sick care focus to a proactive wellness focus and

➢ Shift from institutional care settings to coordinated care that allows the population to age in place (at home).

Though our aging population growth is exploding, the trends (from 2002 to June 2012) in the statistics on care facilities available reflect decreases. [412]

➢ Number of skilled nursing facilities (SNFs) decreased from 16,536 to 15,657.

➢ Licensed beds to occupied beds decreased from 85.9% to 83.1%.

Care provided by SNFs in the post-acute continuum is based on physician orders but follows a nursing model of assessment on activities of daily living (ADLs) and continued monitoring of changes in condition. ADLs are activities done during a normal day, such as getting in and out of bed, dressing, bathing, eating, and using the bathroom. Trends from 2002 to 2012 reflect an increase in both the acuity of patients in SNFs (average resident ADLs increased from 3.85 to 4.11) and the required direct care hours per patient day (3.13 in 2002 to 3.66 in 2012).[413]

Healthcare is a complex continuum of multiple service providers universally driven by reimbursement guidelines. The need for new technologies to support facilities, clinical staff, and administration continues to grow annually. Health IT requirements for the long-term post-acute care (LTPAC) community are growing, but to date, incentives to support procurement, implementation and adoption in this sector that predominantly cares for the elderly has been neglected. Anticipation for inclusion of this sector in Stage 3 of the CMS Meaningful Use of EHRs program lends hope to needed financial incentives for providers in this sector to accelerate plans for health IT adoption. The LTPAC Health IT collaborative (LTPAC-HIT), in its 2012-2014 LTPAC Health IT Road Map, identified five priority areas for the LTPAC healthcare providers. Table 11-2 summarizes these priority areas.

Table 11-2. LTPAC Priority Areas for Action[414]

Priority Area	Description
Care Coordination	Be an enabler of customer-centered longitudinal care planning and coordination.
Quality	Use technology for transparent delivery, measurement, and improvement of care services across care settings.
Business Imperative	Use technology to generate service strategies to assure role in the future of health and wellness delivery.
Consumer-Centered	Use technology to build on legacy of longitudinal person-centered care and services through effective integration of care and hospitality paradigms.
Workforce Acceleration	Prepare workforce to leverage health IT to create great customer relationships, experiences, and outcomes.

Reimbursements from public and private insurers have been the primary traditional funding resource for care providers in this industry segment. Reimbursement is provided from several sources, including private insurance policies typically facilitated through employers;

federally funded Medicare program through CMS; state funded Medicaid programs for the disabled and economically limited; and consumers through co-payments, premiums, and deductibles. Based on 2010 data, the average daily reimbursement per patient for SNF was Medicare $437.47 and Medicaid $172.36.[415] The legislative decisions to continually cut reimbursement rates for both Medicare and Medicaid patients just further threatens this already fragile services sector.

The recent federally funded legislative initiatives can be divided into two categories: health IT and organizational health system reform focused on insurance/reimbursements, structure, and processes of care. Post-acute service providers are unable to directly benefit from either the health IT funding or the Medicare Shared Savings Program.

While post-acute providers are excluded, their services remain a vital component in the delivery continuum especially for the chronically ill and aging population. Ensuring that integrated health IT is implemented and adopted by providers in the LTPAC segment is a priority for improving quality of care, reducing medical errors, and enhancing patient satisfaction for our aging population.

Recent program announcements by the CMS Center for Medicare and Medicaid Innovation lend credibility to the vital role post acute care providers play in creating quality, affordable healthcare. These pilot programs and initiatives will provide evidence and acknowledgement of key areas for this sector of the healthcare industry that funding must be made available on a system-wide basis and not just offer limited program demonstration grants. Examples include:

> **Health Care Innovation Awards**. These projects aim to deliver better health, improved care and lower costs to people enrolled in

Medicare, Medicaid and Children's Health Insurance Program.[416]

➢ **Independence at Home Demonstration.** These demonstrations work with medical practices to test the effectiveness of delivering comprehensive primary care services at home to improve care for Medicare beneficiaries with multiple chronic conditions.[417]

➢ **Initiative to Reduce Avoidable Hospitalizations Among Nursing Facility Residents.** These initiatives implement evidence-based interventions focused on long-stay nursing facility residents with the goal of reducing avoidable inpatient hospitalizations.[418]

➢ **Community-based Care Transitions Program (CCTP).** This program test models for improving care transitions from the hospital to other settings and reducing readmissions.[419]

All of these efforts are supporting the need for long-term innovation initiatives to meet our nation's healthcare quality goals and the aims set forth by the Institute of Medicine. Pilot projects that utilize health IT solutions and target the cost and quality of care for this segment of the population will aid in efforts to achieve those aims.

Health System Complexity

One of the fundamental problems for very complex systems like healthcare is the dilemma and transition of a culture of autonomy that yields challenges in command and control over redesign of the system, as discussed by Paul Starr three decades ago in his seminal work, *The Social Transformation of American Medicine.*[420] Complex adaptive systems tend to have these design and management limitations. Moreover, no one can command or force the US healthcare system to comply with behavioral and performance dictates using any conventional means. The consumers (influential individuals and organizations acting as agents) in complex adaptive systems are sufficiently intelligent to game our complex healthcare system to find workarounds and creatively identify ways to serve their own interests.

Given the challenges with command and control of our complex adaptive healthcare system, management approaches should emphasize *leadership* rather than traditional management techniques— *influence* rather than power. Because none, or very few, of the stakeholder groups (including consumers/patients and families) in the healthcare system are employees, command and control has to be replaced with *incentives* and *inhibitions*. No one can require that stakeholders comply with organizational directives. They must have incentives to behave appropriately. One must think about awarding good behavior or habits, not bad behavior or habits.

Not only are most stakeholders in healthcare independent agents, they are also beyond direct observation. Thus, one cannot manage activities but can only assess the *value of their outcomes*. In a traditional system, one might attempt to optimize efficiency. However, the learning and adaptive characteristics of a complex adaptive system should be leveraged to encourage *agility* as an organizational behavior, rather than a focus on efficiency as a controlling behavior, particularly on out-of-date requirements. This is summarized in Rouse's article, *Health Care as a Complex Adaptive System: Implications for Design and Management*, and in the following Table 11-3.[421]

Table 11-3. Comparison of Organizational Behaviors

Organizational Behaviors	Traditional System	Complex Adaptive System
Roles	Management	Leadership
Methods	Command and control	Incentives and inhibitions
Measurement	Activities	Outcomes
Focus	Efficiency	Agility
Relationships	Contractual	Personal commitments
Network	Hierarchy	Heterarchy
Design	Organizational design	Self-organization

Substantial improvement in the system of healthcare is requiring that stakeholders have greater access to information on the performance of the whole system, any subsystem, and best practices. Dissemination of best practices, unintended consequences encountered, and barriers to advancement would be used to assess current and emerging situations in this complex adaptive system, which would lead to adjustments of incentives and inhibitions to motivate stakeholders to change behaviors to continually increase value.

From an engineering design perspective, Rouse declares in his article, that, as much as possible, complex systems should be designed and not just emerge. Design should begin with the recognition that *the healthcare enterprise—as a system—is a network of relationships* that includes stakeholder organizations, whether they are customers, partners, collaborators, channels, competitors, or regulators. Collaboration efforts that have taken place over the years with the Institute of Medicine and, more recently, with the National Coordinator for Health Information Technology (ONC-HIT)'s convening of its HIT Policy and Standards Committees,[422] have brought together these stakeholders to produce overarching strategies that deal with this challenge of complexity.

Large Scale Health Networks

So what are complex networks and what is network science? Why should we care? Are ACOs networks? Yes, ACOs are networks. They are networks of individuals, organizations, and networks themselves. The Science of Networks, as proposed by Newman, Barabási, and Watts,, looks at the , structure and dynamics of networks as:[423]

➢ A focus on properties of real-world networks,

➢ A view that real-world networks are actually evolving in time, and

➢ A framework for structure and dynamics of networks and how the two relate to each other

It is important to differentiate the following three , types of networks:

➢ **Network (generic)**— , a graph with links and nodes used by network scientists;

➢ **Network Level Collaborative**—, "Network" for short – three or more individuals, organizations, or networks collaborating to achieve a shared goal (requires formal agreement), and

➢ **Technology Network**—, a network of connected technologies.

For a network transition in healthcare, the following is true:

➢ It will involve development of many different network level collaboratives, connected with different technologies, and

➢ There will never be an overarching network for healthcare—rather there will be "networks of networks."

Demand by stakeholders for individual health and population health needs, will require innovation with information and communication technologies(ICT), , to reduce barriers, decrease costs, improve care quality, and access to our nation's health system. However, as noted by Figure 1-3 in Chapter 1, the enactment of recent federal legislative acts with a focus on health information technology—in 2009, ARRA, and HITECH,, and in 2010, the Affordable Care Act, and Meaningful Use of EHRs— Final Rule, set the stage for systemic organizational health system transformation. This was the needed financial incentive to propel the acquisition and adoption of EHRs. The Affordable Care Act led to the final CMS Medicare Shared Savings Program, (MSSP)—Final Rule. It established the framework for public sector ACOs and a framework for private sector ACOs. This, along with the , Supreme Court decision on June 28, 2012 to uphold the Affordable Care Act, has now created a "perfect storm"—a validation of the inevitable transition between fee for-service and capital-global or large-scale health payment systems or networks.

These paradigm-shifting reforms have brought about the opportunity to organize new , large-scale health networks (LSHNs) , that utilize and deploy new healthcare innovations,. Innovative solutions such as mobile devices,, mHealth apps (Chapter 8), , and dedicated Web sites for "health applications-in-the-cloud" , are designed to lower barriers to individual and population health for consumers, families, caregivers, and communities.

Since the early days of computers, interest in the use of ICT, to lower barriers for consumers and patients for health and healthcare services has been rising. Growth in the institutional adoption of. increasingly sophisticated health management systems is an indicator of this rising interest.

However, as already noted, in 2009, the conversation started to shift. The passage of ARRA and HITECH brought incentives for the adoption of health IT, while the Affordable Care Act for transformational reforms, including the MSSP, created the opportunity for public ACOs to develop as LSHNs , including all stakeholders (i.e., consumers/patients and their families, physicians, hospitals and insurers). , This is an exciting time in healthcare in America. For the first time in years, we are challenging and changing the basic approaches to improving quality and access to health and healthcare services in this country.

Building upon the work of Flareau and colleagues, as technologies enable new services and structures, a future transition may occur from ACOs to Accountable Care Networks (ACNs). , Figure 11-3 illustrates this concept.

Figure 11-3. Transition from Clinical Integrated to Accountable Care Networks[424]

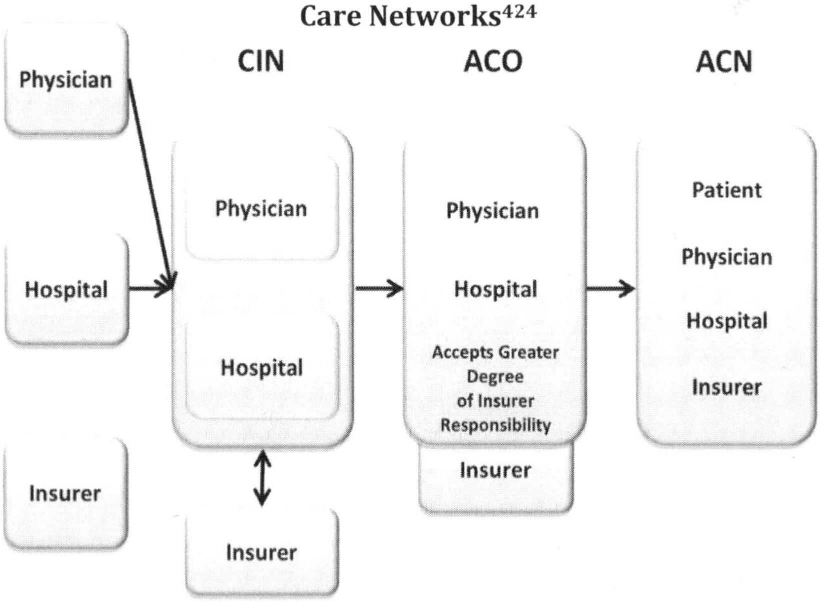

Just as a clinical integration network (CIN) , is a necessary building block of an ACO,, an ACO is a necessary building block for an ACN,. An ACN would be comprised of three or more separate business entities such as a physician group, hospital, and insurer with a formal shared vision, mission, network strategy, and network governance structure,. One can imagine a network of ACNs covering multiple medical trading areas, in one or more regions of the country.

New health ICT, applications in the cloud will bring about fundamental changes in how consumers and patients and their families engage, in their own health and healthcare, how physicians adapt their practices, how hospitals design and implement new services, and how hospitals and physicians are paid for services with the new emerging payment models. However, the large numbers of stakeholders of different types interacting at local, state, national, and even global levels point to a difficult coordination challenge associated with making these kinds of changes required by healthcare reform. As shown in Figure 11-4, at least 12 general types of stakeholders in health can be identified with an interest in—and potential to be affected by—changes in healthcare reform being enabled by the adoption of health information technology.

Figure 11-4. US Health Network Space

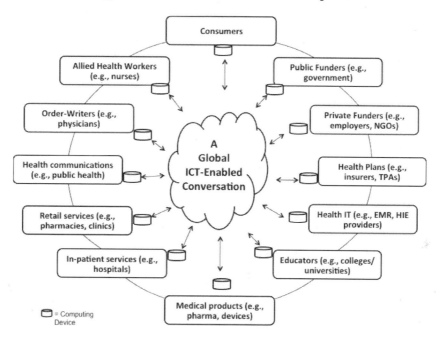

These include consumers, funders, health plans, health IT vendors, educators, medical product companies, patient service providers, retail services, health communications, order writers, and allied health workers. Each of these participant groups has potential to influence the future of healthcare for consumers. At local, state, national and global levels, participants from each of these groups are interacting and in increasing numbers, using local ICTs such as computers, laptops, tablets, smartphones, or cell phones connecting through global ICT platforms such as the Internet, social networks, and multimedia networks. They are making new clinical decisions based on these interactions. One can envision that what is emerging is an ever increasing, rapidly evolving, global conversation that will shape the future of individual and population health for all the stakeholders involved.

Some Overarching Questions

This idea of different participants interacting in an evolving global conversation about health and healthcare reform leads to overarching questions:

➢ How might—or should—these conversations be facilitated?

➢ How might the participants and stakeholders be engaged?

➢ How might conversations be controlled?

➢ How might the effects on individual and population health be measured?

➢ Perhaps most important of all: how might participants be supported so that the best possible health decisions are made for the stakeholders?

A Large Scale Health Network "in the Cloud"

The idea of an LSHN, in the cloud as a technology innovation, is driven by the desire to reduce barriers to improving individual and population health outcomes,. The approach begins with an analysis of the field of individual and population health using perspectives drawn from network sciences,. Such an analysis would find that a network transition, in which all stakeholders in individual and population health—a transition in which end users begin accessing health information and services through networks—appears to be in the early stages of development. It would identify several innovations, including new cloud-computing technologies,, with potential to drive a network transition in individual and population health in the coming years. This analysis could then be used to design LSHNs and design an action research method to support iterative evaluation and improvement of LSHNs as mentioned in Chapter 1 under the section on the dawn of network transition and network level action research (NLAR) ,.

Network Strategic Planning for Health IT

Strategic health IT , planning starts with a vision. A strategic IT vision for a network is created differently from that of an organization. What is different is that it requires a shared vision that is co-created and accepted by all the stakeholders of three or more business entities that comprise any large-scale network collaborative,. If physician practices, hospitals, academic medical centers, and other healthcare organizations are to advance as networks, strategic planning for health IT must be recognized as an essential function. Healthcare leaders are faced with cultural, technical, and financial barriers to accomplishing objectives with identifying and implementing the right health IT initiatives for their organizational networks and the consumers and patients they serve. Collaboration is critical among participants to ensure effectiveness and integration in getting the right innovations to the right places to yield value for the consumers and patients served.[425]

Three points to emphasize in , network strategic planning for health IT are setting priorities, adequate resourcing, and evaluating impact. As federal incentives for health IT sunset, the importance of planning initiatives will continue to grow.

Setting Priorities

As the impact of healthcare reform and policy mandates is assessed, healthcare executives are faced with new care models and payment structures. Organizations are integrating health IT plans as part of the overall strategic plan. Results of the *23rd Annual 2012 HIMSS Leadership Survey*[426] of 302 healthcare executives from across the spectrum of care settings identified three top priorities based on a two-year horizon: (1) achieving Meaningful Use; (2) implementing systems such as CPOE, EHRs and e-prescribing; and (3) leveraging information through the use of , data warehouses, clinical decision support, and , evidence-based medicine practices. To accomplish these priorities, effective IT governance is critical for 21st century healthcare organization as noted by Morrissey in the 2012 *Hospitals & Health Networks Magazine* article titled *"iGovernance."*[427] Establishing accountability for system selection and implementation to ensure adoption by clinical staff is a key element in the IT governance and priority setting process. In the HIMSS survey, less than 3% included cloud computing or telemedicine as priorities, but this can be expected to shift in the coming years. A critical success factor is the establishment of a longitudinal medical record (LMR) across the continuum of care. Supporting the importance of IT governance, more than 80% of the HIMSS survey respondents noted strong guidance was needed in: (1) value from IT investments, (2) overall strategy, (3) enable executive team to improve management through IT, (4) support business and clinical process owners, and (5) processing change management supported by IT.

Resources

Varied initiatives driven by healthcare reform legislation have encouraged organizations to shift financial resources toward IT initiatives. This "carrot and stick" mentality has both short-term and long-term implications. For the first time in several years, the survey respondents cited staffing needs over the lack of adequate financial support as their top barrier. Making the business case provides preliminary assessments for anticipated costs, return on investment, and impact to clinical operations,[428] which can lead to determinations on the amount and number of resources dedicated to implementation, integration and system maintenance efforts. Another barrier is the inability of vendors to deliver products or services effectively. This is quite challenging in the traditional "less technology savvy" silos of long-term care and home health. According to the HIMSS Analytics Database, the average IT operating expense was approximately 2.4% of total expenses for US hospitals in 2011. As expected, 75% of those surveyed had expanded operating budgets for 2012 over 2011. Key initiatives such as achieving Meaningful Use of EHRs and preparing for ICD-10 are requiring substantial capital investments, especially for the hospital sector. Long-term care facilities, critical access, and rural hospitals typically lack technology overall, aside from billing systems. As the industry moves forward, finding and dedicating financial and staff resources for health IT system selection, implementation, and adoption challenges will continue to be a challenge for healthcare executives.

Evaluating Impact

Healthcare reform is contributing to how we assess return on investment (ROI) from health IT initiatives. Upon the expiration of health reform incentives, organizations will be penalized for lack of compliance. As priorities are set and resources dedicated, there is a need to understand the impact of evaluation factors such as patient safety, physician/nursing satisfaction, productivity, and financial savings/revenue impact from implemented systems. As healthcare transitions from fee-for-service reimbursement, IT is being relied upon to improve clinical and quality outcomes. ACOs, both public and private, will be evaluated based on clinical quality and operational performance impact. This will be coupled with organizations measuring their performance against quality measures to reach each stage of the CMS Meaningful Use of EHRs program. The expansion of gathering consumer feedback and experience data for analyzing the effects of strategies continues to emerge across the continuum of care.

The ultimate savings sought since the release of the IOM's 1999 landmark report, *To Err is Human*, is the reduction of medical errors. Health IT has been an enabler of progress toward this goal, but it has been hindered by the occurrence of unintended adverse consequences and "e-iatrogenesis."[429] ACOs bring the opportunity to leverage interconnected systems across their networks. Evaluating financial impact is critical, but, at the end of the day, we place the highest value on lives, and safety comes first with the goal of reducing all medical errors across the network. As organizations evaluate their ROI from implementation of EHRs, HIE, PHRs, CPOE, and other technologies, proper weighting of these evaluation factors is essential to understand and tell the unbiased story of comprehensive ROI.

Implications of the Upheld Affordable Care Act

A "quiet internal" healthcare reform is moving forward regardless of what happens in Washington, DC. The US Supreme Court's ruling on the Affordable Care Act has helped to clear away the remaining uncertainty around federal healthcare reform, but virtually every healthcare leader has a strong commitment to advance care delivery reform initiatives through innovations and quality improvement, regardless of what ultimately happens with the Affordable Care Act. On June 28, 2012, the US Supreme Court issued a landmark ruling on the constitutionality of the Affordable Care Act.[430] Much of the industry's attention was focused on the mandate for individuals to carry health insurance coverage after 2014 or be required to pay a penalty, which the chief justices upheld as constitutional with the reasoning that this penalty would essentially be a tax imposed by the Internal Revenue Service.[431]

Strategically applied health IT will be incredibly important to creating the new healthcare environment our industry leaders are working toward, which is putting Chief Information Officers (CIOs), Chief Medical Information Officers (CMIOs), Chief Medical Officers (CMOs), and other healthcare IT leaders in a position that gives them tremendous responsibility, along with a new level of influence. While this federal ruling did not have a direct impact on any parts of the law related to the CMS Meaningful Use of EHRs program or others that are directly tied to advancement of health IT, it did help reinforce the underpinnings for which health IT is supporting the growth of ACOs, health information exchange, and other transformational elements of the Affordable Care Act.

Another issue of significance that was ruled upon was the law for expansion of Medicaid coverage. This law under the Affordable Care Act would have the potential ramification of dramatically increasing the numbers of Medicaid enrollees that physicians and ACOs would have to care for in the future.[432] However, within its ruling, the court concluded that it was unconstitutional to mandate states to participate in the expanded Medicaid insurance program. Under Section 2001 in the

Affordable Care Act, expanded eligibility is to include enrollees under the age of 65 with income below 133% of the federal poverty level.[433] In addition, Section 2001 increases coverage for participants from the current 50 to 83% of costs up to 100% from 2014 through 2016 and then 90% after 2020. As 26 states opposed this new mandate for participation in the Medicaid program, the court ruled that states would have the option of participation.[434] Even though a recently completed study on states that chose to expand Medicaid coverage provided evidence of a decrease in adult mortality rates, this mandate was not upheld.[435] Part of the concern for physicians, ACOs, and state legislatures alike is the reimbursement of care, given the projected large increases in Medicaid enrollees under this expanded coverage provision. At a macro level, the Congressional Budget Office (CBO) and Joint Committee on Taxation (JCT) estimate, "that fewer people will be covered by the Medicaid program, more people will obtain health insurance through the newly established exchanges, and more people will be uninsured." The CBO and JCT also assessed that the net costs of this insurance provision in the Affordable Care Act would now be $84 billion less over the 2012-2022 period than originally estimated in March 2012.[436]

The bottom line is that a new healthcare environment and culture are emerging, and CIOs, CMIOs, CMOs, and other healthcare executives are leading its transformation. Things will move forward inside healthcare as they were, only now with greater policy certainty. For those chartered with establishing ACOs and the health IT infrastructure necessary to enable their services for improvement of population health, the potential for dealing with a reversal of all the recent years' federal healthcare reforms has subsided. And in this quiet revolution, key players will be creating the new healthcare system. "So the quiet revolution moves forward."[437]

Stakeholders in the New Network Level Ecosystem

There are many stakeholders in the ecosystem that is the US healthcare system. Physicians and care providers, consumers, and healthcare provider organizations are only a few that engage on a daily basis to facilitate transactions, utilize and deliver services, and continuously work toward improving the quality of care experienced.

Physicians and Care Providers

Improving access to primary care services requires having sufficient physician and care providers in place across urban and rural settings. This includes access to preventative services as noted in Title IV—Prevention of Chronic Disease and Improving Public Health, of the Affordable Care Act.[438] Primary care providers fall into three categories based on the population they serve: pediatricians for children, primary care or internists for adults, and geriatricians for seniors. As patients age, the complexity of their health conditions combined with their changing physiology, demands more knowledgeable care providers. The shortage of geriatricians is being addressed by the emergence of state board certified physician extenders. The Kaiser Family Foundation's State Health Facts Web site noted there are only 180,233 nurse practitioners and 83,466 physician assistants.[439] More are needed.

Ensuring adequate physicians and medical extenders are in place is critical, as patients with chronic diseases require medical visits once every 30 days, at a minimum, and even more often based on medical necessity. Access to up-to-date patient information is often a major obstacle, including the need for transportation as patients move back and forth between care settings.

Enhancing access to patient care services will require new remote diagnostic and monitoring capabilities, improvement in electronic patient-provider communications, and expanded use of ePrescribing and PHRs. The aging population has seen an increase of medical extenders in walk-up clinics, long-term care facilities, and, most recently, increased visits at home as care delivery strategies shift to an "age in place" focus.

The ramifications for ACOs and health IT initiatives revolve around the mobility of patient visits and the varied professionals who can benefit from connected clinical information to improve diagnosis and decision making at the time encounters take place. An increased focus by technology vendors in the areas of remote monitoring, mHealth apps (discussed in Chapter 8), and clinical applications for the LTPAC community will enable a stronger connected continuum of care.

Payer Organizations

The economics of healthcare are driven by reimbursement. Since the entity paying for services is typically not the patient who receives them, there is an artificial perception of actual cost. For many consumers, their actual healthcare costs are perceived to be a combination of a portion of premiums for health insurance, co-pays at the time of service, and annual deductibles. A significant portion of healthcare reimbursement is provided by both federal and state government funds and disbursed through CMS, which is the single largest payer in the industry.

Today there are various payment models for each segment of our healthcare system, and the continued development of health IT provides a critical part of the infrastructure that enables exchange of needed clinical and financial patient records. Physicians and clinical professionals are reimbursed on a fee-for-service model, whereby they submit charges for reimbursement to insurance payers as individual services are performed. Diagnosis is determined and assigned a code under the ICD-9 standards that will transition to ICD-10, as discussed in Chapter 4 and impact all physicians, healthcare provider organizations, and ACOs alike, requiring significant investments in planning, training, software, and system upgrades and/or replacements.

Hospitals are reimbursed based on Diagnosis-Related Groups (DRGs) that are based on International Classification of Diseases (ICD) diagnoses, procedures, age, sex, discharge status, and the presence of complications or comorbidities for an episode of care. Skilled nursing facilities (SNFs) are reimbursed on a daily rate. Medicaid rates vary by state in the range of $400 to $750 per day all-inclusive, including medications for services at these organizations. The minimum data set (MDS) is a component of the resident assessment that contains a standardized set of essential clinical and functional status measures. SNFs are required to classify residents into 1 of 44 Resource Utilization Groups (RUGs-III) based on assessment data from the resident assessment. There are 108 MDS elements used in developing the RUG categories for each Medicare resident. The actual number of minutes of therapy services delivered to the resident is a key driver of the RUG reimbursement for Medicare patients. Medicare rates vary based on the RUG score, typically around $550 per day all-inclusive, including medications. Today, new patient admissions received into an SNF require a minimum 3-day stay in the hospital to be covered by Medicare.

Home care falls into two categories: medical and nonmedical. Non-medical includes well-known services like such as Meals on Wheels, personal emergency response alerts, housekeeping, and personal care. Aside from Medicaid waiver programs, most reimbursement is private pay. The process drivers, technology solutions, and varied formats for clinical information within the three distinct reimbursement models— (physicians and diagnostic testing) CPT codes, (hospitals) DRG episodes, and (skilled nursing) RUG assessments—will make sharing risk and bundling payments challenging, while, at the same time, forcing entities to collaborate and share information.

Health IT solutions will need to be able to track information across all platforms and care settings, including consumers being cared for at home. One major hurdle is the cross-referencing medical terminology of diagnosis and treatment plans used by hospitals and physicians with change-in-condition clinical notes kept in nursing environments such as SNFs and home care.

Consumers and the Care Continuum

A key factor for the new horizon is that healthcare is delivered geographically with complete coverage of services existing within a defined radius from where patients live. The concept of a Medical Trading Area (MTA) reflects the economics of how care is delivered and reimbursed within a defined geographic area. All MTAs rely on an emergency life-saving level of care. This service is called a level-one trauma center and, thus, MTAs cover radiuses extending out to the boundary of the next one. Within an MTA are hospitals including urban centers and rural critical access hospitals, as well as post-acute care providers that include both SNFs and long-term care facilities. Nursing homes typically serve both skilled and long-term care residents. SNF residents are rehabilitating to return home and receive up to 100 days paid by Medicare per incident. Long-term care residents are declining in activities for daily living and, thus, need assistance with functions on an ongoing basis.

Measuring Customer Experience Across the MTA

Organizations within each MTA are moving toward transparency with open access to data where consumers can endorse or criticize an organization via social media based on their experience with that organization. Healthcare providers should focus on understanding the customer experience through a multifaceted approach. Today technology solutions can be used to gather and analyze data in real time at various points in the service delivery process to provide current observations and insights from consumers, patients and other stakeholders.

Traditionally, in healthcare, "customer satisfaction benchmarking" surveys have been conducted quarterly or annually, then analyzed for underlying correlations, with results delivered in the form of a quarterly or annual report to the healthcare organization's senior management team members, who use it to validate the need for new initiatives, organizational design changes, and process improvements.

Progressive organizations are beginning to deploy enterprise feedback management (EFM) technology solutions to facilitate immediate and robust customer feedback. Similar to other service related industries, now healthcare organizations can have that data in real time, complete with driver and correlation analysis packaged to support clinical decision making. In the long-term care sector, being able to collect, analyze, and report in a near real-time to real-time manner on this type of customer experience feedback will be essential to meet the needs of value-based purchasing programs and ACOs such as skilled nursing facilities, nursing homes, and others, as they become more integrated within their networks of facilities.[440] Rather than looking at aggregated data to find patterns, you can now look at customer-specific encounters on a prioritized criteria basis and respond immediately.

Within each MTA is the growing importance of eldercare. The 2011 results of the Bureau of Labor Statistics survey *American Time Use Survey*, included statistics on eldercare, revealing how many millions of consumers are involved in providing care for the elderly. Figure 11-5 illustrates the percentage of Americans who are providing eldercare.

Figure 11-5. Eldercare in 2011.[441]

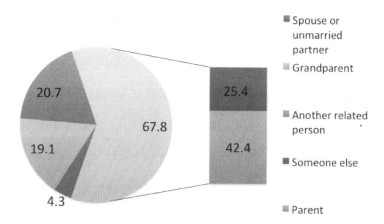

NOTE:
1) Care for a spouse or partner may be underreported.
2) Percent of eldercare providers, civilian non-institutional population, by relationship to care recipient, ages 15 and older, 2011 annual averages.
3) Estimates for relationship categories sum to more than 100 percent because some eldercare providers cared for more than one person.

Source: Bureau of Labor Statistics

Between 22% and 23% of those aged 45 to 64 identify themselves as elder care providers, along with 16% of those older than 65. Almost a third of them are taking care of two older people or more. And 23% also had a minor child in their households. In a great majority of cases, 85%, caregivers and their elders maintained separate households.

A majority of those providing care are women—56%—but that is a smaller majority than past research has found.

Analogy with Banking Industry

One example to consider is that the future of health information exchange may mirror how the financial services industry evolved with ATMs. There are no definitive international or government-compiled numbers totaling the comprehensive number of ATMs in use worldwide, but estimates by the ATM Industry Association place the number of ATMs in use at more than 2.2 million globally.[442] The establishment of standards for an interchange protocol enabled exchange of data on a real-time basis at any hour 365 days per year. The network is linked to a common backbone and, ultimately, transactions take place across the same bank, separate banks, states, and even countries with different currencies.

While the healthcare industry and its requirements are unique and different from the banking industry, as standards for and interoperability continue to mature (Chapter 4), the healthcare industry may one day see similar levels of interoperability, data security, and transaction exchange. Healthcare involves patients' life and death decisions. The future will bring connected technologies through the continued maturation of EHRs with CMS's Meaningful Use of EHRs program. The shift in consumer demographics is disrupting every category of healthcare services and driving the need for innovation. A trend toward aging in place and away from institutional venues for care will continue to drive the adoption of new technologies. Consumer apps, telehealth, social media and the explosion of technology-competent users on the Internet are examples of the healthcare revolution impacting both providers and consumer behavior, along with the growth of plastic surgery, weight management, chiropractors, and medical tourism. This elicits a question of the care continuum that has spawned much of the debate and need for healthcare reform over the past decade.

To better understand this new horizon of healthcare and a transition to networks, it is helpful to explain how things work today. You may have heard the term of "healthcare silos" and, for many, it is quite confusing to clearly delineate the roles of providers and payers. The driving forces of the new horizon are fundamental shifts in both the basis of how providers are paid and, moreover, the actual care delivery system itself. We are slowly transitioning away from fee-for-service toward bundled payments and from silo-based delivery toward shared risk partnership models. This quest to bend the curve or the growth rate in healthcare spending involves reenergizing key principles of fixed "capped" payments for care episodes, while rewarding innovative service models that deliver quality-based outcomes. The demands for and reliance on health information technology is critical for facilitating this new horizon.

How do we provide the best care in the lowest cost settings where the consumer wants it? A dilemma exists and is gradually being addressed through technology and innovation to bridge the gaps that exist in capturing, sharing and analyzing the appropriate information, both clinical and financial) across care settings. Figure 11-6 identifies many of the factors that exist across the continuum of care and the dilemma created.

Figure 11-6. Care Continuum Dilemma—
Interacting Factors

Factor / Care	Acute	Ambulatory	Post Acute	Home
Reimbursement Methods	Fee-for-Diagnosis (DRG codes) episodic	Fee-for-Service (CPT codes) longitudinal	Fee-for-Resource (RUG codes) daily rate	Private Pay & Waiver Programs
Health Information Technologies	HIS (hospital)	EMR (physician practice)	Billing & Charting (nursing facility)	Monitoring Devices (home)
Cost Rates	$4,500-$2,500/day average	$1,500-$1000/day average	$650-$150/day average	$100 or less/day

ACO Bundled Payments — Shared Savings - Balancing Efficiencies & Outcomes

Given these factors an opportunity exists to improve the quality of care for patients by keeping them in their desired setting of care—*right at home.* Figure 11-7 provides an illustration of the continuum and the direction of the industry to move care to lower cost settings.

Figure 11-7. The Care Continuum Opportunity— Moving Care to the Home

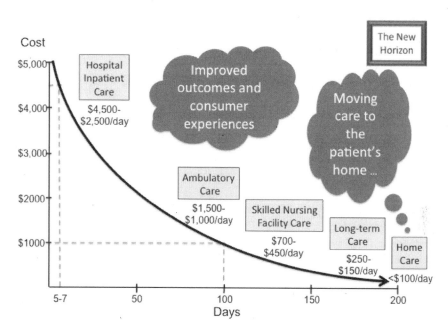

Home care providers include both medical and nonmedical services companies in additional to networks of families and friends. As the Baby Boomer population continues to age, dedication of resources and technological innovations, such as those in the field of remote monitoring, patient portals, and telemedicine, will support industry efforts for providing and moving care to the home.

Looking Ahead: A New Horizon Through Consumer and Innovation Networks

In conclusion, we have recapped topics from many of the chapters and introduced new topics related to consumer and innovation networks. The landscape of healthcare reform is bringing about the dawn of a new era and the continued development of new technologies will only continue to help enable physicians, caregivers, and the healthcare organizations they work within to deliver more efficient, effective, and integrated services each day. Ideally, using comparative effectiveness research (CER) tools (as covered in Chapter 10) and different models (public and private ACOs), ACOs could be compared for different health finance and delivery approaches and help advance the study of healthcare quality, accessibility, and affordability. Health reforms led by the Affordable Care Act are changing the field of CER. Led by demand from nontraditional users (value-based suppliers such as ACOs) and fueled by increasingly sophisticated technology tools, CER is being pushed into innovative territory, where quick results are more important than perfect experimental design.

CER is one kind of research that could be included in Network Level Action Research (NLAR) projects (topic introduced in Chapter 1). Researchers and practitioners could benefit by focusing on relevant problems and lowering barriers to dissemination. Other kinds of research to include in an NLAR project are adoption research (e.g., factors affecting individual or organization-level adoption of health information technologies and use of such innovations and novel medical technologies identified through CER); organizational outcomes research (e.g., effect on organizations trying to implement the innovation), or network research (e.g., effects of network patterns on participation and outcomes).

The Network Transition

There are many valid ways to look at, and theorize about, factors driving change in health in the 21st century. One that offers broad explanatory power is the concept of a *network transition*. This section begins by describing this concept and a tool for assessing it. Results of an assessment of the potential for a network transition in health are then shared. The data suggests the time may be right to form one or more research-driven LSHNs for individual health, healthcare, and population health. Figure 11-8 illustrates a roadmap in a sense of what has transpired through history with the transition to networked organizational structures.

Figure 11-8. The Network Transition[443]

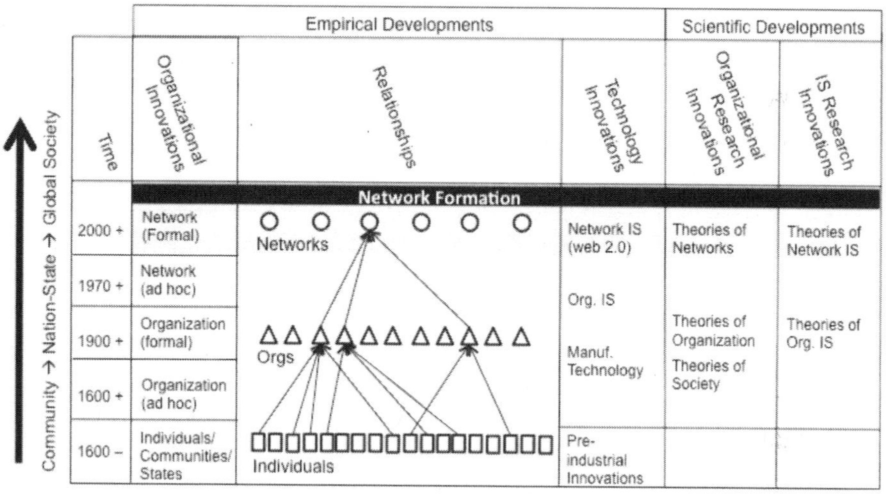

IS = Information Systems

The idea of a network transition is an emerging concept in the academic literature. As described by Raab and colleagues: "Western societies are moving towards a society of networks, i.e. a society, in which the formal, vertically integrated organization that has dominated the 20th century is replaced or at least complemented by consciously created and goal directed networks."[444]

A more formal way to describe the network transition is "a *change of state* within a given *network space* from one in which organizations are the primary drivers of *social and economic change* to one in which *networks* are the primary drivers of social and economic change" (see Table 11-4 for definitions).

Table 11-4. Network Transition—Definition of Terms

Term	Definition
Transition	Change from one position or state to another.
Change of state	Same as *transition.*
Network	Short for *network level collaborative.*
Network level collaborative	Three or more individuals, organizations and/or networks collaborating to achieve a shared goal none can achieve on their own.[445]
Network space	A set of participants (e.g., individuals, organizations, or networks) who connect within a defined social context (e.g., an organization, association, network, city, state, country, industry, sector, or society).
Social and economic change	Changes in laws, customs, and institutions that shape the development, ownership, and exchange of resources among people, organizations, and networks in a social context.[446]

Historical Perspective

According to network scholars, the beginning of the network transition —the emergence of networks as entities formally distinguishable from organizations—begins, empirically, around the year 2000.[447] A brief comparison with the so-called *organizational transition* that has occurred in many societies over the last century helps ground the concept. Starting around 1900, after more than 300 years of trial and error, most Western societies go through a transition in which hierarchically controlled public and private organizations, granted independent legal rights and status under law and custom, became the primary agents of change in society.[448] The unparalleled ability of organizations to aggregate resources and coordinate labor drives innovation and progress in societies and facilitates the organizational transition. For this reason, until very recently, it was assumed that "societies of organizations" would continue to steer society in the future.[449]

Now, some network scholars are questioning this premise. New data suggests that a *network transition*—a transition to a world in which change is primarily influenced by networks—has begun. The argument here is that by binding multiple individuals, organizations, and/or networks together using connections of trust with support from modern ICTs, networks will gain an ability to coordinate change that even the largest, best capitalized organizations or political institutions cannot match.[450] Benkler provides an elegant description of the "network economics" underlying this phenomenon:

> The critical characteristic of the networked economy is a radical decentralization of physical capital necessary for the production, storage,

distribution, and processing of information, knowledge and culture. This decentralization has caused a radical distribution of the practical capability to act in these areas, creating new levels of efficacy for individuals, who increasingly shift from being consumers to being users and producers. Individuals have now become capable of doing much more for themselves and for others, both alone and in vastly more effective loose collaborations with others. [451]

Scholars, healthcare researchers, executives, and policy makers must surmise that the *network transition* for healthcare may develop in a progression similar to that seen in other industries. Unique challenges and barriers to progress in healthcare will be overcome with innovations and adoption of health information technology to enable continued momentum. For, the *pace of change is ever accelerating,* as we start to cross the bridge to the next generation of healthcare in America.

Chapter 11: Takeaways

✓ Healthcare innovation. The introduction of a new concept, idea, service, process, or product aimed at improving treatment, diagnosis, education, outreach, prevention and research, and with the long-term goals of improving quality, safety, outcomes, efficiency and costs.

✓ An accountable care network (ACN) would be comprised of three or more separate business entities such as a physician group, hospital, and insurer with a formal shared vision, mission, network strategy, and network governance structure.

✓ Points to emphasize in network strategic planning for health IT are setting priorities, resourcing, and evaluating impact.

✓ Between 22% and 23% of those aged 45 to 64 identify themselves as elder care providers, along with 16% of those older than 65.

✓ As organizations evaluate their ROI from implementation of EHRs, HIE, PHRs, CPOE, and other technologies, proper weighting of these evaluation factors is essential to understand and tell the unbiased story of comprehensive ROI.

✓ As the Baby Boomer population continues to age, dedication of resources and innovations, such as remote monitoring, patient portals, and telemedicine, will support moving care to the home.

✓ With CER tools, ACOs could be compared for different health finance and delivery approaches to help advance the study of healthcare quality, accessibility, and affordability.

✓ The network transition is "a change of state within a given network space from one in which organizations are the primary drivers of social and economic change to one in which networks are the primary drivers of social and economic change."

[397] Raab J, Kenis P. Heading toward a Society of Networks Empirical Developments and Theoretical Challenges. *J of Manage Inquiry.* Sep 2009;18(3):198-210.

[398] Rogers EM. Chapter 1: Elements of Diffusion. *Diffusion of Innovations. 5th Ed.* New York, NY: Free Press; 2003:1-35.

[399] Flareau B, Yale K, Bohn J, Konshak C. Glossary and Acronyms. In: *Clinical Integration: A Roadmap to Accountable Care.* 2nd Ed. Virginia Beach, VA: Convurgent Publishing; 2011:328.

[400] West MA (Ed), Farr JL (Ed). *Innovation and Creativity at Work: Psychological and Organizational Strategies.* Hoboken, NJ: John Wiley & Sons, Inc.; 1990.

[401] Omachonu VK, Einspruch NG. Innovation in Healthcare Delivery Systems: A Conceptual Framework. *The Innovation Journal.* 2010;15(1):Article 2. Accessed online July 20, 2012, at http://innovation.cc/volumes-issues/vol15-no1.htm.

[402] Omachonu VK, Einspruch NG. 2010.

[403] Konschak C, Jarrell L. Introduction. In: *Consumer-centric Healthcare: Opportunities and Challenges for Providers.* Chicago, IL: Health Administration Press; 2010:4.

[404] Morse G. Ten Innovations That Will Transform Medicine. *Harvard Business Review Blog Network.* March 8, 2010. Accessed online August 2, 2012, at http://blogs.hbr.org/cs/2010/03/health_care_of_the_future.html.

[405] OECD and EuroStat. *Oslow Manual, The Measurement of Scientific and Technological Activities.* 3rd Ed. 2005. Accessed online July 22, 2012, at http://www.oecd.org/dataoecd/35/61/2367580.pdf.

[406] Varkey P, Horne A, Bennet KE. Innovation in Health Care: A Primer. *Am J Med Qual.* 2008 Sep-Oct;23(5):382-388.

[407] Paulus RA, Davis K, Steele GD. Continuous Innovation in Health Care: Implications of the Geisinger Experience. *Health Aff (Millwood).* 2008 Sep-Oct;27(5):1235-1245.

[408] Casalino LP, Rittenhouse DR, Gillies RR, Shortell SM. Specialist Physician Practices as Patient-Centered Medical Homes. *N Engl J Med.* 2010 Apr 29;362(17):1555-8.

[409] Omachonu VK, Einspruch NG. 2010.

[410] Omachonu VK, Einspruch NG. 2010.

[411] Public Broadcasting Service (PBS). The Boomer Century: 1946-2046. Documentary. Accessed online July 25, 2012, at http://www.pbs.org/boomercentury/.

[412] American Health Care Association. Trends in Nursing Facility Characteristics. June 2012. Accessed online July 25, 2012, at http://www.ahcancal.org/research_data/trends_statistics/Documents/Trend_PVNF_FINALRPT_June2012.pdf.

[413] American Health Care Association. June 2012.

[414] LTPAC HIT Collaborative. *A Roadmap for Health IT in Long-Term and Post-Acute Care (LTPAC) 2012-2014.* Accessed online August 4, 2012, at http://ltpachealthit.org/content/2012-2014-roadmap-hit-ltpac.

[415] American Health Care Association. *The State Long-Term Health Care Sector Characteristics, Utilization, and Government Funding: 2011 Update*. September 6, 2011.

[416] CMS Centers for Medicare and Medicaid Innovation. Health Care Innovation Awards. Accessed online July 24, 2012, at http://www.innovations.cms.gov/initiatives/Innovation-Awards/index.html.

[417] CMS Centers for Medicare and Medicaid Innovation. *Independence at Home Demonstration*. Accessed online July 24, 2012, at http://www.innovations.cms.gov/initiatives/Independence-at-Home/index.html.

[418] CMS Centers for Medicare and Medicaid Innovation. *Initiative to Reduce Avoidable Hospitalizations Among Nursing Facility Residents*. Accessed online July 24, 2012, at http://www.innovations.cms.gov/initiatives/rahnfr/index.html.

[419] CMS Centers for Medicare and Medicaid Innovation. *Community-based Care Transitions Program*. Accessed online July 25, 2012, at http://www.innovations.cms.gov/initiatives/Partnership-for-Patients/CCTP/index.html.

[420] Starr P. Introduction: The Social Origins of Professional Sovereignty. In: *The Social Transformation of American Medicine*. New York, NY: Harper Collins, 1982:3-29.

[421] Rouse W. Health care as a complex adaptive system: implications for design and management. *The Bridge*. Spring 2008;17-25.

[422] Office of the National Coordinator for Health Information Technology website. Federal Advisory Committees. Accessed online July 28, 2012, at http://healthit.hhs.gov/portal/server.pt/community/healthit_hhs_gov__federal_advisory_committees_%28facas%29/1149.

[423] Newman M, Barabasi AL, Watts DJ. *The Structure and Dynamics of Networks: Princeton Studies in Complexity*. Princeton, NJ: Princeton University Press. 2006; Watts, DJ. Networks, Dynamics, and the Small-World Phenomenon. *American Journal of Sociology*. 1999;105(2):493-527; Barabasi AL, Bonabeau E. Scale-Free Networks. *Scientific American*. 2003;288(5):60-69.

[424] Flareau B, et. al. Chapter 3: Forming the Clinically Integrated Network. In: *Clinical Integration: A Roadmap to Accountable Care*. 2nd Ed; 2011:69; Original illustration developed based on BDC Advisors presentation to VHA on Clinical Integration (slide 2) referred to on page 69 of the aforementioned work.

[425] Kaplan RS, Norton DP, Rugelsjoen B. Managing Alliances with the Balanced Scorecard. *Harvard Business Review*. January-February 2010;88(2):114-120.

[426] Healthcare Information and Management Systems Society.23rd Annual 2012 HIMSS Leadership Survey: Senior IT Executive Results. February 21, 2012. Accessed online July 31, 2012, at www.himss.org/asp/ContentRedirector.asp?ContentId=79507.

[427] Morrissey J. iGovernance. *Hospitals & Health Networks Magazine*. February 2012. Accessed online July 28, 2012, at http://www.hhnmag.com/hhnmag_app/jsp/articledisplay.jsp?dcrpath=HHNMAG/Article/data/02FEB2012/0212HHN_Coverstory&domain=HHNMAG.

[428] Shortliffe EH. Strategic Action in Health Information Technology: Why the Obvious Has Taken So Long. *Health Aff (Millwood)*. 2005 Sep-Oct;24(5):1222-1233.

[429] Ash JS, Sittig DF, Poon EG, Guappone K, Campbell E, Dykstra RH. The Extent and Importance of Unintended Consequences Related to Computerized Provider Order Entry. *J Am Med Inform Assoc*. 2007;14(4):415-423; Weiner JP, Kfuri T, Chan K, Fowles JB. "e-Iatrogenesis": The Most Critical Unintended Consequence of CPOE and other HIT. *J Am Med Inform Assoc*. 2007;14(3):387-388.

[430] *National Federation of Independent Business v. Sebelius*, 132 S. Ct. 2566 [2012].

[431] Mariner WK, Glantz LH, Annas GJ. Reframing Federalism—The Affordable Care Act (and Broccoli) in the Supreme Court. *N Engl J Med*. 2012 Jul 18.

[432] Flareau B, et. al. History. In: *Clinical Integration: A Roadmap to Accountable Care*, 2nd Ed. Virginia Beach, VA: Convurgent Publishing, 2011:28.

[433] H.R. 3590, Patient Protection and Affordable Care Act, Title II, Subtitle A- Improved Access to Medicaid. §2001(e)(1). Medicaid Coverage for the Lowest Income Populations (2010).

[434] Jost TS, Rosenbaum S. The Supreme Court and the Future of Medicaid. *N Engl J Med*. 2012 Jul 25. [Epub ahead of print].

[435] California Health Line. *States That Expanded Medicaid Saw Drop in Adult Mortality Rates*. July 26, 2012. Accessed online July 28, 2012, at http://www.californiahealthline.org/articles/2012/7/26/study-says-states-that-expanded-medicaid-also-cut-adult-morality.aspx#ixzz21vbxPjHS.

[436] Congressional Budget Office. Estimates for the Insurance Coverage Provisions of the Affordable Care Act Updated for the Recent Supreme Court Decision. July 24, 2012. Accessed online July 28, 2012, at http://www.cbo.gov/publication/43472.

[437] Hagland M. "Quiet" Healthcare Reform Moves Forward. *Healthcare Informatics*. June 29, 2012. Accessed online July 28, 2012 at http://www.healthcare-informatics.com/blogs/mark-hagland/quiet-healthcare-reform-moves-forward-0.

[438] H.R. 3590, Patient Protection and Affordable Care Act, Title IV, Prevention of Chronic Disease and Improving Public Health (2010).

[439] Kaiser Family Foundation's State Health Facts Providers & Service Use. Accessed online July 28, 2012, at http://www.statehealthfacts.org/comparecat.jsp?cat=8&rgn=6&rgn=1.

[440] Smith A. We Need Better Solutions for Customer Loyalty in Long Term Care. *Signature HealthCARE Blog Network*. July 30, 2012. Accessed August 3, 2012 at http://blogs.ltcrevolution.com/customer-experience/2012/07/30/we-need-better-solutions-for-customer-loyalty-in-long-term-care/#comment-19759.

[441] Bureau of Labor Statistics. Eldercare 2011. June 26, 2012. Accessed online July 28, 2012, at http://www.bls.gov/opub/ted/2012/ted_20120626_data.htm#chart1.

[442] ATM Industry Association. *Global ATM Clock*. Accessed online July 28, 2012, at https://www.atmia.com/main/global-atm-clock/.

[443] Thornewill, J. An Exploration of Factors Affecting Participation in U.S. Health Information Exchange Networks: A Dual Network Participation Theory Based Case Study. School of Interdisciplinary and Graduate Studies, University of Louisville, Louisville, Kentucky; 2011.

[444] Raab J, Kenis P. 2009.

[445] Provan KG, Fish A, Sydow J. Interorganizational Networks at the Network Level: A Review of the Empirical Literature on Whole Networks. *Journal of Management.* 2007;33(3):479-516; Thornewill, J. 2011.

[446] North, D. *Understanding the Process of Economic Change.* Princeton, NJ: Princeton University Press,;2005.

[447] Borgatti SP, Foster PC. The Network Paradigm in Organizational Research: A Review and Typology. *Journal of Management.* 2003;29(6):991-1013; Provan KG, et al. 2007; Raab J, Kenis P. 2009; Zaheer A, Gozubuyuk R, Milanov H. It's the Connections: The Network Perspective in Interorganizational Research. *Academy of Management Perspectives.* Feb 2010;24(1):62-77.

[448] Perrow C. A Society of Organizations. *Theory and Society.* Dec 1991;20(6):725-762; Raab J, Kenis P. 2009.

[449] Perrow C. 1991.

[450] Borgatti SP, Foster PC. 2003.

[451] Benkler Y. *The Wealth of Networks: How Social Production Transforms Markets and Freedom* New Haven, CT: Yale University Press; 2006.

Bibliography

Adler KG. Successful EHR implementations: attitude is everything. *Fam Pract Manag.* 2010 Nov-Dec;17(6):9-11.

Akobeng, AK. Understanding Randomised Controlled Trials. *Arch Dis Child.* 2005 August;90(8):840–844.

Arlotte P. 7 Strategies for Improving HITECH Readiness. *Healthc Financ Manage.* 2010 Nov;64(11):90-94, 96.

Ash JS, Sittig DF, Poon EG, Guappone K, Campbell E, Dykstra RH. The extent and importance of unintended consequences related to computerized provider order entry. *J Am Med Inform Assoc.* 2007;14(4):415-423.

Barabasi AL, Bonabeau E. Scale-Free Networks. *Scientific American.* 2003;288(5);60-69.

Bates DW, Bitton A. The Future of Health Information Technology in the Patient-Centered Medical Home. *Health Aff (Millwood).* 2010 Apr;29(4):614–621.

Benkler Y. *The Wealth of Networks: How Social Production Transforms Markets and Freedom.* New Haven, CT: Yale University Press; 2006.

Bernd DL, Fine PS. Electronic Medical Records: A Path Forward. *Front Health Serv Manage.* 2011 Fall;28(1):3-13.

Blumenthal D. Stimulating the Adoption of Health Information Technology. *N Engl J Med.* 2009;360:1477-1479.

Blumenthal D. Wiring the Health System—Origins and Provisions of a New Federal Program. *N Engl J Med.* 2011;365(24):2323-2329.

Blumenthal D, Glasser JP. Information Technology Comes to Medicine. *N Engl J Med.* 2007;356(24):2527-2534.

Blumenthal D, Tavenner M. The "Meaningful Use" Regulation for Electronic Health Records. *N Engl J Med.* 2010 Aug;363(6):501-504.

Bohn J. *Your Next Steps in Healthcare Transformation.* Louisville, KY: Touchcast Press; 2011.

Bonander J, Gates S. Public health in an era of personal health records: opportunities for innovation and new partnerships. *J Med Internet Res.* 2010;12(3):e33.

Borgatti SP, Foster PC. The Network Paradigm in Organizational Research: A Review and Typology. *Journal of Management.* 2003;29(6):991-1013.

Boulos MNK, Wheeler S, Tavares C, Jones R. How smartphones are changing the face of mobile and participatory healthcare: an overview, with an example from eCAALYX. *Biomed Eng Online.* 2011;10:24.

Bowes WA. Assessing readiness for meeting Meaningful Use: identifying electronic health record functionality and measuring levels of adoption. *AMIA Annu Symp Proc.* 2010 Nov 13;2010:66-70.

Campbell EM, Sittig DF, Ash JS, Guappone KP, Dykstra RH. Types of unintended consequences related to computerized provider order entry. *J Am Med Inform Assoc.* 2006;13(5):547-556.

Casalino LP, Rittenhouse DR, Gillies RR, Shortell SM. Specialist Physician Practices as Patient-Centered Medical Homes. *N Engl J Med.* 2010 Apr 29;362(17):1555-1558.

Cebul RD, Love TE, Jain AK, Hebert CJ. Electronic Health Records and Quality of Diabetes Care. *N Engl J Med.* 2011;365(24):825-833.

Center for Medicare and Medicaid Services. National Health Expenditures Aggregate, Per Capita amounts, Percent Distribution, and Average Annual Percent Change: Selected Calendar Years 1960-2010.

Chernew ME, Jacobson PD, Hofer TP, Aaronson KD, Fendrick AM. Barriers to Constraining Health Care Cost Growth. *Health Aff (Millwood).* November 2004 23:122-128.

Chaudhry B, Wang J, Wu S, Maglione M, Mojica W, Roth E, Morton SC, Shekelle PG. 2006. Systematic review: impact of health information technology on quality, efficiency, and costs of medical care. *Annals of Internal Medicine.* 2006 May 16;144(10):742-752.

Christensen CM, Grossman JH, Hwang J. *The Innovator's Prescription. A Disruptive Solution for Health Care.* New York, NY: McGraw-Hill; 2009.

Chute CG, Beck SA, Fisk TB, Mohr DN. The Enterprise Data Trust at Mayo Clinic: a semantically integrated warehouse of biomedical data. *J Am Med Inform Assoc.* 2010 Mar-Apr;17(2):131-135.

Clancy C, Collins FS. Patient-Centered Outcomes Research Institute: The Intersection of Science and Health Care. *Sci Transl Med.* 2010 Jun 23;2(37):37cm18.

Clarke, R. Paul M. Ellwood, MD: reforming health care from Jackson Hole. *HFMA.* November 1, 1994.

Committee on Data Standards for Patient Safety. Institute of Medicine. *Key Capabilities of an Electronic Health Record System: Letter Report.* Washington, DC: National Academies Press. July 31, 2003.

Committee on Identifying and Preventing Medication Errors. Institute of Medicine. Incidence of Medication Errors. In: *Preventing Medication Errors: Quality Chasm Series.* Washington, DC: National Academy Press; 2007.

Committee on Patient Safety and Health Information Technology. Institute of Medicine. *Health IT and Patient Safety: Building Safer Systems for Better Care.* (Prepublication Copy). Washington, DC: The National Academies Press; 2011.

Committee on Quality of Care in America. Institute of Medicine. Chapter 2: Errors in Health Care: A Leading Cause of Death and Injury. In: *To Err is Human. Building a Safer Health System.* Washington, DC: National Academy Press; 1999.

Committee on Quality of Health Care in America. Institute of Medicine. *Crossing the Quality Chasm. A New Health System for the 21st Century.* Washington, DC: National Academies Press; 2001.

Concato J, Lawler EV, Lew RA, Gaziano JM, Aslan M, Huang GD. Observational Methods in Comparative Effectiveness Research. *Am J Med.* 2010 Dec;123(12 Suppl 1):e16-23.

Corrao NJ, Robinson AG, Swiernik MA, Naeim A. Importance of testing for usability when selecting and implementing an electronic health or medical record system. *J Oncol Pract.* 2010 May;6(3):120-124.

Coyle YM, Battles JB. Using antecedents of medical care to develop valid quality of care measures. *Int J Qual Health Care.* 1999 Feb;11(1):5-12.

Cronholm S, Goldkuhl G. Conceptualising Participatory Action Research—Three Different Practices. *Electronic Journal of Business Research Methods.* 2004;1(2):47-58.

Davenport T, Harris J. *Competing on Analytics: The New Science of Winning.* Boston, MA: Harvard Business School Press; 2007.

Davison R, Martinsons MG, Kock N. Principles of Canonical Action Research. *Inform Syst J.* Jan 2004;14(1):65-86.

Davis CK, Stoots M, Bohn JM. Paving the Way for Accountable Care. Excellence in EMR Implementations. *JHIM.* 2012 Winter;26(1):38-45.

Department of Health and Human Services. *Report to Congress: National Strategy for Quality Improvement in Health Care.* March 2011.

Devers K, Berenson R. Can accountable care organizations improve the value of health care by solving the cost and quality quandaries? Robert Wood Johnson policy analysis paper; October 2009.

Dimick, Chris. RECs on a Mission: Assessing the Regional Extension Center Program. *Journal of AHIMA.* 2011 November-December;82(11):26-30.

Donabedian A. Evaluating the Quality of Medical Care. *Milbank Quarterly.* 2005;83(4):691-729. Reprinted from *Milbank Memorial Fund Quarterly.* 1966;44(3):166-203.

Ericson J. Old Priorities, New Urgency. *Health Data Manag.* 2010 Oct;18(10):41-44.

Estimates for the Insurance Coverage Provisions of the Affordable Care Act Updated for the Recent Supreme Court Decision. *Congressional Budget Office.* July 24, 2012.

Etheredge L. Creating a High-Performance System for Comparative Effectiveness Research. *Health Aff (Millwood).* 2010;29(10):1761-1767.

Ferranti JM, Langman MK, Tanaka D, McCall J, Ahmad A. Bridging the Gap: Leveraging Business Intelligence Tools in Support of Patient Safety and Financial Effectiveness. *J Am Med Inform Assoc.* 2010 Mar-Apr;17(2):136-143.

Fisher ES, McClellan MB, Bertko J, et al. Fostering accountable health care: moving forward in Medicare. *Health Aff (Millwood).* 2009;28(2):w219-w231.

Fisher ES, Staiger DO, Bynum JP, Gottlieb DJ. Accountable care organizations: the extended medical staff. *Health Aff (Millwood).* 2007;26(1):w44–w57.

Flareau B, Yale K, Bohn J, Konschak C. *Clinical Integration: A Roadmap to Accountable Care.* 2nd Ed. Virginia Beach, VA: Convurgent Publishing; 2011.

Ford EW, Menachemi N, Peterson LT, Huerta TR. Resistance is futile: but it is slowing the pace of EHR adoption nonetheless. *J Am Med Inform Assoc.* 2009;16(3):274-281.

Fortin J, Zywiak W. Beyond Meaningful Use Getting Meaningful Value from IT. *Healthc Financ Manage.* 2010 Feb;64(2):54-59.

Garrett P, Seidman J. EMR vs. EHR—What is the Difference? *HealthIT Buzz.* January 4, 2011.

Glaser J. HITECH Lays the Foundation for More Ambitious Outcomes-Based Reimbursement. *Am J Manag Care.* 2010 Dec;16(12 Suppl HIT):SP19-23.

Glaser J, Stone J. Effective Use of Business Intelligence. *Healthc Financ Manage.* 2008 Feb;62(2):68-72.

Glaser J, Salzberg C. Information technology for accountable care organizations. *Hospitals and Health Networks.* September 2010.

Goldstein MM, Jane HT. The First Anniversary of the Health Information Technology for Economic and Clinical Health (HITECH) Act: The Regulatory Outlook for Implementation. *Perspect Health Inf Manag.* 2010 Summer;7(Summer):1c.

Gray BH, Gusmano MK, Collins SR. AHCPR and the Changing Politics of Health Services Research. *Health Aff (Millwood).* 2003 Jan-Jun;Suppl Web Exclusives:W3–283–307.

Greenes, R.A. ed. *Clinical Decision Support, the Road Ahead.* Maryland Heights, MO: Academic Press; 2007:207-223.

Hagland M. "Quiet" Healthcare Reform Moves Forward. *Healthcare Informatics.* June 29, 2012.

Hilbert M, Lopez P. The World's Technological Capacity to Store, Communicate, and Compute Information. *Science.* April 2011;332(6025):60-65.

Hirsch MD. Regional extension centers struggling to help docs meet Meaningful Use. *FierceEMR.* November 17, 2011.

Hoffman S, Podgurski A. Improving health care outcomes through personalized comparisons of treatment effectiveness based on electronic health records. *J Law Med Ethics.* 2011 Fall;39(3):425-436.

Holden LM. Complex Adaptive Systems: Concept Analysis. *Journal of Advanced Nursing.* 2005;52(6):651-657.

Holmes C. The Problem List beyond Meaningful Use. Part I: The Problems with Problem Lists. *J AHIMA.* 2011 Feb;82(2):30-33; quiz 34.

Horwitz RI, Viscoli CM, Clemens JD, Sadock RT. Developing improved observational methods for evaluating therapeutic effectiveness. *Am J Med.* 1990;89:630–638.

Hsiao CJ, Hing E, Socey TC, Cai B. Electronic health record systems and intent to apply for Meaningful Use incentives among office-based physician practices: United States, 2001–2011. *NCHS Data Brief.* No 79. Hyattsville, MD: National Center for Health Statistics; 2011.

US Census Bureau. Income, Poverty, and Health Insurance Coverage in the United States: 2010. United States Census Bureau Annual Report.

Javitt JC, Rebitzer JB, Reisman L. Information technology and medical missteps: evidence from a randomized trial. *J Health Econ.* 2008;27(3):585-602.

Javitt JC, Steinberg G, Locke T, Couch JB, Jacques J, Juster I, Reisman L. Using a Claims Data-based, Sentinel System to Improve Compliance with Clinical Guidelines: Results of a Randomized Prospective Study. *Am J Manag Care.* 2005 Feb;11(2):93–02.

Jha A. The Stage 2 Meaningful Use of EHRs Proposed Rules: No Surprises. *Health Affairs Blog.* February 24, 2012.

Jha AK, DesRoches CM, Campbell EG, et al. Use of electronic health records in U.S. hospitals. *N Engl J Med.* 2009;360(16):1628-1638.

Jiang HJ, Lockee C, Bass K, Fraser I. Board engagement in quality: findings of a survey of hospital and system leaders. *J Healthc Manag.* 2008 Mar-Apr;53(2):121-134; discussion 135.

Jones SS, Adams JL, Schneider EC, Ringel JS, McGlynn EA. Electronic health record adoption and quality improvement in US hospitals. *Am J Manag Care.* 2010 Dec;16(12 Suppl HIT):SP64-71.

Joshi MS, Hines SC. Getting the board on board: Engaging hospital boards in quality and patient safety. *Jt Comm J Qual Patient Saf.* 2006 Apr;32(4):179-187.

Jost TS, Rosenbaum S. The Supreme Court and the Future of Medicaid. *N Engl J Med.* 2012 Jul 25.

Kahn JS, Aulakh V, Bosworth A. At the intersection of Health, Health Care and Policy. *Health Affairs.* 2009;28(2):369-376.

Kaiser Family Foundation. How Changes in Medical Technology Affect Health Care Costs. March 2007.

Kaiser Family Foundation and Health Research & Educational Trust. Employer health benefits 2011 summary of findings. September 27, 2011.

Kaplan RS, Norton DP, Rugelsjoen B. Managing Alliances with the Balanced Scorecard. *Harvard Business Review.* January-February 2010;88(2):114-120.

Kaushal R, Jha AK, Franz C, Glasser J, Shetty KD, et al. Return on investment for a computerized physician order entry system. *J Am Med Inform Assoc.* 2006;13(3):261-266.

Kawamoto K, Houlihan CA, Balas EA, Lobach DF. Improving clinical practice using clinical decision support systems: a systematic review of trials to identify features critical to success. *BMJ.* 2005 Apr 2;330(7494):765.

Konschak C, Jarrell L. *Consumer-centric Healthcare: Opportunities and Challenges for Providers.* Chicago, IL: Health Administration Press; 2010.

Kongstvedt, PR, ed. Essentials of Managed Health Care, 5th ed. Sudbury, MA: Jones and Bartlett Publishers; 2007.

Koppel R, Wetterneck T, Telles JL, Karsh BT. Workarounds to Barcode Medication Administration Systems: Their Occurrences, Causes, and Threats to Patient Safety. *J Am Med Inform Assoc.* 2008;15(4):408-423.

Landrigan CP, Parry GJ, Catherine B. Bones CB, Andrew D. Hackbarth AD, et al. Temporal Trends in Rates of Patient Harm Resulting from Medical Care. *N Engl J Med* 2010;363(22):2124-2134.

Laudon K, Laudon J. *Essentials of MIS,* 10th ed. Upper Saddle River, NJ: Prentice Hall; 2012.

Leventhal T, Taliaferro JP, Wong K, Hughes C, Mun S. The patient-centered medical home and health information technology. *Telemed J E Health.* 2012 Mar;18(2):145-149. Epub 2012 Feb 3.

Mariner WK, Glantz LH, Annas GJ. Reframing Federalism—The Affordable Care Act (and Broccoli) in the Supreme Court. *N Engl J Med.* 2012 Jul 18.

McGuire TG, Newhouse JP, Sinaiko AD. An economic history of Medicare Part C. *Milbank Q.* 2011 Jun;89(2):289-332.

Medicare Board of Trustees. *2011 Annual Report of the Boards of Trustees of the Federal Hospital Insurance and Federal Supplementary Medical Insurance Trust Funds.*

Miller J. Aetna Manages Cancer Care. *Managed Healthcare Executive.* July 2011;21(7):18–21.

Miller HD, Yasnoff WA, Burde HA. *Personal Health Records The Essential Missing Element in 21st Century Healthcare.* Chicago, IL: Healthcare Information and Management Systems Society; 2009.

Morrissey J. iGovernance. *Hospitals & Health Networks Magazine.* February 2012.

Morse G. Ten Innovations That Will Transform Medicine. *Harvard Business Review Blog Network.* March 8, 2010.

Morton ME, Wiedenbeck S. A Framework for Predicting EHR Adoption Attitudes: A Physician Survey. *Perspect Health Inf Manag.* 2009 Sep 16;6:1a.

Mosquera M. CMS: Want ACO Savings? *Government Health IT.* April 4, 2011.

Nace DK, Jenrette JE, White A. Creating value: Better health IT. *Better to Best Value-Driving Elements of the Patient Centered Medical Home and Accountable Care Organizations.* Washington, DC: Patient-Centered Primary Care Collaborative; March 2011.

National Federation of Independent Business v. Sebelius, 132 S. Ct. 2566 [2012].

Navathe AS, Conway PH. Optimizing Health Information Technology's Role in Enabling Comparative Effectiveness Research. *Am J Manag Care.* 2010 Dec;16(12 Suppl HIT):SP44–47.

Newman M, Barabasi AL, Watts DJ. *The Structure and Dynamics of Networks: Princeton Studies in Complexity.* Princeton, NJ: Princeton University Press; 2006.

Nguyen J, Choi B. Accountable care: are you ready? *Healthc Financ Manage.* 2011 Aug;65(8):92-100.

North, D. *Understanding the Process of Economic Change.* Princeton, NJ: Princeton University Press; 2005.

Omachonu VK, Einspruch NG. Innovation in Healthcare Delivery Systems: A Conceptual Framework. *The Innovation Journal.* 2010;15(1).

O'Malley AS, Reschovsky JD. Referral and Consultation Communication Between Primary Care and Specialist Physicians: Finding Common Ground. *Arch Intern Med.* 2011 Jan 10;171(1):56–65.

Orszag PR. *Factors Underlying Historical Growth in Healthcare Spending.* CBO Testimony: Growth in Health Care Costs before the Committee on the Budget United States Senate. United States Congressional Budget Office Report. January 31, 2008.

OECD and EuroStat. *Oslow Manual: The Measurement of Scientific and Technological Activities.* 3rd Ed. .2005.

Paulus RA, Davis K, Steele GD. Continuous Innovation in Health Care: Implications of the Geisinger Experience. *Health Aff (Millwood).* 2008 Sep-Oct;27(5):1235-1245.

Perrow C. A Society of Organizations. *Theory and Society.* Dec 1991;20(6):725-762.

Porter ME, Teisberg EO. *Redefining Health Care. Creating Value-Based Competition on Results.* Boston, MA: Harvard Business School Press; 2006.

President's Council of Advisors on Science and Technology. *Realizing the Full Potential of Health Information Technology to Improve Healthcare for Americans: The Path Forward.* December 2010.

Provan KG, Fish A, Sydow J. Interorganizational Networks at the Network Level: A Review of the Empirical Literature on Whole Networks. *Journal of Management* 2007;33(3):479-516.

Raab J, Kenis P. Heading toward a Society of Networks Empirical Developments and Theoretical Challenges. *J Manage Inquiry.* 2009 Sept;18(3):198-210.

Reid RJ, Coleman K, Johnson EA, Fishman PA, Hsu C, Soman MP, Trescott CE, Erikson M, Larson EB. The group health medical home at year 2: Cost savings, higher patient satisfaction, and less burnout for providers. *Health Affairs.* 2010;29(5):835-843.

Reinertsen JL, Gosfield AG, Rupp W, Whittington JW. *Engaging Physicians in a Shared Quality Agenda.* IHI Innovation Series white paper. Cambridge, MA: Institute for Healthcare Improvement; 2007.

Riedel J. Using a Health and Productivity Dashboard: A Case Example. *Am J Health Promot.* 2007 Nov-Dec;22(2):1-10.

Rich EC, Lipson D, Libersky J, Peikes DN, Parchman ML. Organizing Care for Complex Patients in the Patient-Centered Medical Home. *Ann Fam Med.* 2012;10:60-62.

Rittenhouse DR, Shortell SM, Fisher ES. Primary care and accountable care—two essential elements of delivery-system reform. *N Engl J Med.* 2009;361(24):2301–2303.

Rogers, EM. Chapter 1: Elements of Diffusion. *Diffusion of Innovations. 5th Ed.* New York, NY: Free Press; 2003.

Roundtable on Value & Science-driven Health Care. Institute of Medicine. *Digital Infrastructure for the Learning Health System. The Foundation for Continuous Improvement in Health and Health Care.* (Prepublication Copy). Washington, DC: The National Academies Press; 2011.

Rouse WB. Managing complexity: disease control as a complex adaptive system. *Information . Knowledge . Systems Management.* 2000;2(2):143-165.

Rowley R. EHR Data as the Missing Piece of Healthcare Reform. *Practice Fusion* (online resource). February 16, 2012.

Schall M, Coleman E, Rutherford P, Taylor J. *How-to Guide: Improving Transitions from the Hospital to the Clinical Office Practice to Reduce Avoidable Rehospitalizations.* Cambridge, MA: Institute for Healthcare Improvement; June 2011.

Serrat O. Defining Complexity. *Understanding Complexity.* Knowledge Solutions. November 2009;No. 6.

Shanthi D, Sahoo G, Saravanan N. Evolving Connection Weights of Artificial Neural Networks Using Genetic Algorithm with Application to the Prediction of Stroke Disease. *International Journal of Soft Computing.* 2009;4(2):95-102.

Shortliffe EH. Strategic Action in Health Information Technology: Why the Obvious Has Taken So Long. *Health Aff (Millwood).* 2005 Sep-Oct;24(5):1222-1233.

Sittig DF, Singh H. A new sociotechnical model for studying health information technology in complex adaptive healthcare systems. *Arch Intern Med.* 2011 Jul 25;171(14):1281-1284.

Smith A. We Need Better Solutions for Customer Loyalty in Long Term Care. *Signature HealthCARE Blog Network.* July 30, 2012.

Spalding SC, Mayer PH, Ginde AA, Lowenstein SR, Yaron M. Impact of computerized physician order entry on ED patient length of stay. *Am J Emerg Med.* 2011 Feb;29(2):207-211.

Stanford University. Closing the Quality Gap: A Critical Analysis of Quality Improvement Strategies. *AHRQ Technical Review Number 9. Chapter 5. Conceptual Frameworks and Their Application to Evaluating Care Coordination Interventions,* Section 5b. Methodological Approach, Model 2: Donabedian's Quality Framework. June 2007.

Starr P. The Social Origins of Professional Sovereignty. In: *The Social Transformation of American Medicine.* New York, NY: Harper Collins; 1982.

California Healthline. *States That Expanded Medicaid Saw Drop in Adult Mortality Rates.* July 26, 2012.

Tate J. Meaningful Use Attestation and Audits: A Word to the Wise. *Medcity News.* February 10, 2012.

Terry V, Chevendra A, Thind M, Stewart J, Marshall N, Cejic S, Using Your Electronic Medical Record for Research: A Primer for Avoiding Pitfalls. *Family Practice.* 2010;27(1):121-126.

The Joint Commission. Safely Implementing Health information and Converging Technologies. *Joint Commission on Accreditation of Healthcare Organizations, USA.* Sentinel Event Alert. 2008 Dec 11;(42):1-4.

The State Long-Term Health Care Sector Characteristics, Utilization, and Government Funding: 2011 Update. *American Health Care Association.* September 6, 2011.

Thornewill, J. An Exploration of Factors Affecting Participation in U.S. Health Information Exchange Networks: A Dual Network Participation Theory Based Case Study. School of Interdisciplinary and Graduate Studies, University of Louisville. Louisville, Kentucky; 2011.

American Health Care Association. *Trends in Nursing Facility Characteristics*. June 2012.

Tunis SR, Stryer DB, Clancy CM. Practical clinical trials: increasing the value of clinical research for decision making in clinical and health policy. *JAMA*. 2003 Sep 24;290(12):1624-1632.

Varkey P, Horne A, Bennet KE. Innovation in Health Care: A Primer. *Am J Med Qual*. 2008 Sep-Oct;23(5):382-388.

Watson R. *Data Management: Databases and Organizations*, 5th Edition. Hoboken, NJ: John Wiley & Sons, Inc; 2006.

Watts DJ. Networks, Dynamics, and the Small-World Phenomenon. *American Journal of Sociology*. 1999;105(2):493-527.

Weiner JP, Kfuri T, Chan K, Fowles JB. e-Iatrogenesis: The Most Critical Unintended Consequence of CPOE and other HIT. *J Am Med Inform Assoc*. 2007;14(3):387-388.

West MA (Ed), Farr JL (Ed). *Innovation and Creativity at Work: Psychological and Organizational Strategies*. Hoboken, NJ: John Wiley & Sons, Inc.; 1990.

Wilensky GR. The Policies and Politics of Creating a Comparative Clinical Effectiveness Research Center. *Health Aff (Millwood)*. 2009 Jul-Aug;28(4):w719-w29.

Willems JS, Banta HD. Improving the use of medial technology. *Health Aff (Millwood)*. 1982:1(2);86-102.

Wynia MK, Torres MK, Lemieux J. Many physicians are willing to use patients' electronic personal health records, but doctors differ by location, gender and practice. *Health Affairs*. 2011; 30(2):266-273.

Yu P. Why Meaningful Use Matters. *J Oncol Pract*. 2011 Jul;7(4):206-209.

Zaheer A, Gozubuyuk R, Milanov H. It's the Connections: The Network Perspective in Interorganizational Research. *Academy of Management Perspectives*. Feb 2010;24(1):62-77.

Glossary and Acronyms

Glossary

Accountable Care Network—An Accountable Care Network (ACN) is a network level collaborate of three or more organizations and/or networks, including physician groups, hospitals, and insurers collaborating to achieve a shared goal (requires a formal agreement).

Accountable Care Organization—Accountable Care Organizations (ACOs) are collaborations between physicians, hospitals, and other providers of clinical services that will be clinically and financially accountable for healthcare delivery for designated patient populations in a defined geographic market. The ACO has a focus on population-based care management and providing services to patients under both public and private payer programs.

ACO Health Intelligence Hub—Four stakeholder groups (e.g., hospitals, members, health plans, and providers) engaged and interacting with an EHR system through health information exchange across a multilevel technology architecture that drives interconnectivity and efficient flow of information.

Activities of Daily Living—Activities of Daily Living (ADL) are activities done during a normal day, such as getting in and out of bed, dressing, bathing, eating, and using the bathroom.

Association Analysis—A predictive tool used to identify affinities existing among the collection of items in a given set of records.[452]

Baby Boomer Generation—US population demographic group consisting of people born after 1945 who started reaching retirement age in 2010.

Business Intelligence—Applications and technologies for gathering, storing, analyzing, and providing access to large amounts of data that can be paired to provide information in a number of contexts for which healthcare is poised to benefit.[453]

Clinical Data Reporting System—A system that provides the business intelligence for which the ACO needs to operate and manage clinical and financial risk.

Clinical Decision Support—Active clinical knowledge systems designed to integrate a medical knowledge base, patient data, and an inference engine to generate case-specific advice.

Clinically Integrated Network—Legitimate collaborations of otherwise competing providers (hospitals and/or physicians) organized in a way that improves efficiencies in care delivery (including quality improvement and cost reduction) in a way that outweighs any potential anticompetitive effects, such as fixing prices among competitors.[454]

Clinical Data Reporting System—A flexible, adaptable, scalable, and deployable system that adds capabilities incrementally to achieve clinical integration objectives of an ACO.

Clinical Efficacy—Measure of whether a device or drug works better than doing nothing. Determined through tightly structured and controlled clinical trials that compare a new drug or device to a placebo, or, in some situations, compared to existing treatments (such as pre-market notification for certain medical devices).

Clinically Integrated Network—Collections of physicians and hospitals working together as an integrated unit to achieve economies of scale in care delivery, enable joint contracting with insurers, and launch programs designed to increase the quality and coordination of patient care while reducing the cost of that care.

Comparative Effectiveness Research—Any work that compares different medical devices, drugs, and treatment methods to determine which are more effective at treating a disease or condition.

Complex Adaptive System—A system of individual agents, who have the freedom to act in ways that are not always totally predictable, and whose actions are interconnected such that one agent's actions change the context for other agents.[455]

Data Analytics—Facilitates business intelligence and is critical to meeting organizational needs and goals in performance management, system level reporting, and data mining to support research, regulatory requirements, and operational needs.

Data Visualization—The process of enabling users to better assess data in formats of graphics, charts, tables, maps, digital images, three-dimensional presentations, animations, and other digital technologies.

Disruptive Innovation—"A process by which a product or service takes root initially in simple applications at the bottom of a market and then relentlessly moves 'up market', eventually displacing established competitors."[456]

Donabedian Quality Framework—The quality framework developed by Avedis Donabedian, MD, that includes three dimensions to assess healthcare quality: (a) structure of care, (b) process of care, and (c) health outcomes.

e-Iatrogenesis—Patient harm caused at least in part by the application of health information technology. [457]

Electronic Health Record—This is a record in electronic format capable of being shared across multiple care settings. Electronic health records (EHRs) may include data on each patient's demographics, medical history, medications and allergies, laboratory test results, radiology results, vital signs, and billing information. EHRs are intended to feed into health information exchanges and the eventual National Health Information Network (NHIN).

Electronic Medical Record—A health information technology system that includes a clinical data repository, clinical decision support, controlled medical vocabulary, computerized provider order entry, pharmacy order entry, and clinical documentation applications. These systems warehouse patient personal health data for both inpatient and outpatient environments in use by physicians and clinicians to document, monitor, and manage healthcare delivery.

Enterprise Master Patient Index—Enterprise Master Patient Index (EMPI) provides a crosswalk to all of a patient's various identifiers (e.g., medical record numbers) housed in integrated and disparate systems of an ACO.

e-Visits—Evaluation and management service provided by a physician or other qualified health professional to an established patient using a Web-based or similar electronic-based communication network for a single patient encounter.[458]

Financial Analytics—Advanced analytic tools for managing cost and revenue of each ACO partner in an integrated system, as well as providing analytics and insights for physician/facility-wide performance measurement.

Generation X—Demographic group consisting of US citizens born between the mid 1960s and the late 1970s.

Healthcare Innovation—The introduction of a new concept, idea, service, process, or product aimed at improving treatment, diagnosis, education, outreach, prevention, and research, with the long-term goals of improving quality, safety, outcomes, efficiency, and costs.[459]

Health Information Exchange—Health Information Exchange (HIE) can take the form of a noun or verb. As a noun, HIE commonly refers to a third-party nonprofit organization formed to enable information sharing among multiple healthcare entities. As a verb, HIE commonly refers to the activity of exchanging health information across disparate information systems and multiple locations of care, both acute and ambulatory.

HIE Deployment Framework—An HIE infrastructure that is flexible, adaptable, scalable, and deployable that adds capabilities incrementally to achieve the clinical integration objectives and goals of an ACO.

mHealth—"Mobile Health (mHealth) is an area of electronic health (eHealth) and it is the provision of health services and information via mobile technologies such as mobile phones and Personal Digital Assistants (PDAs)."[460]

Medical Trading Area—A Medical Trading Area (MTA) is the economics of how care is delivered and reimbursed within a defined geographic area.

Network (generic)—A graph with links and nodes used by network scientists.

Network Level Action Research—Network Level Action Research (NLAR) is a network-level approach to conducting participatory action research.[461] It brings practitioners and researchers together into a network level collaborative where they work to achieve a shared goal.

Network Level Collaborative—"Network" for short; three or more individuals, organizations, or networks collaborating to achieve a shared goal requiring formal agreement.

Network Transition—A change of state within a given network space from one in which organizations are the primary drivers of social and economic change to one in which networks are the primary drivers of social and economic change.

Neural Network—A predictive analysis tool used to help solve complex problems and poorly understood issues for which large amounts of data have been collected, such as patient or population data in a data warehouse. Used to discover patterns in the data to correct the model continuously.

Observational Studies—A type of clinical study that includes a variety of research designs in which no experiment is set up in advance with random assignment or controls. These studies make conclusions about the effects of the treatment in question based on educated guesses from the data.[462]

Organizational Innovation—Intentional introduction and application (within a group or organization) of ideas, processes, products, or procedures, new to the relevant unit of adoption, designed to significantly benefit the individual, the group, organization, or wider society.[463]

Patient-Centered Outcomes Research Institute—"An independent organization created to help patients, clinicians, purchasers and policy makers make better informed health decisions. PCORI will commission research that is responsive to the values and interests of patients and will provide patients and their caregivers with reliable, evidence-based information for the health care choices they face."[464]

Personal Health Record—A personal health record (PHR) is an electronic record of health related information on an individual that conforms to nationally recognized interoperability standards and that can be drawn from multiple sources while being managed, shared, and controlled by the individual.

Personalized Comparison of Treatment Effectiveness—Personalized Comparison of Treatment Effectiveness (PCTE) is a program that compares similar patient groups (when possible) to identify the best treatment options for a given patient's cohort.[465]

Pioneer ACO Model—An advanced accountable care organization model designed for healthcare organizations and providers that are already experienced in coordinating care for patients across care settings. It will allow these provider groups to move more rapidly from a shared savings payment model to a population-based payment model on a track consistent with, but separate from, the Medicare Shared Savings Program.[466]

Pragmatic Randomized Clinical Trial—A Pragmatic Randomized Clinical Trial (PCT) is a study design set up specifically to address clinical quality and cost issues of interest to decision makers.[467]

Predictive Analysis—Use of statistical techniques such as regression, neural networks, decision trees, and genetic algorithms to predict future values.

Randomized Controlled Trial—A randomized controlled trial (RCT) is an experiment design in which research subjects are chosen and randomly assigned to a treatment group or a control group; the effects of the experiment on the treatment group are then isolated, observed, and compared with the control group.

Revenue Cycle Management—The business process of capturing income and ensuring that customer' bills are paid. For healthcare provider organizations, stages in the process include: scheduling and registration, charge capture and coding, claims and processing, and receivables management.

Semantic Interoperability—The bilateral ability of computer systems to send and receive information and properly interpret the meaning of the data requiring the use of standardized vocabularies. Also, it is the ability to create coherence between systems that do not "speak the same language."

Sequential Patterns—Detecting "frequently occurring sequences or patterns from given records."[468]

Sustaining Innovation—New ideas, services, or products that bring about incremental change.

Telehealth—Use of electronic communications and remote technology-enabled healthcare services for consumers through new channels for communications between patients, physicians, and care provider teams.

Three-Part Aim—Overarching goals of the Medicare Shared Savings Program established as: better care for individuals, better health for populations, and lower growth in expenditures.

Acronyms

Acronym	Meaning
ACN	Accountable Care Network
ACO	Accountable Care Organization
ACORM	ACO Reference Model
AHIMA	American Health Information Management Association
AMA	American Medical Association
ARRA	American Recovery and Reinvestment Act
CAH	Critical Access Hospital
CAP	College of American Pathologists
CCD	Continuity of Care Document
CCHIT	Certification Commission for Health Information Technology
CDA	Clinical Document Architecture
CER	Comparative Effectiveness Research
CHI	Consumer Health Informatics
CIN	Clinically Integrated Network

Acronym	Meaning
CMMI	CMS Center for Medicare and Medicaid Innovation
CMS	Centers for Medicare and Medicaid Services
CPOE	Computerized Provider Order Entry
CQMWG	Clinical Quality Measures Workgroup
DHHS	Department of Health and Human Services
DOD	Department of Defense
DRG	Diagnosis Related Group
DUHS	Duke University Health System
EHR	Electronic Health Record
EMPI	Enterprise Master Patient Index
EMR	Electronic Medical Record
EMRAM	Electronic Medical Record Adoption Model
FFS	Fee For Service
GDP	Gross Domestic Product
GEM	General Equivalence Mappings
HEDIS	Healthcare Effectiveness Data and Information Set
HIE	Health Information Exchange
HIMSS	Health Information Management Systems Society
HIPAA	Health Information Portability and Accountability Act
HITECH	Health Information Technology and Economic and Clinical Health Act
HITSC VTF	HIT Standards Committee's Vocabulary Task Force
HMO	Health Maintenance Organization
IHTSDO®	International Health Terminology Standards Development Organization
IOM	Institute of Medicine
IRS	Internal Revenue Service
KPI	Key Performance Indicator
LIC	Lab Interoperability Cooperative
LOINC	Logical Observation Identifiers Names and Codes
LSHN	Large Scale Health Network
MDS	Minimum Data Set
MedPAC	Medicare Payment Advisory Commission
MTA	Medical Trading Area
NCQA	National Committee for Quality Assurance
NeHC	National eHealth Collaborative
NHE	National Health Expenditure

Acronym	Meaning
NICE	National Institute for Health and Clinical Excellence
NLM	National Library of Medicine
NPRM	Notice of Proposed Rule Making
NwHIN	Nationwide Health Information Network
NYeC	New York eHealth Collaborative
ONC-HIT	Office of the National Coordinator for Health Information Technology
PCORI	Patient Centered Outcomes Research Institute
PCT	Pragmatic Randomized Clinical Trial
PCTE	Personalized Comparison of Treatment Effectiveness
PPE	Potentially Preventable Event
PPO	Preferred Provider Organizations
NAMCS	National Ambulatory Medical Care Survey
PPC-PCMH™	Physician Practice Connections Patient-Centered Medical Home
RCT	Randomized Controlled Trial
REC	Regional Extension Center
RUG	Resource Utilization Group
SNF	Skilled Nursing Facility
SNOMED	Systematized Nomenclature of Medicine
SBAR	Situation, Background, Assessment, and Recommendation
UCUM	Unified Code for Units of Measure

[452] Watson R. 2006.

[453] Glaser J, Stone J. 2008; Fortin J, Zywiak W. 2010.

[454] Flareau B, et al. 2011:18-21.

[455] Plsek P, Lindberg C, Zimmerman B. 1997.

[456] Definition of disruptive innovation from Web site of Clayton Christensen. Accessed online July 29, 2011, at http://www.claytonchristensen.com/.

[457] Weiner JP, et al. 2007.

[458] American Academy of Family Physicians. *e-Visit Policy*. Accessed online August 2, 2012, at http://www.aafp.org/online/en/home/policy/policies/e/evisits.html.

[459] Omachonu VK, Einspruch NG. 2010.

[460] World Health Organization. *Global Observatory for eHealth: Mobile Health (mHealth) definition.* Accessed online August 3, 2012, at http://www.who.int/goe/mobile_health/en/.

[461] Cronholm S, Goldkuhl G. 2004; Davison R, Martinsons MG, Kock N. 2004.

[462] ClinicalTrials.gov. Protocol Registration System. Protocol Data Element Definitions (DRAFT), definition of observational studies. Accessed online September 13, 2011, at http://prsinfo.clinicaltrials.gov/definitions.html.

[463] West MA (Ed), Farr JL (Ed). *Innovation and Creativity at Work: Psychological and Organizational Strategies.* Hoboken, NJ: John Wiley & Sons, Inc.; 1990.

[464] Patient-Centered Outcomes Research Institute. *About Us.* Accessed online August 27, 2012, at http://www.pcori.org/about/.

[465] Hoffman S, Podgurski A. 2011.

[466] Department of Health and Human Services. Press Release. *Pioneer Accountable Care Organization Model: General Fact Sheet.* December 19, 2011. Accessed online May 1, 2012, at http://innovations.cms.gov/initiatives/aco/pioneer/.

[467] Tunis SR, et al. 2003.

[468] Watson R. 2006.

Appendix A: Editor and Author Biographies

Executive Editor Team

Bill Spooner has been Chief Information Officer for the past 15 of his 30 years at Sharp HealthCare. He has led an aggressive IT effort that placed Sharp on the Hospitals and Health Networks 100 Most Wired list for the first 11 years since the list was established. Sharp was an early leader in electronic health records, as the development site for a robust hospital EHR since the mid 1980s. More recently, Mr. Spooner spearheaded the rollout of industry-leading EHRs in both the Sharp hospitals and its medical groups. Sharp has received several awards for its foremost consumer Web site. Sharp recently launched its mySharp portal to engage its patients in their care. IT was cited for its contributions to Sharp's 2007 Malcolm Baldridge National Quality Award.

Recipient of the 2009 John E. Gall Jr. CIO of the Year award, Mr. Spooner is a member of the Healthcare Information Systems Executive Association (HISEA), the Healthcare Information and Management Systems Society (HIMSS), and a Fellow in the College of Healthcare Information Management Executives (CHIME) that he served as Chair in 2006. He has worked with CHIME's Advocacy Leadership Team since its inception in 2004 and chaired the group in 2005. Spooner serves on the Editorial Board of *Healthcare IT News*. He also serves on the California Hospital Association Health Informatics and Technology Committee, as well as a number of industry advisory councils.

Bert Reese is Senior Vice President and Chief Information Officer of Sentara Healthcare, an integrated health system with net revenues of $3.9 billion. Sentara, a not-for-profit healthcare provider in southeastern Virginia and northeastern North Carolina, is comprised of 10 acute care hospitals; a health plan with 432,600 covered lives; 7 nursing centers; 3 assisted living centers; and 600 member physician medical groups. Sentara has continually ranked as one of the most integrated healthcare networks in the United States by *Modern Healthcare* magazine and is the only healthcare system in the nation to be named in the top 10 for 7 consecutive years.

Mr. Reese is responsible for the Information Technology, Process Improvement, Information and Supply Chain Management for the health system. Most recently this group has implemented the Electronic Health Record across the enterprise, resulting in significant financial savings and improved clinical outcomes.

Colin Konschak, MBA, FACHE, FHIMSS, is the managing partner of Divurgent, a healthcare management consulting firm. Mr. Konschak is a registered pharmacist, has an MBA in health services administration, is board-certified in healthcare management, and is a certified Six Sigma Black Belt. Mr. Konschak leads Divurgent's advisory service consulting practice focused on operational and information technology strategies, including those related to accountable care organizations and clinically integrated networks. Colin is the author of several books on the topics of Clinical Integration, Accountable Care and Consumer Centric Care.

Chapter Authors (Chapter Order)

Shane Danaher, MBA (*Chapter 1*) is Client Services Vice President for Divurgent. In this role, he is responsible for developing strategic service offerings, driving client satisfaction, and developing sound marketing strategies. Mr. Danaher brings 8 years of experience to the healthcare technology field and has a proven history of establishing successful relationships with providers and healthcare organizations. Mr. Danaher's strong technology background, combined with a deep understanding of the healthcare market, have helped him create solutions for clients that maximize their project successes.

Mr. Danaher has an Economics degree from Haverford College and a Masters in Business Administration from Virginia Tech. He is the 2012 president for the Virginia chapter of HIMSS and is an accomplished speaker regarding industry topics such as Meaningful Use for professional organizations including MGMA, AAHAM, Workshop on Health IT and Economics (WHITE), and regional physician groups.

David Shiple (*Chapter 1*) leads Divurgent's Advisory Services Practice. In this role, he oversees client relationships, quality assurance, methodology development, and the thought-leadership related to Advisory Services engagements. He is also dedicated to recruiting the best and brightest healthcare professionals to serve as Advisory Services consultants. Divurgent's Advisory Services Practice serves health system CIOs with a range of services, including IT strategic planning, Meaningful Use gap analysis, benefits realization, information services reorganizations, clinical integration, and interim CIO staffing. Mr. Shiple comes from a 27-year background in IT, with 15 of those years dedicated to the healthcare industry. He has a Bachelor of Science in computer science from Clemson University and has worked for companies such as Accenture, Gartner, IBM, and Navigant. Mr. Shiple has contributed to periodicals such as *Modern Healthcare*, *HFM*, and *Bio-IT*.

Richard G. Jung (*Chapter 2 co-author*) is Chief Executive Officer of InTuun, the leading provider of automated care management solutions for provider and hospital-based health plans. He is also Chairman of the Board at Clinicient, an automated revenue cycle management and EHR firm, and a Healthcare IT Advisory Board Member for the University of California at San Diego. Previously, Mr. Jung held senior leadership roles at venture/private equity backed Athenahealth, Medsphere, and MDeverywhere. He began his career on the payer side of the industry with US Healthcare.

J.M. Bohn, MBA (*Corresponding editor and Chapter 2 co-author*) is founder of Clinical Horizons, Inc. and KMI Communications LLC, focusing on publishing and research initiatives in the healthcare and science sectors.

Chon Abraham, PhD, MBA (*Chapter 3*) is an associate professor of Management Information Systems (MIS) at the Mason School of Business, College of William and Mary. She received a BS in Political Science and Systems Engineering and a commission into the US Army from the United States Military Academy at West Point in 1995, an MBA from Old Dominion University with a concentration in MIS in 2000, and a PhD in MIS from the University of Georgia in 2004. She worked as a systems analyst for American Management System in Norfolk, Virginia, after serving on active duty as an Army Finance Officer and prior to entering the PhD program at the University of Georgia in the Terry College of Business. She publishes in various MIS and healthcare information systems oriented journals such as *Journal of Strategic Information Systems; European Journal of Information Systems; Business Intelligence Journal; Communications of the ACM; DataBase; and Decision Support Systems; IBM Center for Healthcare Information Management Publication Series;* and the *Journal of Healthcare Information*

Management. Her research interests mainly focus on implementations of emerging technologies. Ms. Abraham is a 2008-2009 recipient of a Fulbright Research Award to Japan, where she studied healthcare information technology initiatives and served as a visiting assistant professor at Keio University, one of the most prestigious universities in Japan.

Chip Perkins, MBA (*Chapter 4*) is an accomplished healthcare leader with more than 20 years of experience in healthcare information technology advisory services, electronic medical record (EMR) implementations, program management, and clinical transformation engagements. Mr. Perkins began his healthcare career at Cerner Corporation and continued his healthcare consulting career with executive level positions at QuadraMed, Cap Gemini Ernst & Young, Healthlink, IBM Global Business Services, and The College of American Pathologists. Mr. Perkins currently is Vice President of Provider Solutions at OptumInsight, a leading technology, health information, consulting, and outsourcing solutions firm. Mr. Perkins holds an MBA from The Babcock Graduate School of Management and a degree in Business Administration from The College of William and Mary.

Greg Miller (*Chapter 5*) is Senior Vice President at Medicity, Inc., a subsidiary of Aetna Corporation and a leading Health Information Exchange technology provider. For 27 years, Mr. Miller has partnered with hospitals, health systems, and other provider organizations, as they seek to improve the cost, quality, and safety of healthcare delivery, through enabling technologies. Mr. Miller has a wealth of experience helping organizations develop information technology strategic plans, design solutions, deployment plans, project management, and market solutions. His experience spans clinical, financial, and operational areas, across acute and ambulatory care settings, ranging from rural hospitals to nationwide health systems and leading integrated delivery networks nationwide.

Cynthia Davis, MHSA, RN, FACHE (*Chapter 6*) is a Principal with CIC Advisory, Inc. and a recognized technology adoption strategist with more than 25 years of transformational healthcare experience in community and academic based health systems. She has an exceptional record of achievement in consulting, clinical transformation, informatics, strategic planning, and leadership in a large integrated delivery network. Her team's results include high levels of clinical adoption, customer satisfaction, ARRA readiness, and value realization. Ms. Davis has a passion for the application of clinical informatics for efficient and effective care delivery processes and develops strong teams and leaders to support and fully utilize the capabilities of new IT healthcare applications.

She has successfully implemented and provided ongoing customer service, optimization, and support to several multimillion-dollar fast track projects in excess of millions of dollars each on time and within budget using a transformational and process improvement approach. Ms. Davis holds a Master's degree in Health Services Administration from University of Michigan, Bachelor's degree in Nursing from the University of New Mexico, and also is a fellow with the American College of Healthcare Executives.

Mary Sirois, MBA, PT (*Chapter 7*) is the principal responsible for Divurgent's Clinical Transformation practice. Ms. Sirois focuses on the alignment and hardwiring of clinical and business benefits opportunities with improving quality of care in healthcare. Ms. Sirois has nearly 20 years of healthcare operational and strategic planning experience across a wide spectrum of provider and academic environments. A physical therapist by clinical background, she has worked with large and small healthcare systems on the planning necessary for clinical transformation as a result of an electronic health record deployment, organizational governance and change management, medical and clinical staff collaboration on best practice and evidence-based processes, regulatory compliance readiness and issue resolution, organizational budget development and related benefits realization projection, and detailed project planning. Ms. Sirois holds a BS in Physical Therapy from the University of Delaware, an MBA in Healthcare Administration from the University of Dallas, and an Executive Certificate in Strategy and Innovation from MIT.

Tim Webb (*Chapter 8*) is a Partner with InfoArch Consulting and specializes in aligning information technology with business for healthcare payers and providers, resulting in measurable returns to clients such as The Cleveland Clinic, Trinity, BayCare, Blue Cross Blue Shield, and New York Presbyterian. He has 29 years of experience, including 8 years as Chief Information Officer or Director responsible for IT. His consulting career includes Price Waterhouse, First Consulting Group, Healthlink, and Kurt Salmon Associates. His accomplishments include developing IT Strategic Plans, implementing IT governance, managing major IT projects, and day-to-day management of IT organizations of up to 100 staff members. He has conducted numerous IT assessments and service improvement projects; evaluated outsourcing; and conducted all aspects of technology planning, including selection and implementation.

Mr. Webb has spoken in national and regional forums including: CHIME, BICSI, HIMSS (national and regional meetings), and Vendor User Groups. He has previously contributed chapters to two books: *The Internet and Healthcare*, 1999, and *Performance Improvement Through Information Management*, 1998. He has been quoted several times in national periodicals on topics such as technology trends and reducing IT costs. Mr. Webb holds a Bachelor of Science in Electrical Engineering from Purdue University and is a graduate of Eckerd College's Leadership Institute Program, Villanova University's Six Sigma certification program, and the CHIME CIO Boot Camp.

Laishy Williams-Carlson (*Chapter 9*) is a regional Chief Information Officer for Bon Secours Health System, a not-for-profit Catholic health system that owns, manages, or joint ventures 18 acute-care hospitals, nursing care facilities, assisted living facilities, and home care and hospice programs. Bon Secours employs more than 21,000 people in seven states. In her current role, Mrs. Carlson co-directs Bon Secours' ConnectCare electronic medical record project, responsible for technical aspects of the implementation. The hospitals that are live on ConnectCare have reached HIMSS EMRAM Stage 6 status, "Most Wired" designation, and Stage 1 of Meaningful Use. In addition, Mrs. Carlson is the Chief Information Officer for the Bon Secours Hampton Roads system. She has worked in healthcare finance and Information Systems for more than 25 years in various roles, including Controller, Director of I.S., and CIO.

Ken Yale, DDS, JD (*Chapter 10*) is vice president of Clinical Solutions at ActiveHealth Management. Previously, he built and launched innovative health technologies and business models for a variety of health organizations, including clinically integrated networks, patient-centered medical homes, accountable care organizations, health plans, medical management companies, and health information technology companies. Before building innovative health businesses, he was chief of staff of the White House Office of Science and Technology, served as a special assistant to the President, and executive director of the White House Domestic Policy Council. He provided legislative counsel to the US Senate and was a commissioned officer in US Public Health Service.

John P. Reinhart, CPA, MBA (Candidate 2012) *(Chapter 11)* is the Founder and Chief Executive Officer of the International Center for Long Term Care Innovation (InnovateLTC). InnovateLTC is a for-profit business accelerator focused on disruptive products, service models, and technologies aimed at the global aging population. InnovateLTC was formed in February 2010 in collaboration with Signature Healthcare and the University of Louisville. Prior to the launch, Mr. Reinhart was Chief Innovation Officer for Signature Healthcare and led its Intra-Preneurship Pillar strategy. Mr. Reinhart is a serial entrepreneur and founding partner of Commonwealth Leverage Group, a partnership of accomplished entrepreneurial executives focused on providing strategic services to emerging ventures in the healthcare and technology sectors. From 1999 through 2003, he was President and Chief Operating Officer of Advanced Imaging Concepts, Inc., an ambulatory sector healthcare software company subsequently acquired by Allscripts Healthcare Solutions, Inc., where he then served as Executive Vice President, Clinical Solutions Group until 2006. Mr. Reinhart was recognized as an Ernst Young Entrepreneur of the Year in 2004 for Emerging Businesses. Early in his career, he was a CPA with Coopers and Lybrand, after graduating from the University of Kentucky in 1987, and he is currently completing an MBA in Health Sector Management and Policy at the University of Miami in Florida (2012).

Robert Esterhay, MD *(Chapter 11)* has a research interest in network participation theory as it applies to individuals, organizations, and networks. He has been at the informatics crossroads of individual health, healthcare, and population health for more than 35 years in his education, work experience, and, most recently, his academic setting. He is the chair of the Department for Health Management and Systems Sciences in the School of Public Health and Information Sciences at the University of Louisville. His 1969 medical school thesis involved computer-assisted learning utilizing computer-simulated patients for training medical students, medical residents, and medical school faculty. This was prior to personal computers, the Internet, and the World Wide Web. In the mid 1970s, he led an early implementation of an electronic medical record information system at the University of Maryland Cancer Center and, in the mid 1990s, a nationwide implementation of an electronic medical record system in 60 long-term, acute care hospitals, and 300 nursing homes for Kindred Healthcare (formerly Vencor). Some of his accomplishments include: taking the ideas and concepts for a cancer information system for the National Cancer Institute (NCI) and creating NCI's PDQ®—a comprehensive cancer database that continues to be used over the Internet today; serving as a member of the Kentucky TeleHealth Network Board; and serving as the first co-chair of the Kentucky e-Health Board; analyzing community Health Information Exchanges (HIEs) (funded by the Kentucky Science & Engineering Foundation) and using the developed governance model to create the Louisville HIE. In summary, Dr. Esterhay has a record of successful and productive teaching, research, and service projects in an area of high relevance for the challenge of designing and implementing data-driven and health information sciences research.

Appendix B: Medicare Shared Savings Program Quality Measures[469]

Domain	Measure # and Title	NQF Measure #/Steward	Data Source
AIM: Better Care for Individuals			
Patient/Caregiver Experience	#1. CAHPS: Getting timely care, appointments, and information	NQF #5, AHRQ	Survey
Patient/Caregiver Experience	#2. CAHPS: How well your doctors communicate	NQF #5, AHRQ	Survey
Patient/Caregiver Experience	#3. CAHPS: Patient's rating of doctor	NQF #5, AHRQ	Survey
Patient/Caregiver Experience	#4. CAHPS: Access to specialists	NQF #5, AHRQ	Survey
Patient/Caregiver Experience	#5. CAHPS: Health promotion and education	NQF #5, AHRQ	Survey
Patient/Caregiver Experience	#6. CAHPS: Shared decision making	NQF #5, AHRQ	Survey
Patient/Caregiver Experience	#7. CAHPS: Health status/functional status	NQF #6, AHRQ	Survey
Care Coordination/ Patient Safety	#8. Risk-standardized, all condition readmission	NQF TBD, AHRQ	Claims
Care Coordination/ Patient Safety	#9. Ambulatory sensitive conditions admissions: Chronic Obstructive Pulmonary Disease [AHRQ Prevention Quality Indicator (PQI) #5]	NQF #275, AHRQ	Claims
Care Coordination/ Patient Safety	#10. Ambulatory sensitive conditions admissions: Congestive heart failure [AHRQ Prevention Quality Indicator (PQI) #5]	NQF #277 AHRQ	Claims

Domain	Measure # and Title	NQF Measure #/Steward	Data Source
Care Coordination/ Patient Safety	#11. Percent of PCPs who successfully qualify for an EHR incentive program payment	CMS	EHR Incentive Program reporting
Care Coordination/ Patient Safety	#12. Medication reconciliation: Reconciliation after discharge from an inpatient facility	NQF #97 AMA-PCPI / NCQA	GPRO Web interface
Care Coordination/ Patient Safety	#13. Falls: screening for fall risk	NQF #101 NCQA	GPRO Web interface
AIM: Better Health for Populations			
Preventive Health	#14. Influenza immunization	NQF #41 AMA-PCPI	Preventive Health
Preventive Health	#15. Pneumococcal vaccination	NQF #43 NCQA	Preventive Health
Preventive Health	#16. Adult weight screening and follow-up	NQF #421 CMS	Preventive Health
Preventive Health	#17. Tobacco use assessment and tobacco cessation intervention	NQF #28 AMA-PCPI	Preventive Health
Preventive Health	#18. Depression screening	NQF #418 CMS	Preventive Health
Preventive Health	#19. Colorectal cancer screening	NQF #31 NCQA	Preventive Health
Preventive Health	#20. Mammography screening	NQF #31 NCQA	Preventive Health
Preventive Health	#21. Proportion of adults 18+ who had their blood pressure measured within the preceding 2 yrs	CMS	Preventive Health
At-risk population— diabetes	#22. Diabetes composite (all or nothing scoring): hemoglobin A1c control (<8%)	NQF #0729 MN Community Measurement	At-risk population— diabetes

Domain	Measure # and Title	NQF Measure #/Steward	Domain
At-risk population—diabetes	#23. Diabetes composite (all or nothing scoring): low density lipoprotein (<100)	NQF #0729 MN Community Measurement	At-risk population—diabetes
At-risk population—diabetes	#24. Diabetes composite (all or nothing scoring): blood pressure (<140/90)	NQF #0729 MN Community Measurement	At-risk population—diabetes
At-risk population—diabetes	#25. Diabetes composite (all or nothing scoring): tobacco non-use	NQF #0729 MN Community Measurement	At-risk population—diabetes
At-risk population—diabetes	#26. Diabetes composite (all or nothing scoring): Aspirin use	NQF #0729 MN Community Measurement	At-risk population—diabetes
At-risk population—diabetes	#27. Diabetes Mellitus: hemoglobin A1c pool control (>9%)	NQF #59 NCQA	At-risk population—diabetes
At-risk population—hypertension	#28. Hypertension (HTN): blood pressure control	NQF #18 NCQA	At-risk population—hypertension
At-risk population—ischemic vascular disease	#29. Ischemic vascular disease (IVD): complete lipid profile and LDL control (<100 mg/dL)	NQF #75 NCQA	At-risk population—ischemic vascular disease
At-risk population—ischemic vascular disease	#30. Ischemic vascular disease (IVD): use of aspirin or another antithrombotic	NQF #68 NCQA	At-risk population—ischemic vascular disease
At-risk population—heart failure	#31. Heart failure: beta-blocker therapy for left ventricular systolic dysfunction (LVSD)	NQF #83 NCQA	At-risk population—heart failure

Domain	Measure # and Title	NQF Measure #/Steward	Domain
At-risk population—coronary artery disease	#32. Coronary artery disease (CAD) composite (all or nothing scoring): drug therapy for lowering LDL-cholesterol	NQF #74 CMS (composite) / AMA-PCPI (individual component)	At-risk population—coronary artery disease
At-risk population—coronary artery disease	#33. Coronary artery disease (CAD) composite (all or nothing scoring): Angiotensin-Converting Enzyme (ACE) Inhibitor or Angiotensin Receptor Blocker (ARB) therapy for patients with CAD and diabetes and/or Left Ventricular Systolic Dysfunction (LVSD)	NQF #74 CMS (composite) / AMA-PCPI (individual component)	At-risk population—coronary artery disease

[469] Centers for Medicare and Medicaid Services. Improving Quality of Care for Medicare Patients: Accountable Care Organizations. Accessed online March 27, 2012 at https://www.cms.gov/MLNProducts/downloads/ACO_Quality_Factsheet_ICN907407.pdf; Centers for Medicare and Medicaid Services. *Accountable Care Organization 2012 Program Analysis: Quality Performance Standards Narrative Measure Specifications Final Report.* December 12, 2011. Accessed online March 27, 2012 at http://www.cms.gov/SharedSavingsProgram/downloads/ACO_QualityMeasures.pdf.

Appendix C: Stage 1 Meaningful Use Measures

Objective	Measure
Core Set	
Domain: Improve quality, safety, efficiency, and reduce health disparity	
Use CPOE for medication orders directly entered by any licensed healthcare professional who can enter orders into the medical record per state, local and professional guidelines.	More than 30% of all unique patients with at least one medication in their medication list admitted to the EH's or inpatient or ED (POS 21 or 23) have at least one medication order entered using CPOE.
Implement drug-drug and drug allergy interaction checks	The EP/eligible hospital CAH has enabled this functionality for the entire EHR reporting period.
Record demographics: preferred language, gender, race, ethnicity, date of birth, date of preliminary cause of death in the event of mortality in the eligible hospital or CAH.	More than 50% of all unique patients seen by the EP or admitted to the eligible hospital's or CAH's inpatient or emergency department (POS 21 or 23) have demographics recorded as structured data.
Maintain an up-to-date problem list of current and active diagnoses.	More than 80% of all unique patients seen by the EP or admitted to the eligible hospital's or CAH's inpatient or ED (POS 21 or 23) have at least one entry or an indication that no problems are known for the patient recorded as structured data.
Maintain active medication list.	More than 80% of all unique patients seen by the EP or admitted to the eligible hospital's or CAH's inpatient or ED (POS 21 or 23) have at least one entry (or an indication that the patient is not currently prescribed any medication) recorded as structured data.
Maintain active medication allergy list.	More than 80% of all unique patients seen by the EP or admitted to the eligible hospital's or CAH's inpatient or ED (POS 21 or 23) have at least one entry (or an indication that the patient has no known medication allergies) recorded as structured data.

Objective	Measure
Record and chart changes in vital signs: height, weight, blood pressure, calculate and display BMI, plot and display growth charts for children 2-20 years including BMI.	For more than 50% of all unique patients age 2 and older seen by the EP or admitted to eligible hospital's or CAH's inpatient or ED (POS 21 or 23), height, weight, and blood pressure are recorded as structured data.
Record smoking status for patients 13 years old or older.	More than 50% of all unique patients 13 years or older seen by the EP or admitted to the eligible hospital's or CAH's inpatient or ED (POS 21 or 23) have smoking status recorded as structured data.
Implement one clinical decision support rule related to a high priority hospital condition along with the ability to track compliance with that rule.	Implement one clinical decision support rule.
Report clinical quality measures to CMS or the states.	For 2011, provide aggregate numerator, denominator, and exclusions through attestation. For 2012, electronically submit the clinical quality measures data.
Domain: Engage patients and families	
Provide patients with an electronic copy of their health information (including diagnostic test results, problem list, medication lists, medication allergies, discharge summary, procedures) upon request.	More than 50% of all patients of the EP or the inpatient or ED of the eligible hospital or CAH (POS 21 or 23) who request an electronic copy of their health information are provided it within 3 business days.
Provide patients with an electronic copy of their discharge instructions at time of discharge, upon request.	More than 50% of all patients discharged from an eligible hospital or CAH's inpatient department or ED (POS 21 or 23) and who request an electronic copy of their discharge instructions are provided a copy.
Provide clinical summaries for patients for each office visit (EP).	Clinical summaries provided to patients for more than 50% of all office visits within 3 business days.
Domain: Improve care coordination	
Capability to exchange key clinical information (for example, discharge summary, procedures, problem list,	Performed at least one test of certified EHR technology's capacity to electronically exchange key clinical

Objective	Measure
medication list, medication allergies, diagnostic test results), among providers of care and patient-authorized entities electronically.	information.

Domain: Ensure adequate privacy and security protections for personal health information

Objective	Measure
Protect electronic health information created or maintained by the certified EHR technology through the implementation of appropriate technical capabilities.	Conduct or review a security risk analysis per 45 CFR 164.308 (a)(1) and implement security updates, as necessary, and correct identified security deficiencies as part of its risk management process.

Menu Set

These objectives allow for eligible professionals and hospitals/critical access hospitals to choose five measures to complete their Stage 1 requirements, one of which must be from the population and public health domain.

Domain: Improve quality, safety, efficiency, and reduce health disparity

Objective	Measure
Implement drug-formulary checks.	The EP/eligible hospital/CAH has enabled this functionality and has access to at least one internal or external drug formulary for the entire EHR reporting period.
Record advance directives for patients 65 years or older.	More than 50% of all unique patients 65 years or older admitted to the eligible hospital's or CAH's inpatient department (POS 21) have an indication of an advance directive status recorded.
Incorporate clinical lab test results into certified EHR technology as structured data.	More than 40% of all clinical lab tests results ordered by the EP or by an authorized provider of the eligible hospital or CAH for patients admitted to its inpatient or ED (POS 21 or 23) during the EHR reporting period whose results are either in a positive/negative or numerical format are incorporated in certified EHR technology as structured data.
Generate lists of patients by specific conditions to use for quality improvement, reduction of disparities, research, or outreach.	Generate at least one report listing patients of the EP, eligible hospital, or CAH with a specific condition.
Send reminders to patients per patient preference for preventive/follow-up care (EP).	More than 20% of all unique patients 65 years or older or 5 years or younger were sent an appropriate reminder during the

Objective	Measure
	EHR reporting period.
Domain: Engage patients and families	
Provide patients with timely electronic access to their health information (including lab results, problem list, medication lists, medication allergies) within 4 business days of the information being available to the EP (EP).	More than 10% of all unique patients seen by the EP are provided timely (available to the patient within 4 business days of being updated in the certified EHR technology) electronic access to their health information subject to the EP's discretion to withhold certain information.
Use certified EHR technology to identify patient-specific education resources and provide those resources to the patient if appropriate.	More than 10% of all unique patients seen by the EP or admitted to the eligible hospital's or CAH's inpatient or ED (POS 21 or 23) are provided patient-specific education resources.
Domain: Improve care coordination	
The EP, eligible hospital, or CAH who receives a patient from another setting of care or provider of care or believes an encounter is relevant should perform medication reconciliation.	The EP, eligible hospital or CAH performs medication reconciliation for more than 50% of transitions of care in which the patient is transitioned into the care of the EP or admitted to the eligible hospital's or CAH's inpatient or ED (POS 21 or 23).
The EP, eligible hospital or CAH who transitions its patient to another setting of care or provider of care or refers their patient to another provider of care should provide summary of care record for each transition of care or referral.	The EP, eligible hospital, or CAH who transitions or refers its patient to another setting of care or provider of care provides a summary of care record for more than 50% of transitions of care and referrals.
Domain: Improve population and public health	
Capability to submit electronic data on reportable (as required by state or local law) lab results to public health agencies and actual submission in accordance with applicable law and practice for eligible hospitals and critical access hospitals.	Performed at least one test of certified EHR technology's capacity to provide electronic submission of reportable lab results to public health agencies and follow-up submission if the test is successful (unless none of the public health agencies to which eligible hospital or CAH submits such information have the capacity to receive the information electronically).
Capability to submit electronic syndromic surveillance data to public health agencies and actual submission in accordance with applicable law and practice.	Performed at least one test of certified EHR technology's capacity to provide electronic syndromic surveillance data to public health agencies and follow-up submission if the test is successful (unless none of the public health agencies to which an EP, eligible hospital or CAH

Objective	Measure
	submits such information have the capacity to receive the information electronically).
Capability to submit electronic data to immunization registries or immunization information systems and actual submission in accordance with applicable law and practice.	Performed at least one test of the certified EHR technology's capacity to submit electronic data to immunization registries and follow-up submission if the test is successful (unless none of the immunization registries and follow-up submission if the test is successful (unless none of the immunization registries to which the EP, eligible hospital, or CAH submits such information have the capacity to receive the information electronically).

Appendix D: Changes to Stage 1 Meaningful Use Measures Per Final Stage 2 Rule[470]

Stage 1 Objective	Final Changes	Effective Year (CY/FY)
Use CPOE for medication orders directly entered by licensed healthcare professional who enters orders into the medical record per state, local and professional guidelines.	Change: Addition of an alternative measure. More than 30% of medication orders created by the EP or authorized providers of the eligible hospital's or CAH's inpatient or ED (POS 21 or 23) during the EHR reporting period are recorded using CPOE.	2013 - Onward (Optional)
Generate and transmit permissible prescriptions electronically (eRx).	Change: Addition of an additional exclusion. Any EP who: does not have a pharmacy within their organization and there are no pharmacies that accept electronic prescriptions within 10 miles of the EP's practice location at the start of his/her EHR reporting period.	2013 - Onward (Optional)
Record and chart changes in vital signs.	Change: Addition of alternative age limitations. More than 50% of all unique patients seen by the EP or admitted to the eligible hospital's or CAH's inpatient or ED (POS 21 or 23) during the EHR reporting period have blood pressure (for patients age 3 and over only) and height and weight (for all ages) recorded as structured data.	2013 - Onward (Optional)
Record and chart changes in vital signs.	Change: Addition of alternative exclusions. Any EP who (1) Sees no patients 3 years or older is excluded from recording blood pressure; (2) Believes that all 3 vital signs of height, weight, and blood pressure have no relevance to their scope of practice is excluded from recording them; (3) Believes that height and weight are relevant to their scope of practice, but blood pressure is not, is excluded from recording blood pressure; or (4) Believes that blood pressure is relevant to scope of practice, but	2013 - Onward (Optional)

Stage 1 Objective	Final Changes	Effective Year (CY/FY)
	height and weight are not, is excluded from recording height and weight.	
Record and chart changes in vital signs.	Change: Age limitations on height, weight and blood pressure. More than 50% of all unique patients seen by the EP or admitted to the eligible hospital's or CAH's inpatient or ED (POS 21 or 23) during the EHR reporting period have blood pressure (for patients age 3 and over only) and height and weight (for all ages) recorded as structured data.	2014 – Onward (Required)
Record and chart changes in vital signs.	Change: Changing the age and splitting the EP exclusion. Any EP who: (1) Sees no patients 3 years or older is excluded from recording blood pressure; (2) Believes that all 3 vital signs of height, weight, and blood pressure have no relevance to their scope of practice is excluded from recording them; (3) Believes that height and weight are relevant to their scope of practice, but blood pressure is not, is excluded from recording blood pressure; or (4) Believes blood pressure is relevant to scope of practice, but height and weight are not, is excluded from recording height and weight.	2014 – Onward (Required)
Capability to exchange key clinical information (for example, problem list, medication list, medication allergies, and diagnostic test results), among providers of care and patient authorized entities electronically.	Change: Objective is no longer required.	2013 – Onward (Required)
Report ambulatory	Change: Objective is incorporated	2013 – Onward

Stage 1 Objective	Final Changes	Effective Year (CY/FY)
(hospital) clinical quality measures to CMS or the states.	directly into the definition of a meaningful EHR user and eliminated as an objective under §495.6.	(Required)
EP and Hospital Objectives: Provide patients with electronic copy of their health information (including test results, problem list, medication lists, medication allergies, discharge summary, procedures) upon their request. **Hospital Objective:** Provide patients with electronic copy of discharge instructions at time of discharge, upon their request. **EP Objective:** Provide patients with timely electronic access to their health information (including lab results, problem list, medication lists, and allergies) within 4 business days of the information being available to the EP.	**Change:** Replace these 4 objectives with the Stage 2 objective and one of the two Stage 2 measures. **EP Objective:** Provide patients the ability to view online, download, and transmit their health information within 4 business days of the information being available to the EP. **EP Measure:** More than 50% of all unique patients seen by the EP during the EHR reporting period are provided timely (within 4 business days after the information is available to the EP) online access to their health information subject to the EP's discretion to withhold certain information. **Hospital Objective:** Provide patients the ability to view online, download, and transmit information about a hospital admission. **Hospital Measure:** More than 50% of all patients who are discharged from the inpatient or emergency department (POS 21 or 23) of an eligible hospital or CAH have their information available online within 36 hours of discharge.	2014 – Onward (Required)
Public Health Objectives:	Change: Addition of "except where prohibited" to the objective regulation text for the public health objectives under §495.6	2013 – Onward (Required)
Stage 1 Policy Changes		
Meeting an exclusion for a menu set objective counts toward the number of menu set objectives that must be satisfied to meet	Meeting an exclusion for a menu set objective does not count towards the number of menu set objectives that must be satisfied to meet meaningful use.	2014 – Onward (Required)

Stage 1 Objective	Final Changes	Effective Year (CY/FY)
Meaningful Use.		

---

[470] Centers for Medicare & Medicaid Services. 42 CFR Parts 412, 413, and 495. Medicare and Medicaid Programs; Electronic Health Record Incentive Program--Stage 2. Final Rule. August 23, 2012. Section 3 (b). Changes to Stage 1 Criteria for Meaningful Use. p. 41-43.

Appendix E: Final Stage 2 Core and Menu Set Objectives and Measures Per Final Stage 2 Rule[471]

Health Outcomes Policy Priority	Stage 2 Objectives		Stage 2 Measures
	EPs	EHs and CAHs	
CORE SET			
Improving quality, safety, efficiency, and reducing health disparities	Use computerized provider order entry (CPOE) for medication, laboratory and radiology orders directly entered by any licensed healthcare professional who enters orders into the medical record per state, local and professional guidelines.	Use computerized provider order entry (CPOE) for medication, laboratory and radiology orders directly entered by any licensed healthcare professional who enters orders into the medical record per state, local and professional guidelines.	More than 60% of medication, 30% of laboratory, and 30% of radiology orders created by the EP or authorized providers of the eligible Hospital's or CAH's inpatient or emergency Department (POS 21 or 23) during the EHR reporting period are recorded using CPOE.
	Generate and transmit permissible prescriptions electronically (eRx).		More than 50% of all permissible prescriptions, or all prescriptions written by the EP and queried for a drug formulary and transmitted electronically using CEHRT
	Record the following demographics: Preferred language, sex, race, ethnicity, date of birth.	Record the following demographics: preferred language, sex, race, ethnicity, date of birth, date of preliminary cause of death in the event of mortality in the eligible hospital or CAH.	More than 80% of all unique patients seen by the EP or admitted to the eligible hospital's or CAH's inpatient or emergency department (POS 21 or 23) during the EHR reporting period have demographics recorded as structured data.
	Record and chart changes in vital signs: Height/length, weight, blood pressure (age 3 and over), calculate and display BMI, plot and display growth charts for patients 0-20 years, including BMI.	Record and chart changes in vital signs: Height/length, weight, blood pressure (age 3 and over), calculate and display BMI, plot and display growth charts for patients 0-20 years, including BMI.	More than 80% of all unique patients seen by the EP or admitted to the eligible hospital's or CAH's inpatient or emergency department (POS 21 or 23) during the EHR reporting period have blood pressure (for patients age 3 and over only) and height/length and weight (for all ages) recorded as structured data.
	Record smoking status for patients 13 years old or older.	Record smoking status for patients 13 years old or older.	More than 80% of all unique patients 13 years old or older seen by the EP or admitted to the eligible hospital's or

Health Outcomes Policy Priority	Stage 2 Objectives		Stage 2 Measures
	EPs	**EHs and CAHs**	
			CAH's inpatient or emergency departments (POS 21 or 23) during the EHR reporting period have smoking status recorded as structured data.
	Use clinical decision support (CDS) to improve performance on high priority health conditions.	Use clinical decision support (CDS) to improve performance on high priority health conditions.	1. Implement 5 clinical decision support interventions related to four or more clinical quality measures at a relevant point in patient care for the entire EHR reporting period. Absent four clinical quality measures related to an EP, eligible hospital or CAH's scope of practice or patient population, the clinical decision support interventions must be related to high-priority health conditions. It is suggested that one of the 5 CDS interventions be related to improving healthcare efficiency. 2. The EP, eligible hospital, or CAH has enabled and implemented the functionality for drug-drug and drug-allergy interaction checks for the entire EHR reporting period.
	Incorporate clinical lab-test results into Certified EHR Technology as structured data.	Incorporate clinical lab-test results into Certified EHR Technology as structured data.	More than 55% of all clinical lab tests results ordered by the EP or by authorized providers of the eligible hospital or CAH for patients admitted to its inpatient or emergency department (POS 21 or 23) during the EHR reporting period whose results are either in a positive/negative affirmation or numerical format are incorporated in certified EHR Technology as structured data.
	Generate lists of patients by specific	Generate lists of patients by specific	Generate at least one report listing patients of

Health Outcomes Policy Priority	Stage 2 Objectives		Stage 2 Measures
	EPs	**EHs and CAHs**	
	conditions to use for quality improvement, reduction of disparities, research, or outreach.	conditions to use for quality improvement, reduction of disparities, research, or outreach.	the EP, eligible hospital or CAH with a specific condition.
	Use clinically relevant information to identify patients who should receive reminders for preventive/follow-up care and send these patients the reminder, per patient preference.		More than 10% of all unique patients who have had two or more office visits with the EP within the 24 months before the beginning of the EHR reporting period were sent a reminder, per patient preference when available.
		Automatically track medications from order to administration using assistive technologies in conjunction with an electronic medication administration record (eMAR).	More than 10 percent of medication orders created by authorized providers of the eligible hospital's or CAH's inpatient or emergency department (POS 21 or 23) during the EHR reporting period for which all doses are tracked using eMAR.
Engage patients and families in their health care.	Provide patients the ability to view online, download, and transmit their health information within 4 business days of the information being available to the EP.		1. More than 50% of all unique patients seen by the EP during the EHR reporting period are provided timely (within 4 business days after the information is available to the EP) online access to their health information subject to the EP's discretion to withhold certain information. 2. More than 5% of all unique patients seen by the EP during the EHR reporting period (or their authorized representatives) view, download, or transmit to a third party their health information.
		Provide patients the ability to view online, download, and transmit information about a hospital admission.	1. More than 50% of all patients who are discharged from the inpatient or emergency department (POS 21 or 23) of an eligible hospital or CAH have their information available online within 36 hours of discharge

Health Outcomes Policy Priority	Stage 2 Objectives		Stage 2 Measures
	EPs	EHs and CAHs	
			2. More than 5% of all patients (or their authorized representatives) who are discharged from the inpatient or emergency department (POS 21 or 23) of an eligible hospital or CAH view, download or transmit to a third party their information during the reporting period.
	Provide clinical summaries for patients for each office visit.		Clinical summaries provided to patients or patient-authorized representatives within 1 business day for more than 50% of office visits.
	Use Certified EHR Technology to identify patient-specific education resources and provide those resources to the patient.	Use Certified EHR Technology to identify patient-specific education resources and provide those resources to the patient.	Patient-specific education resources identified by CEHRT are provided to patients for more than 10% of all unique patients with office visits seen by the EP during the EHR reporting period. More than 10 percent of all unique patients admitted to the eligible hospital's or CAH's inpatient or emergency departments (POS 21 or 23) are provided patient- specific education resources identified by Certified EHR Technology.
	Use secure electronic messaging to communicate with patients on relevant health information.		A secure message was sent using the electronic messaging function of Certified EHR Technology by more than 5 percent of unique patients (or their authorized representatives) seen by the EP during the EHR reporting period.
Improve care coordination	The EP who receives a patient from another setting of care or provider of care or believes an encounter is relevant should perform	The eligible hospital or CAH who receives a patient from another setting of care or provider of care or believes an encounter is	The EP, eligible hospital or CAH performs medication reconciliation for more than 50% of transitions of care in which the

Health Outcomes Policy Priority	Stage 2 Objectives		Stage 2 Measures
	EPs	EHs and CAHs	
	medication reconciliation.	relevant should perform medication reconciliation.	patient is transitioned into the care of the EP or admitted to the eligible hospital's or CAH's inpatient or ED (POS 21 or 23).
	The EP who transitions their patient to another setting of care or provider of care or refers their patient to another provider of care provides a summary care record for each transition of care or referral.	The eligible hospital or CAH who transitions their patient to another setting of care or provider of care or refers their patient to another provider of care provides a summary care record for each transition of care or referral.	1. The EP, eligible hospital, or CAH that transitions or refers their patient to another setting of care or provider of care provides a summary of care record for more than 50% of transitions of care and referrals. 2. The EP, eligible hospital or CAH that transitions or refers their patient to another setting of care or provider of care provides a summary of care record for more than 10% of such transitions and referrals either— (A) electronically transmitted using EHRT to a recipient or (B) where the recipient receives the summary of care record via exchange facilitated by an organization that is a NwHIN Exchange participant or in a manner that is consistent with the governance mechanism ONC establishes for the nationwide health information network. 3. An EP, eligible hospital or CAH must satisfy one of the two following criteria: (A) Conducts one or more successful electronic exchanges of a summary of care document, as part of which is counted in "measure 2" (for EPs the measure at §495.6(j)(14)(ii)(B) and for eligible hospitals and

Health Outcomes Policy Priority	Stage 2 Objectives		Stage 2 Measures
	EPs	EHs and CAHs	
			CAHs the measure at §495.6(l)(11)(ii)(B)) with a recipient who has EHR technology that was developed designed by a different EHR technology developer than the sender's EHR technology certified to 45 CFR 170.314(b)(2); or (B) Conducts one or more successful tests with the CMS designated test EHR during the EHR reporting period.
Improve population and public health	Capability to submit electronic data to immunization registries or immunization information systems except where prohibited, and in accordance with applicable laws and practices.	Capability to submit electronic data to immunization registries or immunization information systems except where prohibited, and in accordance with applicable laws and practices.	Successful ongoing submission of electronic immunization data from Certified EHR Technology to an immunization registry or immunization information system for the entire EHR reporting period.
		Capability to submit electronic reportable laboratory results to public health agencies, except where prohibited, and in accordance with applicable laws and practices.	Successful ongoing submission of electronic reportable laboratory results from Certified EHR Technology to public health agencies for the entire EHR reporting period.
		Capability to submit electronic syndromic surveillance data to public health agencies, except where prohibited, and in accordance with applicable laws and practices.	Successful ongoing submission of electronic syndromic surveillance data from Certified EHR Technology to a public health agency for the entire EHR reporting period.
Ensure adequate privacy and security protections for personal health information	Protect electronic health information created or maintained by the Certified EHR Technology through the implementation of appropriate technical capabilities	Protect electronic health information created or maintained by the Certified EHR Technology through the implementation of appropriate technical capabilities.	Conduct or review a security risk analysis in accordance with the requirements under 45 CFR 164.308(a)(1), including addressing the encryption/security of data stored in CEHRT in accordance with requirements under 45 CFR 164.312 (a)(2)(iv) and 45 CFR 164.306(d)(3), and

Health Outcomes Policy Priority	Stage 2 Objectives		Stage 2 Measures
	EPs	EHs and CAHs	
			implement security updates as necessary and correct identified security deficiencies as part of the provider's risk management process.
MENU SET			
Improving quality, safety, efficiency, and reducing health disparities		Record whether a patient 65 years old or older has an advance directive.	More than 50% of all unique patients 65 years old or older admitted to the eligible hospital's or CAH's inpatient department (POS 21) during the EHR reporting period have an indication of an advance directive status recorded as structured data.
	Imaging results consisting of the image itself and any explanation or other accompanying information are accessible through Certified EHR Technology.	Imaging results consisting of the image itself and any explanation or other accompanying information are accessible through Certified EHR Technology.	More than 10% of all tests whose result is one or more images ordered by the EP or by an authorized provider of the eligible hospital or CAH for patients admitted to its inpatient or ED (POS 21 and 23) during the EHR reporting period are accessible through Certified EHR Technology.
	Record patient family health history as structured data.	Record patient family health history as structured data.	More than 20 percent of all unique patients seen by the EP or admitted to the eligible hospital or CAH's inpatient or ED (POS 21 or 23) during the EHR reporting period have a structured data entry for one or more first-degree relatives.
		Generate and transmit permissible discharge prescriptions electronically (eRx).	More than 10% of hospital discharge medication orders for permissible prescriptions (for new, changed, and refilled prescriptions) are queried for a drug formulary and transmitted electronically using Certified EHR Technology.

Health Outcomes Policy Priority	Stage 2 Objectives		Stage 2 Measures
	EPs	EHs and CAHs	
	Record electronic notes in patient records.	Record electronic notes in patient records.	Enter at least one electronic progress note created, edited and signed by an eligible professional for more than 30% of unique patients with at least one office visit during the EHR reporting period.
			Enter at least one electronic progress note created, edited and signed by an authorized provider of the eligible hospital's or CAH's inpatient or ED (POS 21 or 23) for more than 30% of unique patients admitted to the eligible hospital or CAH's inpatient or ED during the EHR reporting period.
			Electronic progress notes must be text-searchable. Nonsearchable notes do not qualify, but this does not mean that all of the content has to be character text. Drawings and other content can be included with searchable text notes under this measure.
		Provide structured electronic lab results to ambulatory providers.	Hospital labs send structured electronic clinical lab results to the ordering provider for more than 20% of electronic lab orders received.
Improve Population and Public Health	Capability to submit electronic syndromic surveillance data to public health agencies, except where prohibited, and in accordance with applicable laws and practices.		Successful ongoing submission of electronic syndromic surveillance data from Certified EHR Technology to a public health agency for the entire EHR reporting period.
	Capability to identify and report cancer cases to a public health central cancer registry, except where		Successful ongoing submission of cancer case information from CEHRT to a public health central cancer

Health Outcomes Policy Priority	Stage 2 Objectives		Stage 2 Measures
	EPs	EHs and CAHs	
	prohibited, and in accordance with applicable laws and practices.		registry for the entire EHR reporting period.
	Capability to identify and report specific cases to a specialized registry (other than a cancer registry), except where prohibited, and in accordance with applicable laws and practices.		Successful ongoing submission of specific case information from Certified EHR Technology to a specialized registry for the entire EHR reporting period.

---

471 Centers for Medicare & Medicaid Services. 42 CFR Parts 412, 413, and 495. Medicare and Medicaid Programs; Electronic Health Record Incentive Program--Stage 2. Final Rule. August 23, 2012. Table B5. Stage 2 Objectives and Measures. pp. 294-301.

Index

B

C